Terahertz Biomedical and Healthcare Technologies

Materials to Devices

Terahertz Biomedical and Healthcare Technologies

Materials to Devices

Edited by

AMIT BANERJEE, PHD
Scientist
Microelectronic Technologies & Devices
Department of Electrical and Computer Engineering
National University of Singapore
Singapore

BASABI CHAKRABORTY, PHD
Professor and Head
Pattern Recognition and Machine Learning Laboratory
Department of Software and Information Science
Iwate Prefectural University
Japan

HIROSHI INOKAWA, PHD
Professor
Doctor of Engineering
Research Institute of Electronics
Shizuoka University
Hamamatsu, Shizuoka, Japan

JITENDRA NATH ROY, PHD
Professor and Dean (Science)
Department of Physics
Kazi Nazrul University
Asansol, West Bengal, India

ELSEVIER

Elsevier
Radarweg 29, PO Box 211, 1000 AE Amsterdam, Netherlands
The Boulevard, Langford Lane, Kidlington, Oxford OX5 1GB, United Kingdom
50 Hampshire Street, 5th Floor, Cambridge, MA 02139, United States

Library of Congress Cataloging-in-Publication Data

A catalog record for this book is available from the Library of Congress

British Library Cataloguing-in-Publication Data

A catalogue record for this book is available from the British Library

ISBN: 978-0-12-818556-8

For information on all Elsevier publications visit our website at https://www.elsevier.com/books-and-journals

Publisher: Matthew Deans
Acquisitions Editor: Kayla Dos Santos
Editorial Project Manager: Mariana C. Henriques
Production Project Manager: Sreejith Viswanathan
Cover designer: Miles Hitchen

Typeset by TNQ Technologies

Contributors

Amit Banerjee, PhD
Scientist
Microelectronic Technologies & Devices
Department of Electrical and Computer Engineering
National University of Singapore
Singapore

Sourav Banerjee, PhD
Assistant Professor
Kalyani Government Engineering College
Kalyani, West Bengal, India

Suranjana Banerjee, PhD, MTech, BTech, BSc
Electronics
Dum Dum Motijheel College
Kolkata, West Bengal, India

Electronics & Telecommunication Engineering
Indian Institute of Engineering
Science & Technology
Kolkata, West Bengal, India

Tanmoy Basu, PhD
Research Fellow
Centre for Advanced 2D Materials
National University of Singapore
Singapore

Centre for Ion Beam Applications
Department of Physics
National University of Singapore
Singapore

Nurnihar Begum, PhD
Research Scholar
Department of Engineering & Technological Studies
University of Kalyani
Kalyani, West Bengal, India

Basabi Chakraborty, PhD
Professor and Head
Pattern Recognition and Machine Learning Laboratory
Department of Software and Information Science
Iwate Prefectural University
Japan

Chinmay Chakraborty, PhD
Doctor
Birla Institute of Technology
Electronics & Communication Engineering
Deoghar, Jharkhand, India

Sulagna Chatterjee, MSc, MTech, PhD (Tech)
Adamas University
Kolkata, West Bengal, India

Debashis Das, MTech
Student Member
Kalyani Government Engineering College
Kalyani, West Bengal, India

Subal Kar, MTech, PhD (Tech)
Fulbright Scholar, Former Professor and Head
Institute of Radio Physics and Electronics
University of Calcutta
Kolkata, West Bengal, India

Bright Keswani, PhD
Professor
Department of Computer Applications
Suresh Gyan Vihar University
Jaipur, Rajasthan, India

Poonam Keswani, PhD
Assistant Professor
Akashdeep PG College
Jaipur, Rajasthan, India

Ilya Krasnikov, PhD
Department of Physics
Amur State University
Blagoveshchensk, Russia

Hannover Centre for Optical Technologies
Hannover, Germany

Yogeenth Kumaresan, PhD
School of Materials Science and Engineering
Gwangju Institute of Science and Technology
Gwangju, Republic of Korea

Ashis Kumar Mandal
Department of Software and Information Science
Iwate Prefectural University
Morioka, Japan

Ambarish G. Mohapatra, PhD
Senior Assistant Professor and Head
Department of Electronics and Instrumentation Engineering
Silicon Institute of Technology
Bhubaneswar, Odisha, India

Rahul Mondal, PhD
Research Scholar
Department of Engineering & Technological Studies
University of Kalyani
Kalyani, West Bengal, India

M. Mukherjee, MSc, MTech, PhD (Tech), PDF
Adamas University
Kolkata, West Bengal, India

Nilesh Mukherjee, PhD
Research Scholar
Department of Engineering & Technological Studies
University of Kalyani
Kalyani, West Bengal, India

Yutaka Oyama, PhD
Tohoku University
Sendai, Japan

Praveen Kumar Poola, PhD
Electronics and Communication Engineering
K L H Deemed to be University
Off-campus Hyderabad
Hyderabad, Telangana, India

Srinivasa Rao Ragam, PhD
Advance Materials and Device Metrology
CSIR-National Physical Laboratory
New Delhi, India

Megha Rathi, Sr., PhD
Doctor
Department of Computer Science & IT, Jaypee Institute of Information Technology
Noida, Uttar Pradesh, India

P. Soni Reddy, PhD
Research Scholar
Department of Engineering & Technological Studies
University of Kalyani
Kalyani, West Bengal, India

Partha Pratim Sarkar, PhD
Professor
Department of Engineering & Technological Studies
University of Kalyani
Kalyani, West Bengal, India

Sushanta Sarkar, PhD
Assistant Professor
Department of Engineering & Technological Studies
University of Kalyani
Kalyani, West Bengal, India

Rikta Sen
Department of Software and Information Science
Iwate Prefectural University
Morioka, Japan

Aleksei Seteikin, PhD
Associate Professor
Department of Physics
Amur State University
Blagoveshchensk, Russia

Department of Fundamental and Applied Photonics
Immanuel Kant Baltic Federal University
Kaliningrad, Russia

Saumitra Vajandar, PhD
Centre for Ion Beam Applications
Department of Physics
National University of Singapore
Singapore

Lokesh Vijay, MBBS
Consultant Surgery
Delhi Multi Specialty Hospital
Delhi, India

Prity Vijay, PhD
Data Scientist
Zessta Software Private Limited
Hydrabad, Telangana, India

Pu Zhao, PhD
Lehigh University
Pennsylvania, PA, United States

Thorlabs
Shanghai, China

About the Editors

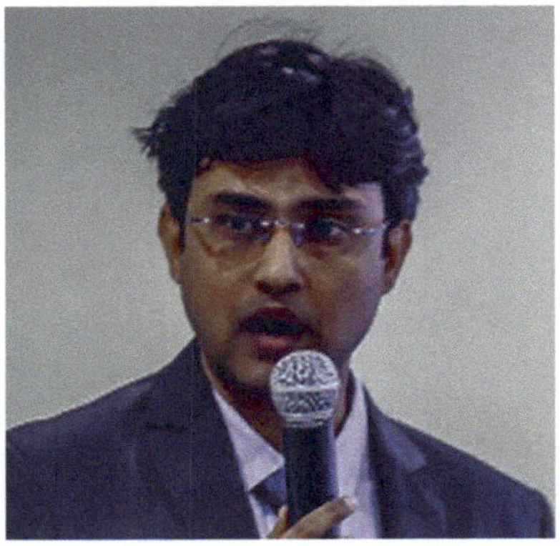

Dr. Amit Banerjee
Scientist, Microelectronic Technologies & Devices,
Department of Electrical and Computer Engineering,
National University of Singapore,
Singapore
Email: amitbanerjee.nus@gmail.com; eleami@nus.edu.sg

Short Biography: Amit Banerjee joined the Advanced Device Research Division, Research Institute of Electronics, National University Corporation, Japan, as a Scientific Researcher in 2016 and was also part of the Innovative Photonics Evolution Research Center at Hamamatsu, Japan. He later joined the Microelectronic Technologies & Devices, Department of Electrical and Computer Engineering of the prestigious National University of Singapore, as Scientist in 2017. Currently, Amit is a member of 30+ international advisory boards, technical program committees in various countries, acted as panel editor, reviewer for reputed journals and scientific book volumes, member of Japan Society of Applied Physics, Indian Physical Society; External Adviser, Bioelectronics and Biomedical Technologies, Ocuro Science and Technology (Biomed-startup); Adviser and Lead Contributor: Semiconductor Devices and Process Technologies, EDGE196, Entrepreneur Development Global Ecosystem; Adviser, Entrepreneurs Face, Singapore, Global Venture Capital and Entrepreneurs Network, Singapore; Technical Adviser to ULVAC Technologies; among various others. Amit has coauthored several scientific papers, edited books, presented in several international conferences as plenary and keynote speakers, received awards including young physicist award and honorary life-membership from Indian Physical Society, award by the Metrology Society of India, Indian Institute of Chemical Engineers, award by Department of Atomic Energy, his work on nanodiamonds was also awarded and featured as a key scientific article contributing to excellence in engineering, scientific, and industrial research, by Advances in Engineering, USA; recently, their work related to on-chip integrable terahertz detectors was awarded by Quality in Research, Indonesia, along with Professor Hiroshi Inokawa, RIE, Japan. Alongside the pursuit of research and administrative ambitions, Amit is keenly engaged in consulting futuristic technologies for business firms, educational ventures, and universities. Amit received PhD degree in Semiconductor Technology from Energy Research Unit, Indian Association for the Cultivation of Science (Government of India), and extensively worked on design and development of high vacuum plasma CVD reactors, which are used in industrial manufacturing of solar cells, coatings, and TFTs. He also developed low-cost high vacuum MW-PECVD units and conceived the process for cost-effective commercial grade antireflection coating synthesis for solar cells by nanocrystalline diamonds. His current work is on Terahertz Technology, including THz sensors and sources, design, and fabrication, aiming at biomedical imaging applications. His recent work on antenna-coupled microbolometer arrays is compatible with the state-of-the-art medium-scale semiconductor device fabrication processes and technologically competitive with commercial viability as on-chip integrable detector arrays for terahertz imaging.

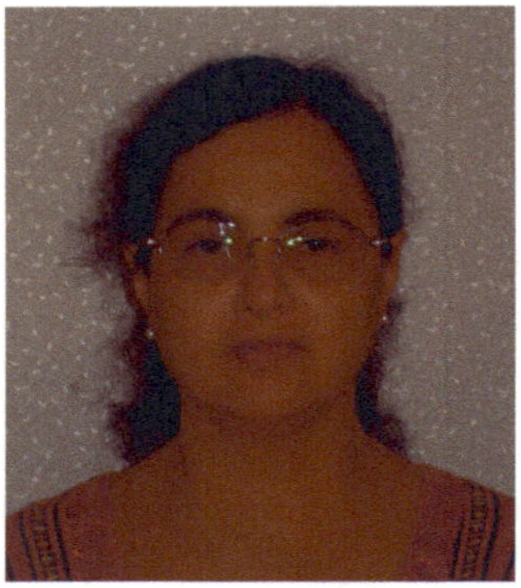

Dr. Basabi Chakraborty
Professor and Head, Pattern Recognition and Machine Learning Laboratory
Faculty of Software and Information Science, Iwate Prefectural University, Japan
Email: basabi@iwate-pu.ac.jp

Short Biography: Basabi Chakraborty received B. Tech, M. Tech, and PhD degrees in RadioPhysics and Electronics from Calcutta University, India, and worked in Indian Statistical Institute, Calcutta, India, until 1990. From 1991 to 1993, she worked as a part-time researcher in Advanced Intelligent Communication Systems Laboratory in Sendai, Japan. She received another PhD in Information Science from Tohoku University, Japan, in 1996. From 1996 to 1998, she worked as a postdoctoral research fellow in Research Institute of Electrical Communication, Tohoku University, Japan. In 1998, she joined as a faculty in Software and Information Science Department of Iwate Prefectural University, Iwate, Japan. Currently, she is serving as Professor and Head of Pattern Recognition and Machine Learning Laboratory in the same department. Her main research interests are in the area of Pattern Recognition, Machine Learning, Soft Computing Techniques, Biometrics, Data Mining, and Social Media Data Mining. She is a senior member of the Institute of Electrical and Electronics Engineers (IEEE), member of ACM, Japanese Neural Network Society, Japanese Society of Artificial Intelligence, and executive committee member of ISAJ (Indian Scientists Association in Japan). She served as the chair of IEEE JC WIE (Women in Engineering) during 2010–2011. She also served as the founder chair of IEEE WIE Sendai section during 2017–2018. Currently, she is executive committee member of IEEE R10 WIE, IEEE JC WIE, and Sendai WIE.

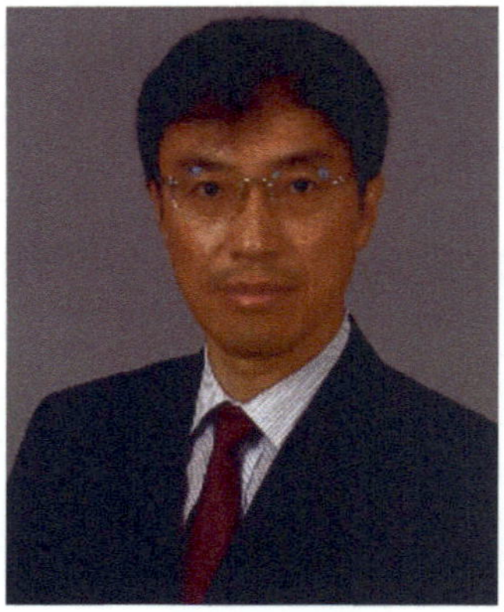

Dr. Hiroshi Inokawa
Professor
Research Institute of Electronics,
Shizuoka University
Hamamatsu, Japan
Email: inokawa.hiroshi@shizuoka.ac.jp

Short Biography: Hiroshi Inokawa received BS, MS, and PhD degrees in electrical engineering from Kyoto University, Japan, in 1980, 1982, and 1985, respectively. In 1985, he joined the Atsugi Electrical Communications Laboratories, Nippon Telegraph and Telephone Corporation (NTT), Kanagawa, Japan. Since then, he has been engaged in the research and development of scaled-down CMOS devices and silicon single-electron devices. During the course of his research, he invented the basic structure of FinFET in 1989 and single-electron multiple-valued logic in 2001 and received IEEE International Symposium on Multiple-Valued Logic Outstanding Contributed Paper Awards in 2004 and 2006, Director's Award of NTT Basic Research Laboratories in 2004, 28th JSAP Award for the Best Original Paper in 2006, etc. In 2006, he became a professor of the Research Institute of Electronics, Shizuoka University, Hamamatsu, Japan, where he has been studying nanodevices for advanced circuits and systems. His recent work on SOI MOSFET single-photon detector was introduced by IEEE Photonics Journal in 2012 as a Breakthrough in Photonics. Professor Inokawa is a member of IEEE, the Japan Society of Applied Physics (JSAP), the Institute of Electronics, Information and Communication Engineers of Japan, and the Institute of Electrical Engineers of Japan (IEEJ). He has served as a JSAP board member of representative in 2001–03, an editor of JJAP in 2007–13, the chair of the IEEJ survey committee of silicon nanosystem integration technology in 2009–11, an advisory committee member of NICT Japan Trust International Research Cooperation Program in 2006–09, a researcher of National Institute of Science and Technology Policy in 2002-present, etc.

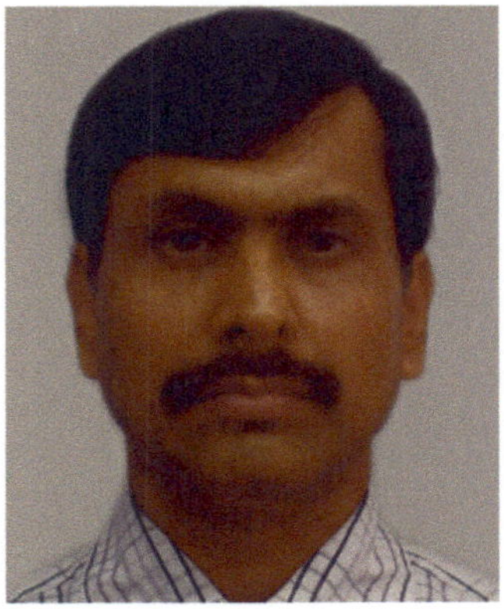

Dr. Jitendra Nath Roy
Professor and Dean (Science)
Department of Physics,
Kazi Nazrul University, C H Kalla,
Asansol, West Bengal, India
Email: jnroys@yahoo.co.in

Short Biography: Jitendra Nath Roy received MSc and PhD degree in Physics from Vidyasagar University, India. He had joint research program at Department of Electrical and Computer Engineering, Light Wave Communications Research Group, Xanthi, Greece. Professor Roy received International Sardar Patel Award from Sardar Vallabhbhai Patel Foundation for significant contribution in physical science. Dr. Roy has 20 years of experience in teaching research and administration. Presently, Dr. Roy is working as a Professor and Dean (science) in Department of Physics at Kazi Nazrul University, Asansol, WB, India. He has already published more than 123 research papers in peer-reviewed journals and conference proceedings. Dr. Roy received research grant from AICTE, Government of India, under FRS Scheme for research in "Designing of an all-optical conversion scheme from binary to its Modified Trinary Number." Dr. Roy is member of many International Advisory Committees, Technical Program Committees in various countries, acted as Panel Editor, Reviewer for reputed journals. Professor Roy has produced nine PhD students in different topics of applied optics and photonics, linear and nonlinear optical material, and laser. His current research interest is in Terahertz Optical Asymmetric Demultiplexer-based switch in Computing, Communication, and Control.

Contents

CHAPTER 1

THz Solid-State Source Based on IMPATT Devices

SURANJANA BANERJEE, PHD, MTECH, BTECH, BSC

INTRODUCTION

The terahertz (THz) region of the electromagnetic spectrum lies between the traditional millimeter wave and optical bands in the frequency range of 0.1–10 THz and wavelength range of 3–0.03 mm. It is also popularly called "THz gap" lying between microwave and infrared frequency band as shown in Fig. 1.1. THz science and technology are attracting the attention of researchers in recent times mainly due to the emergence of time-domain spectroscopy using pulse laser of extremely narrow width as sources. The researchers are now able to carry out time-resolved "far-infrared" studies and explore spectroscopy and imaging applications in the THz frequency regime.

THz technology can be used in information science, biology, medicine, astronomy, and environmental science. THz sources have numerous applications in surveillance, bioterrorist attack, and pathogen detection where THz wave is used to detect airborne anthrax particles. Some of THz semiconductor sources are $GaAs_{1-x}N_x$-based Gunn-like diodes, quantum well (QW), negative effective mass (NEM) oscillators, and quantum cascade lasers (QCLs). THz current oscillation in doped n^+nn^+ $GaAs_{1-x}N_x$ diodes driven by DC electric field has been theoretically studied by Feng and Cao [1]. Self-oscillation is associated with the negative differential velocity effect in the highly nonparabolic conduction band of this unique material system. They observed that impurity and phonon scattering mechanisms are responsible for current self-oscillation in QW NEM p^+pp^+ diodes. The NEM p^+pp^+ diode may be used as an electrically tunable THz source. The first THz QC laser with photon energy less than the semiconductor optical phonon energy was demonstrated at 4.4 THz. The optimization of device parameters of resonant-phonon THz QCLs can be done by using Monte Carlo method.

A lot of research interest has generated for the research and development of THz components, sources, and detectors due to their various applications in astronomy, spectroscopy, bioimaging, biosensing, quality inspection in industrial products, and medical and pharmaceutical research areas. Bioimaging using tera ray shows better resolution of carcinoma cells in human body as compared with that using X-ray (Fig. 1.2).

In recent years, the development of THz solid-state source with appreciable power is attracting the attention of researchers due to their important applications in short range terrestrial and airborne communication and space-based communication. Some of the THz sources reported in the literature are electron beam, optically pumped far-infrared gas lasers, semiconductor QCLs, resonant tunneling diode, TUNNETT diode, and Gunn diode.

Recently, cascaded frequency multipliers have been reported which can generate 10–2 μW power at 1.9–2.7 GHz for application as local oscillators in an astronomical receiver. However, some semiconductor devices such as QCLs, high electron mobility transistors, and heterojunction bipolar transistors have emerged as potential sources to generate THz signals. These solid-state sources can be tuned to appropriate THz frequency at 300 K. But the power generated by these sources at THz is not high enough to use them in the transmitter section of the system. The generation of THz signal with appreciable power is indeed a challenging area of research. The researchers are therefore exploring to search for an alternative solid-state source at THz frequency band which should be compact, cost-effective, efficient, and powerful. In this respect, the development of impact avalanche transit time (IMPATT) devices based on wide bandgap (WBG) semiconductor like GaN is worthwhile to note.

Terahertz Biomedical and Healthcare Technologies. https://doi.org/10.1016/B978-0-12-818556-8.00001-X

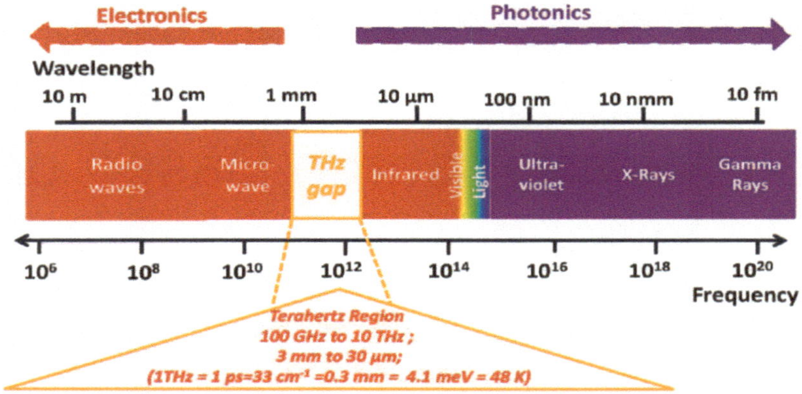

FIG. 1.1 Terahertz region.

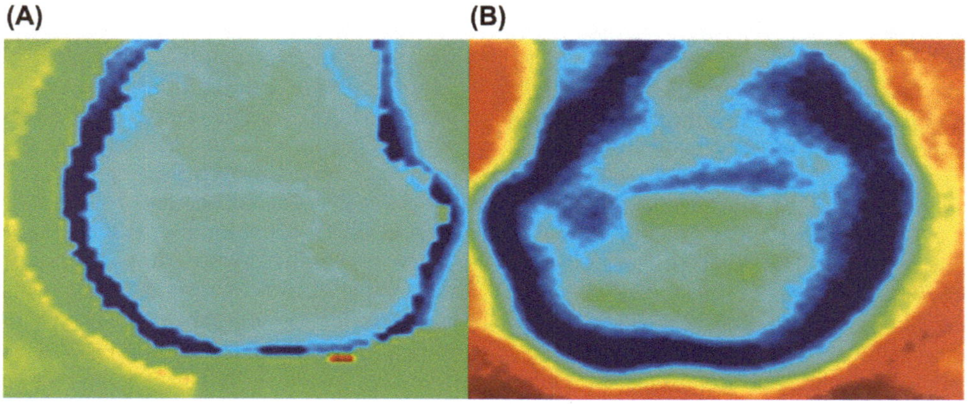

FIG. 1.2 **(A)** X-ray view, **(B)** tera view.

POTENTIAL THZ SOLID-STATE SOURCE USING IMPATT DIODES

Various solid-state sources are available for generation of RF power at microwave and millimeter wave frequency bands. Among these sources, IMPATT and mixed tunneling transit time (MITATT) devices have already emerged as high-power, high efficiency solid-state sources both at lower microwave (3–30 GHz) and higher mm-wave and sub-mm-wave (30–300 GHz) frequency bands. Most of the research activities for mm-wave systems using IMPATT sources are concentrated on window frequencies, i.e., 35, 94, 140, and 220 GHz, where atmospheric attenuation is relatively low.

IMPATT devices based on Si are reported to provide high power at different mm-wave window frequencies [2,3]. Although these devices have been realized at lower microwave and higher mm-wave frequency bands, no significant progress has yet been reported to practically realize this source for operation at THz frequencies. In recent years, the potentiality of IMPATT devices based on WBG semiconducting materials such as SiC, GaN, and type-IIb diamond as high-power sources has been reported at THz frequencies [4–10]. This chapter will provide a comprehensive review on the physical phenomena responsible for generation of THz wave from IMPATT devices and the design and development of these devices as compact, low-cost, efficient, and powerful THz sources.

The Basic Concepts of IMPATT Operation

IMPATT devices are basically reverse biased p-n junction diodes operated at avalanche breakdown voltage. Embedded in a resonant cavity, they exhibit oscillation at microwave and millimeter wave frequencies to generate power. These devices excel metal semiconductor field-effect transistors (MESFETs) and Gunn diodes in terms of output power, DC to RF conversion efficiency at higher mm-wave frequencies. These devices are highly attractive and reliable sources for mm-wave power generation due to their wide frequency coverage, high-power output and high conversion efficiency coupled with tuning capability, low cost, and simple circuit arrangement. They find wide applications in satellite communication systems, tracking radars and missile guidance for both civilian and defense applications.

In 1954, Shockley [11] showed that the transit time (TT) delay of an electron bunch in a forward biased p-n junction diode is responsible to produce negative resistance at microwave frequencies. The origin of negative resistance in IMPATT device is ideally a phase lag of 180° between the input RF voltage and external current. Under avalanche breakdown condition, the phenomena of impact ionization and avalanche multiplication in the depletion layer of the device give rise to an avalanche phase delay of 90°. The carriers injected from the avalanche layer require a finite TT to cross the drift layer and arrive at the terminal which introduces another delay called TT delay. When the avalanche delay added to TT delay is equal to half-cycle time, the diode resistance becomes negative at the corresponding frequency. W. T. Read in 1958 [12] showed that the combined effects of avalanche and TT delay in a reverse biased p^+-n i n^+ diode under avalanche breakdown produces an appropriate phase delay of 180° between input voltage and external current to produce negative resistance at microwave frequencies. Johnson et al. [13] in 1965 first observed microwave oscillation from a simple p^+nn^+ device. T. Misawa [14] showed from small-signal analysis the existence of negative resistance of an avalanche diode of arbitrary doping profile.

Commercially available millimeter wave IMPATTs are mostly based on Si due to matured processing technology of Si. Although IMPATTs made of GaAs are also practically realized, the available reports indicate that their RF performance as regard high-power delivery with high conversion efficiency is limited above 50 GHz. IMPATTs based on InP and 4H-SiC have been designed and fabricated. WBG semiconductors like 4H-SiC, GaN, and type-IIB diamond show great promise as base semiconductors for fabrication of IMPATTs, MITATTs, and TUNNETTs at higher millimeter wave up to THz frequency bands [4–8,15,16]. Further IMPATTs based on heterojunctions of Gr. IV-IV and Gr. III-V semiconductors are reported to be useful sources to deliver sufficient power with low noise level at sub-mm-wave frequencies above 100 GHz.

Significant progress in output power and efficiency has been achieved with IMPATT diodes and oscillators at frequencies from 30 to 300 GHz over the past decades. Silicon IMPATTs have emerged as premier solid-state sources of RF power in both continuous wave (CW) and pulsed modes of operation at mm-wave frequency bands. Flat profile single drift and double-drift silicon IMPATTs operating in the CW mode have produced output powers of 2.25 W at 40 GHz, 600 mW at 94 GHz, 110 mW at 140 GHz, 50 mW at 220 GHz, and 1.2 mW at 301 GHz. Similarly, pulsed output powers of 23 W at 35 GHz, 42 W at 96 GHz, 3 W at 140 GHz, and 520 mW at 220 GHz have been reported [17,18] from silicon IMPATT devices. Above 50 GHz, the RF performance of Si IMPATTs excels that of GaAs IMPATTs. Some efforts have been made to improve the performance of GaAs IMPATTs at mm-wave V-band (60 GHz) and W-band (94 GHz) frequencies taking the advantages of improved device design and process technology.

Apart from Si and GaAs IMPATTs, indium phosphide IMPATTs have been realized providing good RF performance at X- and V-bands. J. J. Berenz et al. in 1978 [19] reported the fabrication of single drift p^+nn^+ structure of InP IMPATTs by ion-implantation technique and showed that the devices provide a CW power of 1.6 W with 11.1% efficiency at 9.78 GHz. Vassilevsky et al. and Yuan et al. [8,20] reported fabrication of single drift region (SDR) IMPATTs based on 4H-SiC with flat and high-low doping profile at X- and Ku-bands, respectively. A maximum output power of 300 mW and breakdown voltage of 290 V was reported from these devices at a bias current density of $0.95 \times 10^7\ Am^{-2}$. The high breakdown field and electron saturation velocity of SiC is ideally suited to fabricate high-power IMPATTs from this semiconductor. The power-frequency product (pf^2) of IMPATT diode is proportional to $(E_mV_{sn})^2$. The breakdown field or critical field of SiC is about 10 times higher than that of Si or GaAs and the saturation velocity is about 2 times higher. Thus, the power-frequency product (in the electronic limit) of SiC IMPATTs is expected to be 400 times higher than Si or GaAs IMPATTs.

Practical IMPATT diodes are intermediate between Read and Misawa diodes in the sense that the avalanche zone is well defined, neither too thin nor too wide. The avalanche charge pulse is injected from a well-defined avalanche zone into the drift zone approximately 90° behind the RF voltage and the injected charge travels with a saturated drift velocity in the drift region. The SDR IMPATT diode having p^+nn^+ structure and double-drift region (DDR) IMPATT diode having p^+pnn^+ structure are mostly used as practical structures of the device.

Some Landmarks in the Development of IMPATTs

The first ever practical structure of IMPATTs realized experimentally is SDR p^+-n-n^+/n^+-p-p^+ structure with a SDR for electrons or holes and an avalanche region of narrow width located at one end of the depletion layer near the metallurgical junction. Schematic diagrams of the structure, doping profile, and electric field profile at breakdown of p^+nn^+ SDR IMPATT diode are shown in Fig. 1.3A–C, respectively. The field profile shown in Fig. 1.3C indicates that the device is just punched through at operating temperature and the avalanche zone width is a fraction of the depletion layer width. Flat profile SDR IMPATT diodes using Si/GaAs/InP/4H-SiC as base semiconductors have been experimentally realized. A punched through structure of IMPATT diode avoids positive resistance due to undepleted epitaxy. It may be noted in this context that SDR p^+nn^+ structure of Si IMPATTs is better than its complementary n^+pp^+ structure so far as high power delivery from the device is concerned.

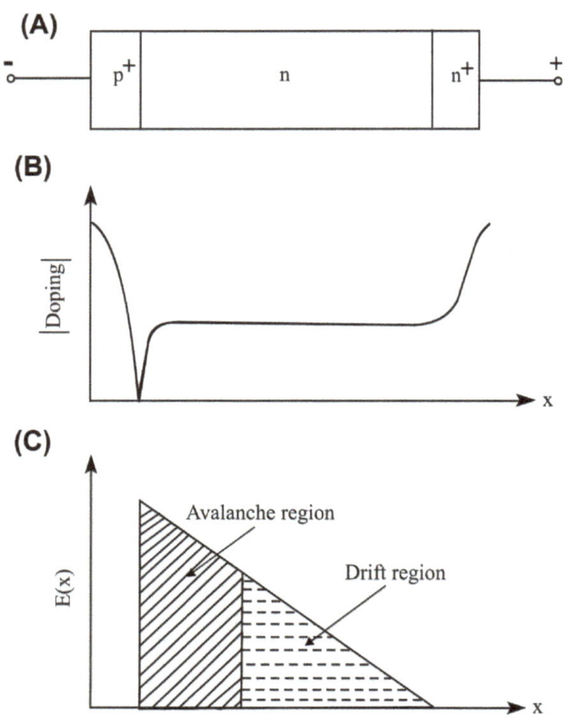

FIG. 1.3 **(A)** Single drift region (SDR) IMPATT diode structure, **(B)** doping profile and **(C)** field at breakdown showing the avalanche and drift regions.

A Double-Drift Region (DDR) structure (p^+-p-n-n^+) of IMPATTs with two drift regions, one for electrons and another for holes on either side of a central avalanche region, was first proposed by Scharfetter et al. [21] in 1970. In this type of structure, both electrons and holes take part equally to deliver microwave power while drifting in opposite directions through two drift regions on either side of the central avalanche region. It is quite evident that two drift regions in the case of DDR IMPATT diodes should provide higher output power, higher efficiency, and higher impedance per unit area, compared with SDR IMPATT diode in which microwave power is contributed by the drift of only one type of carrier, either electron or hole. DDR structure of IMPATT diode performs better than its SDR counterpart not only with respect to RF power output but also with respect to DC to RF conversion efficiency. DDR IMPATT diode is capable of delivering both high-power and high-efficiency at mm and sub-mm-wave frequency bands. The schematic diagrams of the structure, doping profile, and field profile of DDR n^+-n-p-p^+ IMPATT diode are shown in Fig. 1.4A–C, respectively. A high field avalanche region located centrally near the metallurgical junction and two low relatively low field drift regions on either side of the avalanche zone constitute the active region of a DDR IMPATT diode. In the central avalanche zone, carriers are generated by impact ionization due to sufficiently high field in the avalanche layer.

The equivalent circuit of IMPATT device may be considered to consist of a negative resistance R_D in series with a reactance X_D, where R_D is usually small compared with X_D. The width of the active region (W) DDR structure is larger than that of SDR structure of IMPATT diode resulting in a smaller capacitance $\left(C = \frac{\epsilon A}{W}\right)$ and hence a larger capacitive reactance per unit area $\left(X_c = \frac{1}{jwc}\right)$ of the device. The power-frequency product of an IMPATT diode is a constant at higher millimeter wave frequencies. The impedance and the breakdown voltage of DDR IMPATTs are both almost double that of SDR IMPATTs. The area of the DDR device can be increased to maintain the same value of capacitive reactance as that of comparable SDR device, in order to derive maximum output power from DDR diode. Simultaneously, the increased area reduces the series resistance associated with n^+ and p^+ contact regions. Also the degradation of efficiency due to the effect of minority carrier storage is not significant in a DDR diode because the avalanche zone is centrally located.

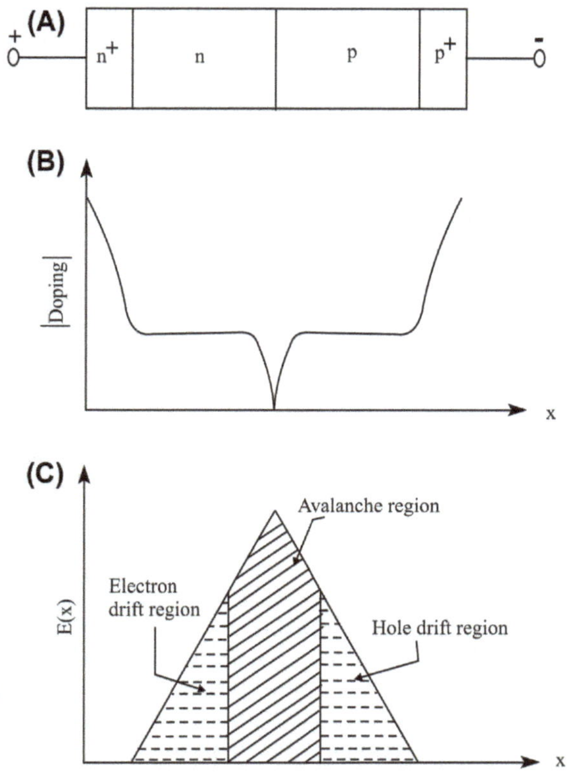

FIG. 1.4 **(A)** Double-drift region (DDR) IMPATT diode structure, **(B)** doping profile, and **(C)** Field at breakdown showing the avalanche and drift regions.

According to Scharfetter-Gummel formula, the DC to RF power conversion efficiency of a DDR IMPATT diode is given by

$$\eta = \frac{1}{\pi} \frac{V_D}{1 + \frac{V_D}{V_A}} \tag{1.1}$$

where V_A and V_D are the voltage drops across the avalanche and drift zones of DDR diode. The ratio of drift region voltage drop (V_D) to avalanche zone voltage drop is higher in DDR diode as compared with that in SDR diode which leads to higher conversion efficiency of DDR IMPATT diode.

The magnitude of peak electric field at the p-n junction of DDR diode is less than that of SDR diode under identical operating conditions. Further, the depletion region of a DDR diode is wider than that of an SDR diode. The effect of tunneling of charge carriers on the high-frequency properties of DDR device is less pronounced since the depletion layer width is wider in DDR diode. Scharfetter et al. [21] first demonstrated mm-wave power generation from experimental flat profile DDR Si IMPATT diode. Seidel et al. in 1971 [22] reported that an ion-implanted flat profile DDR Si IMPATT device delivers high CW output power of 1 W at 50 GHz with 14.2% conversion efficiency. A CW power of 0.53 W with 10.3% conversion efficiency at the same frequency was reported by the same worker [22] from corresponding Si flat profile SDR diode. Later several researchers confirmed the superiority of DDR diodes over their SDR counterparts at both microwave and mm-wave frequencies.

HETEROJUNCTION IMPATT DIODE

The conduction band discontinuity properties of abrupt heterojunctions formed between two semiconductors of different bandgaps, incorporated in IMPATT structure, lead to improved RF performance of the device at higher mm-wave frequency bands. The important feature of HJ-IMPATT is the sharpness of the peak electric field at the junction. The use of a heterojunction in place of the conventional p-n junction in an IMPATT structure leads to its superior DC characteristics, better RF properties, and less phase noise [23–25]. For given doping levels, and assuming no interface charge, the maximum field at the interface is found to be larger in a heterojunction based on $GaAs/Al_{0.3}GaAs_{0.7}$ than that in a standard GaAs p-n homojunction [26,27]. The avalanche noise characteristics of InP/GaInAs ($Ga_{0.47}$ $in_{0.53}$ As) and InP/GaInAsP ($Ga_{0.33}$ $In_{0.67}$ $As_{0.7}$ $P_{0.3}$) DDR heterojunction IMPATTs are reported to be better than their homojunction counterparts [28,29]. But HJ-IMPATTs require a high applied voltage to initiate breakdown due to low reverse leakage current. Further heterojunction IMPATTs exhibit sharper breakdown than homojunction device. The sharp avalanche breakdown observed in the HJ-IMPATT devices is due to narrow region of leakage current generation and reduced diffusion current. Mishra et al. [25] studied the RF properties of heterojunction IMPATTs and predicted that these devices excel homojunction IMPATTs as regard high power, low noise, and high efficiency. In spite of the improved performance of HJ-IMPATTs over standard IMPATTs, few experimental results have yet been reported in the literature.

IMPATTS BASED ON MATERIALS OTHER THAN SILICON

In early 1970s, silicon was extensively used as a base material for fabrication of IMPATT diodes. Luy et al. in 1987 [30] experimentally realized MBE grown DDR Si IMPATT devices and reported an output power of 600 mW at 94 GHz. Wollitzer et al. in 1996 [2] also reported that DDR Si IMPATT device can deliver 300 mW power at 140 GHz. However, at mm-wave frequencies higher than 300 GHz, the performance of silicon DDR IMPATTs degrades sharply.

Several researchers carried out theoretical and experimental research on IMPATTS based on GaAs at lower microwave frequency. Huang [31] studied a modified structure of GaAs IMPATTs and showed that there is a trade-off between efficiency and noise performance of the device. Goldwasser and Rosztoczy [32] in 1974 realized a low-high-low structure of GaAs IMPATT diode and showed that the device is capable of providing higher efficiency. Bozler et al. [33] in 1976 fabricated a low-high-low GaAs IMPATT diode by ion-implantation method and showed that DC to RF conversion efficiency of the device is considerably improved. In the same year, several researchers reported the suitability of GaAs IMPATT diodes for operation at lower mm-wave frequencies. Thus, GaAs emerged as an alternative base material of IMPATTs. Later in 1989, Eisele [34] reported 270 mW RF power output with 5.7% conversion efficiency from GaAs IMPATT oscillator at 94 GHz. H. Eisele [35] in 1990 showed that the noise figure of GaAs SDR IMPATT diode is lower than Si SDR diode operating at W-band frequencies. Eisele and Haddad [36] reported in 1992 that GaAs IMPATTs are capable of delivering 15 mW power with 1.5% conversion efficiency at 135.3 GHz. Kearney et al. [37] proposed a low-noise GaAs IMPATT diode as an alternative to Gunn diode for microwave power generation. They reported that proper design of the device may lead to a conversion efficiency greater than 20% with lower FM noise. In 1994, Curow [38] proposed a GaAs-based low noise IMPATT structure operating at D-band. The results showed that an output power up to 400 mW can be achieved around 150 GHz operations. Tschernitz et al. [39] in 1994 reported that Read-type GaAs IMPATT device delivers 75 mW power at 120 GHz and 8 mW power at D-band around 144 GHz. Tschernitz and Freyer [40] in 1995 investigated the high-frequency performance of GaAs double-Read IMPATT diodes at 140 GHz.

InP was later used as the base material for fabrication of IMPATT diode. Berenz et al. [19] in 1978 fabricated SDR InP IMPATT diode with flat doping profile for the first time by using ion-implantation method. They obtained an output power of 1.1 W at 9.78 GHz with 11.5% efficiency from the experimental device. Since then several theoretical reports were published showing the distinct advantages of InP IMPATTs over Si IMPATTs particularly at mm-wave frequency bands. Banerjee et al. [41] reported comparative studies on the high-frequency performance of DDR IMPATT diodes based on InP and GaAs. They showed that InP IMPATTs excel their silicon counterparts at higher mm-wave frequencies and their GaAs counterparts at lower mm-wave frequencies. Simulation studies reported in Refs. [42–44] also revealed that InP IMPATTs are promising candidates for power generation at higher mm-wave and THz frequency bands.

POTENTIALITY OF IMPATT DIODES BASED ON WIDE BANDGAP SEMICONDUCTORS AS THz SOURCES

The design and simulation studies on THz IMPATTs based on some WBG semiconductors such as 4H-SiC, WZ-GaN, and type-IIb diamond are reported in Refs. [4–7]. Some reports on the fabrication and RF characterization of 4H-SiC IMPATTs are available at lower microwave X-band [8,45] frequency, but not at higher mm-wave and THz frequency bands. Although the material properties of both WZ-GaN and type-IIb diamond are highly suitable to realize high-power IMPATTs at these frequency bands, experimental reports on the same are not yet available in the literature so far as the author's knowledge is concerned. This may be due to lack of accurate design data and availability of high-quality GaN wafer. The recent development of the epitaxial growth technique of type-IIb diamond and its favorable opto-electronic, mechanical, and thermal properties has aroused a lot of research interest to use this material for fabrication of high-power, high-frequency semiconductor devices. Trew et al. in 1991 [9,10] reported the good prospect of diamond-based MESFET, IMPATT diode, and bipolar junction transistor as efficient sources for microwave power generation. However, at mm-wave and THz frequencies, WZ-GaN and type-IIb diamond-based IMPATTs would emerge as high-power sources.

AVALANCHE RESPONSE ANALYSIS FOR THz OPERATION ON IMPATT DIODE

The prospect of IMPATT device made of different semiconductors such as GaAs, Si, InP, 4H-SiC, and Wz-GaN for THz operation depends mainly on two factors: (i) avalanche response time (ART) and (ii) tunneling. These two factors determine the upper cut-off frequency for IMPATT action. In this section, an analytical method based on ART of IMPATTs based on different semiconductors including the WBG ones will be presented to predict the cut-off frequency of operation. A comparison of the ART and TT of charge carriers in IMPATTs based on different materials leads to finding out the limiting or cut-off frequency for IMPATT operation. This method gives a firsthand physical insight regarding the potentiality of IMPATTs as THz sources. The avalanche response analysis is a useful tool to predict the operation of IMPATT diodes at THz frequency.

The avalanche response analysis when compared with the TT of carriers in the drift layer at a particular frequency provides the limiting frequency for IMPATT operation based on different semiconductors at that frequency. The material parameters which strongly influence the DC and RF properties of IMPATTs are field-dependent ionization rates (α_n, α_p) and saturated drift velocities (v_{sn}, v_{sp}) of charge carriers. The impact ionization rates of electrons and holes in a semiconductor determine the response time for the growth of avalanche current in an IMPATT diode based on the particular semiconductor. IMPATTs based on a particular material will cease to oscillate and deliver power when the operating frequency is more than the upper cut-off frequency in which case the ART of charge carriers is longer than their TT. The ART depends on the carrier ionization rates and TT depends on the saturated drift velocity of charge carriers and the operating frequency. Thus, both ART and TT depend very much on the base semiconductor of IMPATT diode. The upper cut-off frequency beyond which IMPATT oscillation ceases can be estimated by calculating ART and TT from the following analysis.

The ARTs initiated by electrons, τ_{An}, and holes, τ_{Ap}, are expressed as

$$\tau_{An} = \frac{1}{(v_{sn} + v_{sp})} \int_{-x_{A_1}}^{x_{A_2}} \exp\left[- \int_{-x_{A_1}}^{x} (\alpha_n - \alpha_p) dx' \right] dx \quad (1.2)$$

$$\tau_{Ap} = \tau_{An} \exp\left[\int_{-x_{A_1}}^{x_{A_2}} (\alpha_n - \alpha_p) dx \right] \quad (1.3)$$

When avalanche process is initiated by a mixture of electrons and holes, then the corresponding response time τ_A is given by

$$\tau_A = \tau_{An} \left\{ (1-k) + k \cdot \exp\left[- \int_{-x_{A_1}}^{x_{A_2}} (\alpha_n - \alpha_p) dx \right] \right\}^{-1}, \quad (1.4)$$

where the parameter $k = J_{ps}/J_s$ and $(1-k) = J_{ns}/J_s$.

In Eq. (1.4), J_{ns} and J_{ps} are the reverse saturation current components of thermally generated electrons and holes, respectively, and $J_s = J_{ps} + J_{ns}$ is the total reverse saturation current. The ARTs can be calculated using Eqs. (1.2)–(1.4) by taking the realistic material parameters from Ref. [46–49].

Some Results Based on ART Analysis of DDR IMPATTs

ARTs (τ_A) of DDR IMPATTs based on different semiconductors are calculated by using Eq. (1.4).The spatial variations of ionization rates of electrons ($\alpha_n(x)$) and holes ($\alpha_p(x)$) in the depletion layer of DDR IMPATTs based on different semiconductors are first obtained from the DC simulation results. Eqs. (1.2) and (1.3) are then solved numerically to determine ART (τ_A) initiated by electrons and holes, respectively. The TTs (τ_T) of carriers to cross the drift layers of DDR IMPATT devices based on different semiconductors depend on the operating frequency and can be estimated using the simple relation obtained from Ref. [50].

Figs. 1.5 and 1.6 show the variations of τ_A and τ_T with optimum frequency for DDR IMPATT diodes made of conventional (Si, GaAs) and WBG (4H-SiC, WZ-GaN, InP), semiconductors respectively. Within the operating frequency range, ART is less than TT in DDR IMPATT diodes and this can be determined for different base semiconducting materials from Figs. 1.5 and 1.6. ART (τ_A) depends on two important material parameters viz. saturated drift velocity and ionization rate of electrons and holes (v_{sn}, v_{sp} and α_n, α_p) in the base semiconductor of IMPATT device. Thus, τ_A is a function of base material.

It is observed from Fig. 1.5 that ART(τ_A) in DDR GaAs IMPATTs is longer than that in DDR Si device by factors of 1.47 and 2.15 at frequencies of 94 and 220 GHz, respectively. The cut-off frequencies of double-drift IMPATTs based on Si and GaAs are estimated as 500 and 220 GHz, respectively, by determining the frequency above which ART exceeds TT from Fig. 1.5.

It is observed from Fig. 1.6 that the ARTs, τ_A of both Wz-GaN and 4H-SiC DDR IMPATTs, are orders of magnitude shorter than of DDR InP devices. For example, at 94 GHz, τ_A of Wz-GaN and 4H-SiC DDR IMPATTs are 9.18×10^{-4} and 6.26×10^{-3} times of τ_A of InP DDR IMPATTs, respectively. At 1.0 THz, the above factors are 2.82×10^{-4} and 8.58×10^{-3}, respectively. DDR IMPATT diode based on GaN has the shortest τ_A as compared with DDR devices based on 4H-Sic, InP, Si, and GaAs. Fig. 1.6 shows further that GaN DDR IMPATT device can operate up to a frequency of 5.0 THz at since its ART is of the order of 10^{-16} s and its TT is approximately 5 orders of magnitude longer. The results indicate that Si- and GaAs-based DDR devices can deliver significant RF power at 0.22 and 0.50 THz, respectively, while those based on 4H-SiC and InP can deliver power at much higher frequency of 1 THz.

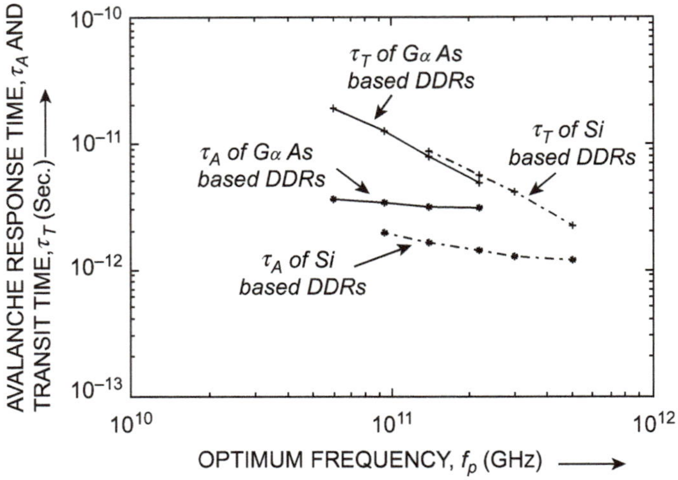

FIG. 1.5 Plots of avalanche response time and transit time against operating optimum frequency of double-drift region (DDR) IMPATTs made of Si and GaAs.

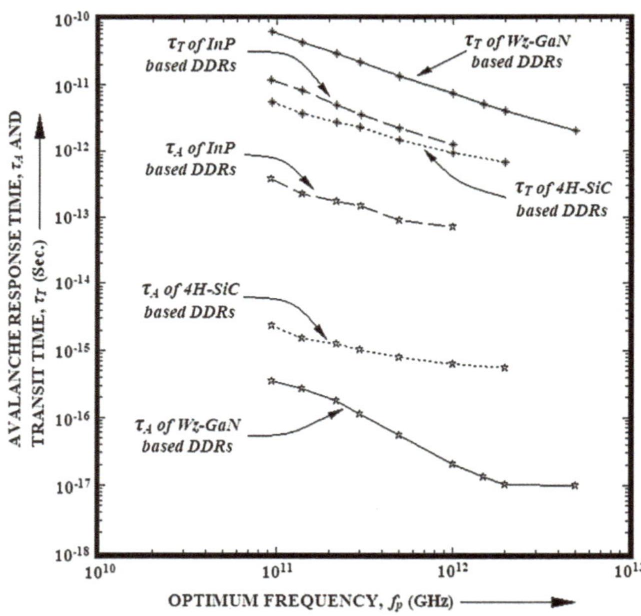

FIG. 1.6 Plots of avalanche response time and transit time against operating optimum frequency of double-drift region (DDR) IMPATTs based on GaN, InP, and 4H-SiC.

ART Analysis to Determine the Optimum Operating Frequencies of Si- and Diamond-Based DDR IMPATT Devices

Eq. (1.4) is used to calculate ART (τ_A) of both Si- and diamond-based DDR devices at different operating optimum frequencies. The electron and hole ionization rates (α_n, α_p) depend strongly on electric field (E) and hence on the spatial coordinate (x) in the active layer of the device. Thus, α_n (x) and α_p (x) in Eq. (1.4) can be obtained once the electric field profile in the active region of the device is simulated. The field profile is obtained through simultaneous numerical solution of fundamental device equations subject to appropriate boundary conditions at depletion layer edges. The carrier TTs in the drift layers of DDR devices at different operating frequencies are calculated using the simplified formula reported in Ref. [50].

Fig. 1.7 shows the plots of τ_A and τ_T for diamond and Si DDR IMPATTs versus optimum frequency. Above a

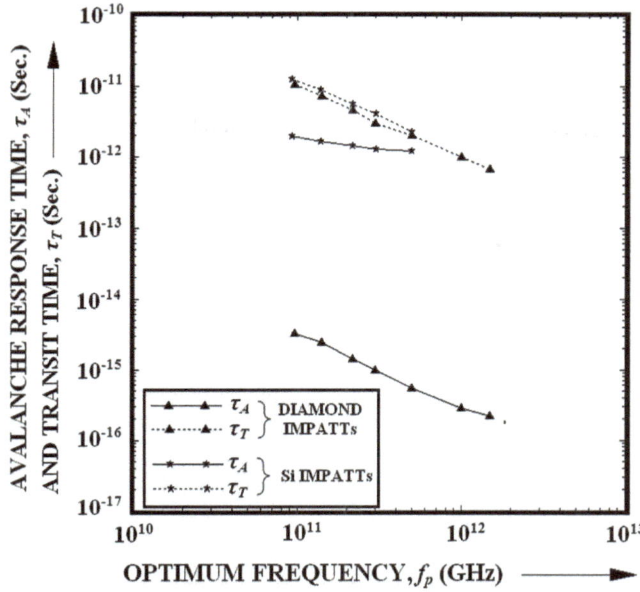

FIG. 1.7 Plots of avalanche transit time and transit time versus optimum frequency of diamond- and Si-based IMPATTs.

certain high frequency, the carrier transit time (τ_T) becomes shorter than the ART (τ_A) due to which the RF performance of the device becomes limited [7,44]. It is quite evident from Eq. (1.4) that τ_T depends on the terms $\alpha_n(x)$ and $\alpha_p(x)$. Thus, the ART, τ_A at a fixed operating frequency is very much dependent on the base semiconductor material. Fig. 1.7 shows that τ_A of Si DDR device at 94 GHz is 5.99×10^2 times higher than that of diamond DDR device, whereas at 0.5 THz, τ_A of Si DDR is 2.21×10^3 times higher than τ_A of diamond DDR. The results clearly indicate that compared with Si DDR IMPATTs, diamond-based IMPATTs can be operated for power generation at higher frequency of 1.5 THz. Above 1 THz, ART (τ_A) of diamond IMPATTs is in the range of femtosecond ($1.0-0.1 \times 10^{-15}$ s), about 4 orders shorter than that of Si devices. ART analysis carried out for Si DDR devices shows that their RF performance is avalanche response limited above 0.5 THz frequency.

AN OVERVIEW OF DESIGN, SIMULATION, AND ANALYSIS OF IMPATTS

A generalized double-iterative field maximum computer method free from any simplifying assumption was proposed by Roy et al. [51] in 1979 to study the DC properties of IMPATTs of any arbitrary doping profile. This method provides electric field profile, current density profile, avalanche region width, voltage drops across the avalanche and drift zones, breakdown voltage, and efficiency of DC to RF conversion. Small-signal analysis and simulation of IMPATTs was later reported by Roy et al. [52]. This analysis takes into account the effect of mobile space charge and realistic field-dependent ionization rates and drift velocities of charge carriers. The small-signal admittance characteristics, negative resistivity, and reactivity profiles of the device were obtained from the small-signal simulation based on Gummel-Blue approach. Banerjee et al. in 1991 [53] studied the small-signal properties and RF performance of simple flat and complex low-high-low doping profiles of DDR Si IMPATTs at V-band by carrying out small-signal simulation. The design results were used to fabricate the devices by silicon molecular beam epitaxy. A close agreement between theoretical and experimental results showed the accuracy of the method.

The effect of temperature on the small-signal admittance characteristics of IMPATT diode was studied by Y. Takayama [54] in 1975. Hirachi et al. [55] fabricated Si IMPATT device for operation at mm-wave frequency and showed that the DC to RF conversion efficiency of the device can be improved if the ohmic contact of the device is made with the help of ion-implanted technique. The effect of carrier diffusion on the static and microwave performance of IMPATT diode was studied theoretically by M. S. Gupta [56]. The effect of tunneling on the high-frequency performance of IMPATT diode was studied by Chive et al. [57]. Some reports are available on the experimental realization of IMPATT devices. K. B. Winterbon [58] fabricated IMPATT device by ion-implantation technique and reported the range of ion beam energy used in the process. The high-frequency limitation of silicon IMPATT diodes was studied by Doumitria et al. [59]. Wan et al. [60] in 1975 reported a multilayer epitaxial growth process for fabrication of silicon IMPATT diode at mm-wave frequencies.

Design of Structural and Doping Parameters

The operating frequency of DDR IMPATT diode depends on the transit time (τ_T) of charge carriers to cross the depletion layer of the device. The structural and doping parameters of the device depend on the design frequency (f_d). The following simple design formula [50] is used to obtain the depletion layer widths of n and p regions of the device:

$$W_{n,p} = 0.37 v_{sn,sp}/f_d \tag{1.5}$$

where $v_{sn,sp}$ are the saturation velocities of electrons and holes, respectively. The background doping concentrations of n- and p-depletion regions (N_D, N_A) are initially chosen according to the design frequency. The doping concentration of n^+- and p^+-layers are normally taken to be same, i.e., $N_{n+} = N_{p+} = 10^{26}\ \text{m}^{-3}$. These parameters are used as input data for DC simulation. The electric field profile in the depletion layer and the respective punch through factor can be obtained. The doping parameters and the doping profile are suitably adjusted so that the electric field just punches through the depletion layer of the device at a particular design frequency, f_d, and a particular bias current density (J_0). Small-signal simulation is carried out to obtain the admittance characteristics of the device. Various useful information on the RF properties of IMPATT oscillator such as optimum frequency (f_p), avalanche resonance frequency, Q-factor, and bandwidth can be extracted from the admittance plots.

The optimum frequency f_p is that frequency at which the negative conductance of IMPATTs reaches a peak under oscillating condition. This frequency can be obtained from the admittance (conductance-susceptance) plots of the device. The design should take care of bringing the value of f_p closer to the design frequency, f_d. This can be done by adjusting the bias current within the operating range. The bias current density is then fixed for a particular design frequency. The simulation is done by taking realistic doping profile of DDR IMPATTs using appropriate doping functions in different regions of the device. The design parameters of the device made of different semiconductors, obtained from the aforementioned method, are given in Table 1.1. Various material parameters such as field-dependent ionization rates (α_n, α_p), drift velocities (v_n, v_p) of charge carriers, bandgap (E_g), intrinsic carrier concentration (n_i), effective density of states of conduction and valence bands (N_c, N_v), diffusion coefficients (D_n, D_p), mobilities (μ_n, μ_p), and diffusion lengths (L_n, L_p) of the semiconductors can be obtained from Refs. [48,61–63]. The junction diameter of IMPATT device at a particular frequency (D_j) can be obtained from a rigorous thermal analysis considering appropriate heat sink arrangement. The report [64,65] shows that the value of D_j is 35 μm for CW operation of Si DDR IMPATTs at 94 GHz.

Some reports on the DC properties of IMPATT diode

The important DC parameters of the device can be obtained from modeling and simulation program described in Refs. [51]. These parameters are (i) peak electric field at the metallurgical junction (ξ_P), (ii) breakdown voltage (V_B), (iii) voltage across the avalanche layer (V_A), (iv) efficiency of DC to microwave conversion (η), (v) width of avalanche zone (x_A), and (vi) fractional value of avalanche zone width with respect to total width of active layer (x_A/W). Table 1.2 shows the aforementioned DC parameters. The variations of ξ_P, V_B, and η with operating frequency are shown in Figs. 1.8–1.10 for DDR IMPATTs based on Si, GaAs, InP, Wz-, and 4H-SiC. The simulated DC parameters of the device made of different materials can be compared by using Table 1.2 and Figs. 1.8–1.10 at different operating frequencies. It is observed that the peak field (ξ_P) at the p-n junction of DDR IMPATTs increases with increasing frequency (Table 1.2). Table 1.2 shows that with increasing frequency, the reverse voltage at breakdown (V_B), width of avalanche layer (x_A), and voltage drop across the avalanche zone (V_A) of the device decrease. It is also observed from the table that with increasing frequency, the DC to RF conversion efficiency (η) of DDR IMPATTs based on different semiconductors decreases. The DC properties of IMPATTs depend very much on the material properties and therefore vary with the change of base material of IMPATTs. At a particular operating frequency, the peak electric field (ξ_P) in 4H-SiC DDRs is found to highest as compared with DDRs based on other materials. The peak electric field, ξ_P, in GaN DDR IMPATTs is of the same order as that in 4H-SiC DDRs, but its magnitude in DDR

TABLE 1.1
Design Parameters of Double-Drift Region IMPATTs at mm-Wave and THz Frequencies.

Semiconductor	f_d (GHz)	J_0 ($\times10^8$ Am^{-2})	W_n (μm)	W_p (μm)	N_D ($\times10^{23}$ m^{-3})	N_A ($\times10^{23}$ m^{-3})	N_{n+} ($\times10^{25}$ m^{-3})	N_{p+} ($\times10^{25}$ m^{-3})	D_j (μm)
Wz-GaN	94	1.050	1.5800	1.5800	0.590	0.600	5.000	2.700	35.00
	140	2.250	1.0500	1.0500	0.690	0.710	5.000	2.700	25.00
	220	4.275	0.7350	0.7350	1.050	1.100	5.000	2.700	20.00
	300	8.700	0.5350	0.5350	1.550	1.600	5.000	2.700	15.00
	500	18.375	0.3300	0.3300	2.860	2.900	5.000	2.700	10.00
	1000	45.000	0.1850	0.1850	6.840	7.200	5.000	2.700	5.00
	1500	55.500	0.1300	0.1300	9.800	10.50	5.000	2.700	2.50
	2000	72.000	0.1020	0.1020	13.500	14.500	5.000	2.700	1.20
	5000	88.500	0.0520	0.0520	35.500	36.500	5.000	2.700	0.70
InP	94	4.500	0.3200	0.3200	1.900	1.900	5.000	2.700	35.00
	140	7.700	0.2100	0.2100	3.400	3.400	5.000	2.700	25.00
	220	12.000	0.1300	0.1300	5.200	5.200	5.000	2.700	20.00
	300	20.000	0.1000	0.1010	7.200	7.200	5.000	2.700	15.00
	500	47.000	0.0650	0.0650	13.500	13.500	5.000	2.700	10.00
	1000	60.000	0.0285	0.0285	28.000	28.000	5.000	2.700	5.00
Type-IIb diamond (C)	94	4.000	0.7800	0.7200	0.460	0.530	5.000	2.700	35.00
	140	7.500	0.5300	0.5300	0.810	0.870	5.000	2.700	25.00
	220	13.000	0.3200	0.3200	1.350	1.490	5.000	2.700	20.00
	300	17.000	0.2200	0.2200	2.050	2.220	5.000	2.700	15.00
	500	25.000	0.1200	0.1200	3.750	4.100	5.000	2.700	10.00
	1000	39.000	0.0520	0.0520	9.500	10.000	5.000	2.700	5.00
	1500	48.000	0.0300	0.0300	36.000	37.000	5.000	2.700	2.50
4H-SiC	94	2.100	0.5800	0.5800	2.800	2.900	5.000	2.700	35.00
	140	4.300	0.4000	0.4000	4.900	5.000	5.000	2.700	25.00
	220	9.300	0.3000	0.3000	6.900	7.000	5.000	2.700	20.00
	300	16.600	0.2500	0.2500	9.500	10.500	5.000	2.700	15.00
	500	60.000	0.1600	0.1600	14.500	16.500	5.000	2.700	10.00
	1000	210.000	0.0900	0.0900	37.000	43.000	5.000	2.700	5.00
Si	94	3.400	0.4000	0.3800	1.200	1.250	5.000	2.700	35.00
	140	5.800	0.2800	0.2450	1.800	2.100	5.000	2.700	25.00
	220	14.500	0.1800	0.1600	3.950	4.590	5.000	2.700	20.00
	300	24.500	0.1320	0.1120	6.000	7.300	5.000	2.700	15.00
	500	55.000	0.0720	0.0720	15.000	16.200	5.000	2.700	10.00

TABLE 1.2
DC Parameters.

Base Material	Serial Number	J_0 ($\times 10^8$ Am^{-2})	ξ_P ($\times 10^7$ V m^{-1})	V_B (V)	V_A (V)	η (%)	x_A (nm)	x_A/W (%)
GaAs	1	2.20	5.6067	28.87	17.06	13.02	376.0	40.00
	2	5.60	6.0442	22.67	15.57	9.97	332.0	55.33
	3	11.50	7.3067	15.78	11.41	8.82	208.0	54.74
	4	24.50	9.1317	11.61	9.49	5.77	146.0	66.36
Si	1	3.40	6.0115	24.27	16.21	10.58	352.0	46.32
	2	5.80	6.6617	18.98	13.52	9.16	268.0	53.07
	3	13.0	8.1990	13.74	10.29	7.99	170.0	53.10
	4	17.2	9.3490	11.29	9.07	6.25	134.0	59.82
	5	52.0	12.1760	9.06	7.75	4.59	90.0	67.16
InP	1	1.40	7.3904	28.82	14.42	15.90	230.0	33.72
	2	2.90	7.9279	19.78	10.44	15.02	156.0	33.91
	3	5.00	8.5904	13.30	7.48	13.93	104.0	37.01
	4	7.80	8.9205	10.71	6.29	13.13	84.0	41.79
	5	19.0	9.7447	7.08	4.56	11.35	56.0	46.67
	6	40.5	10.6450	4.43	3.34	7.82	38.0	67.85
4H-SiC	1	4.00	35.9060	226.08	111.09	16.19	382.0	33.81
	2	9.00	38.9163	158.19	79.82	15.77	252.0	32.31
	3	21.0	40.6251	121.47	69.46	14.62	212.0	36.55
	4	51.0	42.6311	107.72	60.73	13.89	178.0	37.08
	5	135.0	45.2179	86.32	53.26	12.19	152.0	50.67
	6	460.0	51.7022	51.54	36.35	9.38	92.0	61.33
Wz-GaN	1	0.05	15.9820	251.61	123.12	16.25	904.0	28.43
	2	0.30	16.2877	215.59	106.21	16.15	758.0	35.09
	3	1.00	17.0345	155.13	81.57	15.49	560.0	39.16
	4	1.50	17.8712	118.13	62.21	15.07	408.0	38.49
	5	3.00	19.2765	76.34	41.42	14.56	252.0	39.38
	6	10.8	21.4739	41.76	24.28	13.32	134.0	40.61
	7	16.0	22.4766	31.43	19.31	12.27	102.0	45.95
	8	23.5	23.3778	25.21	16.13	11.46	82.0	48.81
	9	30.0	26.3812	11.92	9.72	5.88	44.0	67.69

IMPATTs based on InP, Si, and GaAs is one order lower in DDRs based on WBG semiconductors such as GaN and SiC. The magnitude of electric field, ξ_P, at the metallurgical junction of DDR InP IMPATT device is highest and that of DDR GaAs device is lowest. In this context, it is worthwhile to note that the magnitude of peak field ξ_P increases with the increasing frequency (Table 1.2). It is observed that ξ_P in 4H-SiC DDR IMPATTs increases from 3.59×10^8 at 94 GHz to 5.17×10^8 Vm^{-1} at 1.0 THz.

It is observed from Table 1.2 that the reverse voltage at breakdown (V_B) is highest in DDR GaN devices among all other DDR devices. The breakdown voltages of DDRs based on WBG semiconductors like 4H-SiC and Wz-GaN are found (Table 1.2, Figs. 1.8 and 1.10) to be larger than those based on conventional semiconductors like Si, GaAs, and InP. Between Si and InP DDR IMPATTs operating at the same frequency, the reverse breakdown occurs at higher voltage (V_B) in InP DDR devices (Table 1.2, Figs. 1.8 and 1.10).

The difference of breakdown voltage (V_B) and avalanche zone voltage (V_A) of DDR device is the voltage drop across its drift zone, i.e., $V_D = V_B - V_A$. According to Scharfetter-Gummel semiquantitative formula [66], the DC to RF conversion efficiency of IMPATT device is given by $\eta = (2m/\pi) \times (V_D/V_B)$ where the voltage modulation factor, m, is taken to be 0.5. Therefore, $\eta = (1/\pi) \times (V_D/V_B)$. This means that higher the ratio (V_D/V_B), higher is the efficiency of DC to RF conversion. Figs. 1.8 and 1.10 show that with increasing frequency, the conversion efficiency decreases for all DDR devices due to the decrease of the ratio, V_D/V_B.

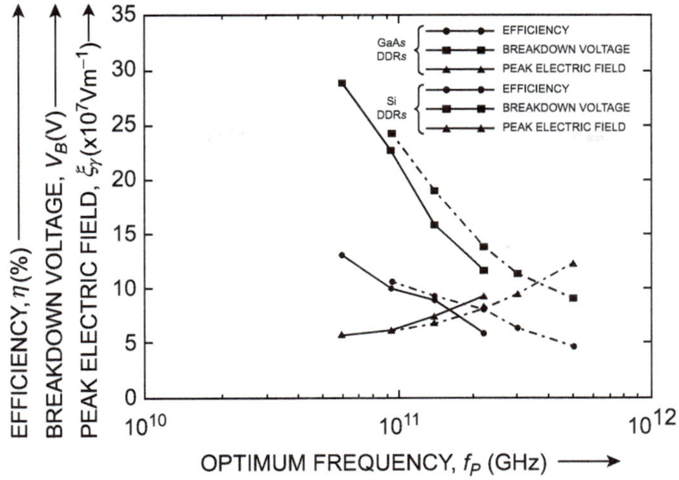

FIG. 1.8 Plots of η, V_B, and ξ_P of double-drift region (DDR) Si and GaAs IMPATTs versus optimum frequency.

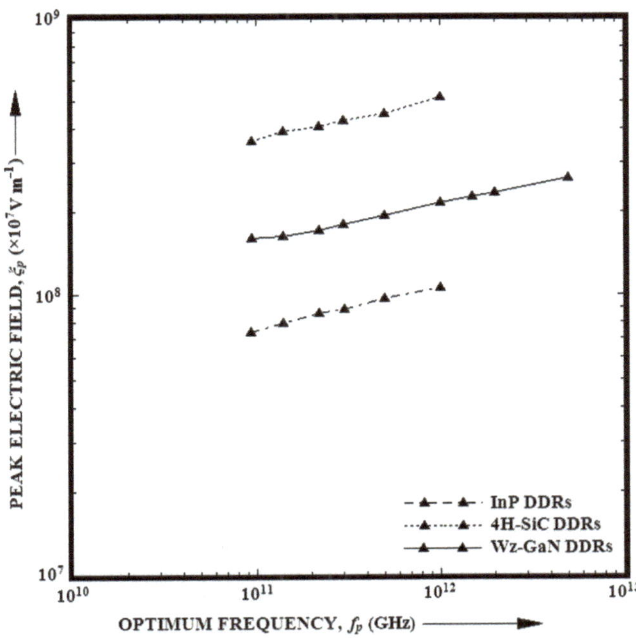

FIG. 1.9 Plots of peak junction field ξ_P of double-drift region (DDR) IMPATTs based on InP, 4H-SiC, and Wz-GaN against optimum frequency.

Fig. 1.10 shows that at 94 GHz, the efficiency versus frequency curves of double-drift IMPATTs based on 4H-SiC and Wz-GaN intersect each other. This means that 4H-SiC and GaN DDR devices will have same efficiency at 94 GHz frequency. However, at 1 THz, 4H-SiC DDR IMPATTs will have much lower efficiency than GaN DDR devices. The DC to microwave conversion efficiency is highest in InP DDR IMPATTs followed by Si and GaAs DDR devices (Figs. 1.8 and 1.10).

The RF performance of Si and GaAs DDR devices with respect to their efficiency (η) can be compared at different frequencies in the range of 94–500 GHz from Fig. 1.8. It is observed that the efficiency of Si DDRs is higher than GaAs DDRs within the frequency

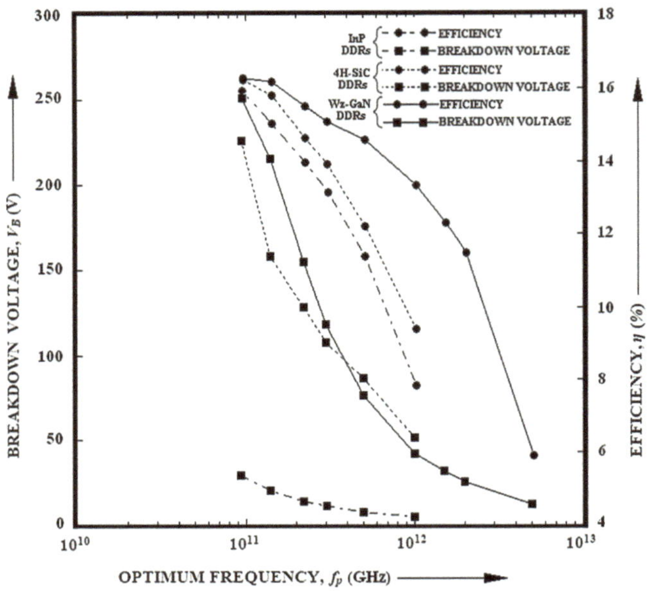

FIG. 1.10 Plots of V_B and η versus optimum frequency for double-drift region (DDR) IMPATT devices based on InP, 4H-SiC, and Wz-GaN.

range of 150–220 GHz. At 140 GHz, the efficiencies of Si and GaAs DDRs are nearly the same. It is observed from Fig. 1.10 that DDRs based on WBG semiconductors like Wz-GaN and 4H-SiC should provide higher efficiency than those made of conventional semiconductors like Si and GaAs (Fig. 1.8 and Table 1.2). The aforementioned results clearly indicate that GaN DDR devices excel all other DDRs with respect to achieving high efficiency in the THz frequency band. It is interesting to note that the rate of decrease of efficiency with increasing frequency ($d\eta/df$) is lower in GaN DDRs than that in 4H-SiC and InP DDRs up to a maximum frequency of 1 THz. Thus, GaN DDRs have an edge over other DDRs as regard high-power delivery and high conversion efficiency in the THz frequency band.

Table 1.2 shows that the ratio of avalanche zone width to total drift layer width (x_A/W) increases for each base material of DDR IMPATTs as one moves from serial number 1 to higher serial number which corresponds to increasing frequency (Table 1.3). This indicates that the avalanche zone widens with increasing frequency. Thus, the voltage across the avalanche zone (V_A) increases and consequently the voltage across the drift zone (V_D) decreases with increasing frequency. The ratio V_D/V_B decreases and correspondingly the conversion efficiency (η) decreases with increasing frequency. The ratio x_A/W of GaAS DDR IMPATTs increases from 40.0% to 66.36% as frequency increases from 60 to 220 GHz and the DC to RF conversion efficiency η decreases to a low value of 5.77% in GaAs DDR IMPATTs at 220 GHz. Similarly, in case of Si DDR IMPATTs, x_A/W increases from 53.10% to 67.16% and η decreases from 7.99% to 4.55% as the frequency increases from 220 to 500 GHz (Table 1.2). It is further observed that x_A/W of DDRs based on InP, 4H-SiC, and Wz-GaN increases from 41.79% to 67.85%, 37.08% to 61.33%, and 38.49% to 40.61%, respectively, as frequency increases from 300 GHz to 1 THz. It is interesting to note that in the range of frequency 0.3–1 THz, x_A/W of GaN DDRs remains almost constant without appreciable increase in contrast with that of 4H-SiC and InP DDRs (vide serial numbers 4, 5, 6 of Tables 1.2 and 1.3). But x_A/W of GaN devices increases appreciably above 1 THz. With the increase of frequency from 1–5 THz, x_A/W of GaN DDR IMPATTs increases sharply from 40.61% to 67.69% (column 9, serial numbers 6–9 of Tables 1.2 and 1.3). This increase of x_A/W causes increase of V_A/V_B and decrease of V_D/V_B, leading to sharp decrease of conversion efficiency from 13.32% to 5.88% (column 7, serial numbers 6–9, Tables 1.2 and 1.3). Similarly the conversion efficiency of 4H-SiC DDR device decreases from 13.13% to 7.82% and that of InP DDRs decreases from 13.89% to 9.38% with increase of frequency from 0.3 to 1 THz. All the aforementioned DC results indicate that GaN DDR IMPATTs can emerge as useful sources of power generation in the THz frequency regime.

TABLE 1.3
High-Frequency Parameters.

Base Material	Serial Number	f_p (GHz)	G_p ($\times 10^7$ Sm^{-2})	B_p ($\times 10^7$ Sm^{-2})	$Q_p = -(B_p/G_p)$	Z_R ($\times 10^{-9}$ Ωm^{-2})	P_{RF} (mW)	D_j (μm)
GaAs	1	60	−2.9548	3.5293	1.19	−13.9461	1828.47	55.0
	2	94	−5.8886	7.8662	1.34	−6.0988	909.89	35.0
	3	140	−10.4730	19.4641	1.86	−2.1438	400.04	25.0
	4	220	−17.1452	56.7970	3.31	−0.4871	226.89	20.0
Si	1	94	−4.0002	6.5654	1.64	−6.7679	708.43	35.0
	2	140	−8.0772	15.4697	1.92	−2.6524	446.35	25.0
	3	219	−18.0334	38.7885	2.15	−0.9855	334.23	20.0
	4	302	−26.2239	80.1598	3.05	−0.3686	184.59	15.0
	5	500	−67.5571	222.3756	3.29	−0.1251	136.10	10.0
InP	1	94	−8.2457	6.8436	0.83	−7.1811	2059.17	35.0
	2	140	−26.6945	13.7556	0.52	−2.9599	1602.12	25.0
	3	220	−49.3589	47.2443	0.96	−1.0573	857.17	20.0
	4	300	−78.9689	72.7609	0.92	−0.6849	500.22	15.0
	5	501	−278.1512	213.6971	0.77	−0.2268	342.21	10.0
	6	1000	−598.7561	703.7719	1.17	−0.0701	72.10	5.0
4H-SiC	1	95	−1.9711	0.5574	0.28	−46.9756	30,290.98	35.0
	2	140	−4.2152	1.3511	0.32	−21.5132	16,180.81	25.0
	3	220	−9.1919	3.7236	0.41	−9.3454	13,315.09	20.0
	4	300	−20.4917	8.3277	0.41	−4.1883	13,130.85	15.0
	5	500	−51.1584	14.3506	0.28	−1.8121	9355.78	10.0
	6	1000	−121.6192	46.1491	0.38	−0.7187	1982.31	5.0
Wz-GaN	1	95	−0.1638	1.7788	10.86	−5.1361	3117.78	35.0
	2	140	−0.3953	3.7869	9.58	−2.7262	2818.41	25.0
	3	220	−1.1101	9.1187	8.21	−1.3155	2622.73	20.0
	4	300	−2.3439	16.9007	7.21	−0.8051	1806.27	15.0
	5	500	−8.1282	46.6598	5.74	−0.3632	1162.62	10.0
	6	1000	−47.1109	180.2237	3.82	−0.1358	504.16	5.0
	7	1500	−126.7654	408.2341	3.22	−0.0693	192.09	2.5
	8	2000	−211.6412	730.3715	3.45	−0.0366	47.54	1.2
	9	5000	−445.7865	1045.0674	2.34	−0.0345	7.62	0.7

High-frequency properties of IMPATT diode

High-frequency parameters can be obtained from small-signal simulation of DDR IMPATTs made of conventional and WBG semiconducting materials. Table 1.3 shows these parameters, i.e., optimum frequency (f_p), peak negative conductance (G_p), positive susceptance (B_p), quality factor or Q-factor (Q_p), negative resistance (Z_R), and RF power output (P_{RF}) of the devices.

Fig. 1.11 shows the small-signal admittance, i.e., conductance versus susceptance (G-B) plots for GaAs and Si DDR IMPATTs. These plots show that the optimum frequencies for GaAs devices are 94, 140, 220, and 300 GHz, while those for Si devices are 94, 140, 220, 300, and 500 GHz. The admittance plots shown in Fig. 1.11 clearly indicate that Si DDR IMPATTs can be used up to 0.5 THz in contrast to GaAs IMPATTs.

Figs. 1.12 and 1.13 show the admittance curves of InP and 4H-SiC DDR IMPATTs, respectively. The optimum frequencies obtained from these plots are 94, 140, 220, 300, 500, and 1000 GHz for both InP and 4-H SiC devices.

The Q-factor ($Q_p = -B_p/G_p$) is an indicator of conversion efficiency and growth rate of oscillation in IMPATT devices. This factor should be close to and slightly less than 1 ($Q_p \approx 1$) to obtain stable oscillation and higher efficiency from IMPATT devices. Table 1.3 shows that the Q-factor of InP DDR IMPATTs is the lowest close to unity (Table 1.3) followed by 4H-SiC DDR device and others. Table 1.3 also shows Q-factors of DDR IMPATTs based on different materials at mm-wave and THz frequencies. The optimum frequencies obtained from the admittance plots of DDR

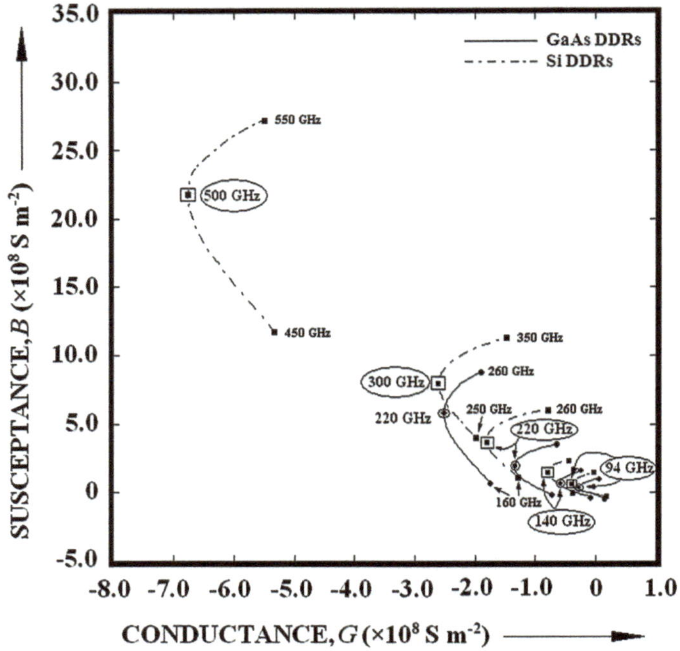

FIG. 1.11 Admittance characteristics (G-B) plots of double-drift region (DDR) IMPATTs made of GaAs and Si.

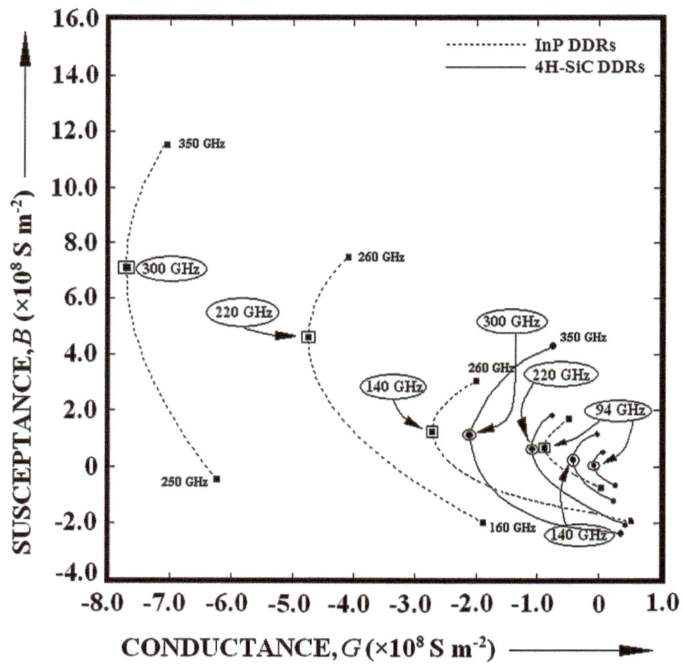

FIG. 1.12 G-B plots for double-drift region (DDR) IMPATTs based on InP and 4H-SiC (optimum frequencies are shown).

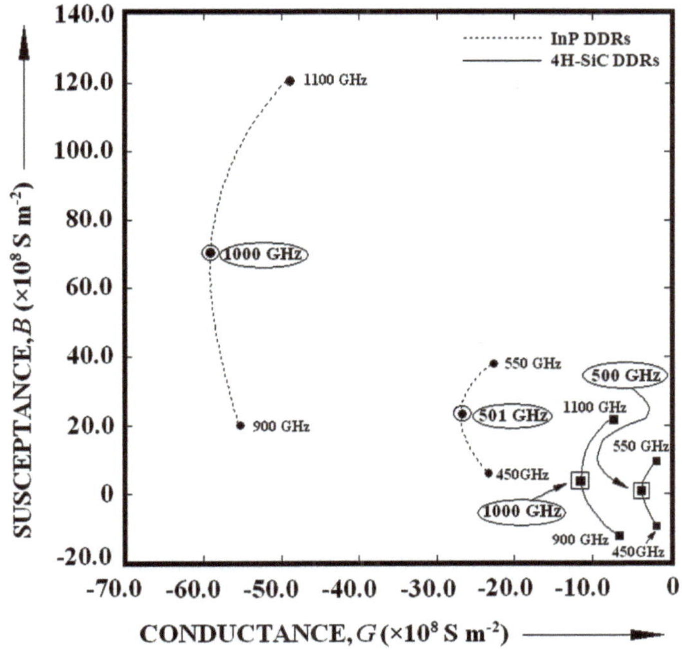

FIG. 1.13 Admittance (G-B) plots of double-drift region (DDR) IMPATT devices made of InP and 4H-SiC (optimum frequencies in THz band as marked).

IMPATTs based on medium and WBG semiconductors play the decisive role to select the proper base material of IMPATTs and design the same for THz operation. Fig. 1.14 shows the admittance plots of DDR IMPATTs based on GaN at the optimum frequencies of 94, 140, 220 and 300 GHz which are incidentally the window frequencies in the millimeter wave region. Fig. 1.15 shows similar plots at the optimum frequencies of 500, 1000, 1500, 2000 and 3000 GHz ie, 0.5, 1, 1.5, 2.0 and 3.0 THz.

Device negative resistance (Z_R) is an important parameter to estimate the RF power output from the device. Table 1.3 shows the simulated values of Z_R, obtained from the real part of device impedance. It decreases with increasing frequency for different base materials of DDR IMPATTs under consideration. It is observed from Table 1.3 that 4H-SiC DDR IMPATTs exhibit highest negative resistance (Z_R) among all other DDR devices for the frequency range of 94 GHz to 1 THz. The highest negative resistance of 4H-SiC DDR IMPATTs implies that these devices deliver highest RF power at the optimum frequency as compared with DDR devices based on other materials.

Fig. 1.16 shows the variations of RF power output (P_{RF}) with optimum frequency for all types of DDR IMPATTs. It is observed that P_{RF} decreases nonlinearly with increasing frequency in all cases. Table 1.3 gives the output power from IMPATTs based on different semiconductors at different optimum frequencies. It is observed from both Fig. 1.16 and Table 1.3 that Si DDR IMPATTs deliver higher output power than GaAs IMPATTs at 140 and 220 GHz window frequencies. The cut-off frequencies above which their it may be noted that the RF performances of Si and GaAs DDRs are limited above 500 and 220 GHz, respectively. These cut-off frequencies are obtained from avalanche response analysis. The simulated output powers from different DDR devices are shown in Table 1.3 and Fig. 1.16. As regard power delivery at 94, 140, and 220 GHz window frequencies, InP DDRs should be preferred to Si and GaAs DDRs. Moreover, InP IMPATTs are capable of delivering power up to 1 THz frequency. The avalanche response limits the operating frequencies of both Si and GaAs DDR IMPATTs below 1 THz. It is worthwhile to observe from Fig. 1.16 as well as Table 1.3 that DDR IMPATTs based on WBG semiconductors like 4H-SiC and Wz-GaN are excellent candidates for THz operation. The reported results indicate that these devices are capable of delivering high power with high conversion efficiency at THz frequencies. It may be concluded from the aforementioned results that IMPATT devices based on Wz-GaN are without any competition above 1 THz as regard delivering high power with high conversion efficiency.

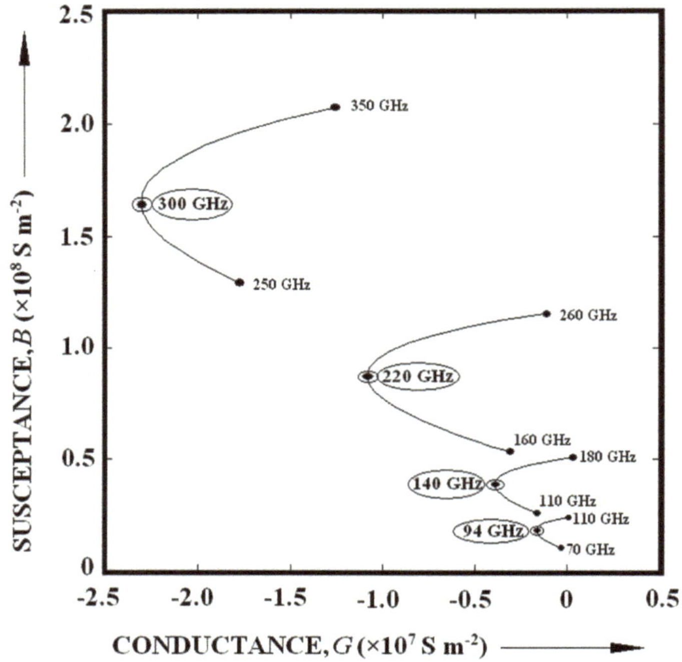

FIG. 1.14 Admittance (G-B) plots for double-drift region (DDR) devices based on Wz-GaN (optimum frequencies are marked).

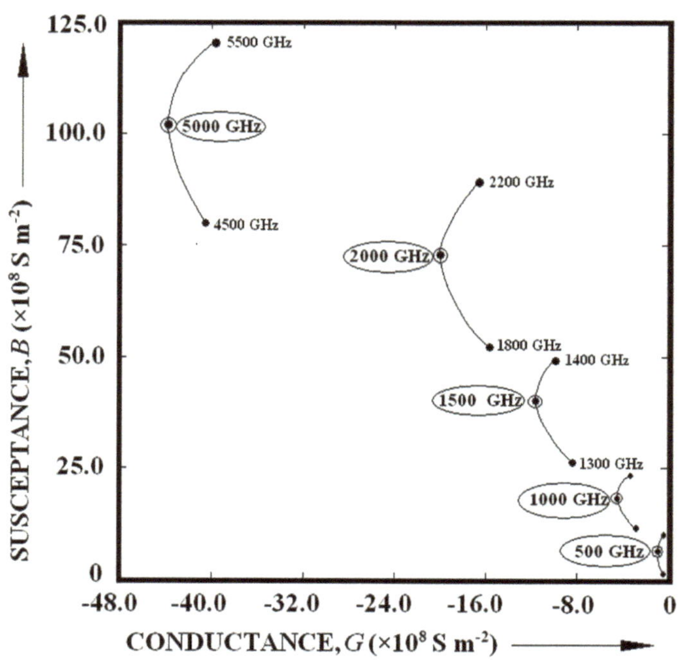

FIG. 1.15 Conductance-susceptance (G-B) plots for double-drift region (DDR) devices made of Wz-GaN operating at THz frequency bands (optimum frequencies are marked).

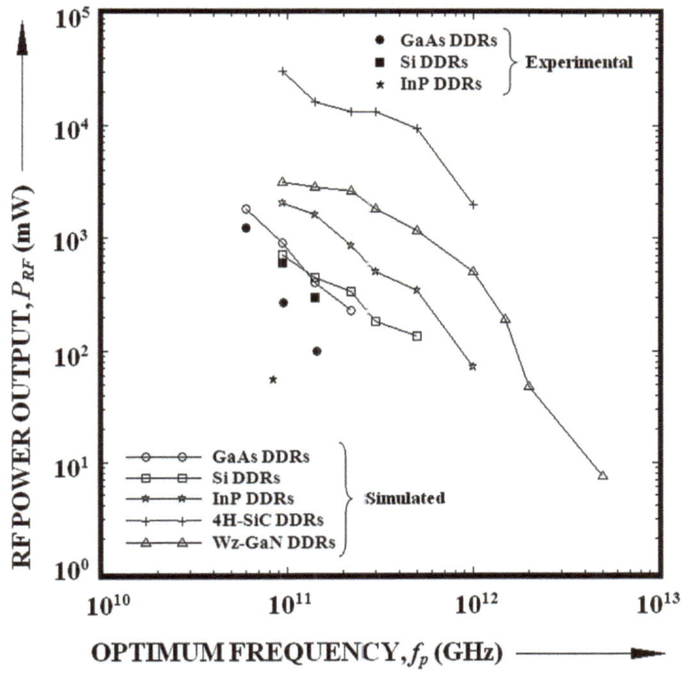

FIG. 1.16 Power-frequency curves for different double-drift region (DDR) devices (available experimental data shown in the inset).

RF power output (P_{RF}) of DDR IMPATT devices based on different semiconductors are obtained at different operating frequencies from the breakdown voltage (V_B), RF voltage modulation (m_x), negative conductance at the optimum frequency (G_p), and diameter of circular mesa-etched device (D_j). With increasing frequency, all dimensions of the device decrease and so also the parameter (D_j). It is observed from a rigorous steady-state thermal analysis of the device reported in Ref. [64,65] that D_j should decrease from 55 μm at 60 GHz to 0.7 μm at 500 GHz to restrict the rise of junction temperature above 500 K. The values of junction diameter of DDR IMPATTs, based on five different semiconductors and operating at various mm-wave and THz frequency bands, are given in Table 1.3.

Comparison of simulated RF properties of IMPATTs with experimental data

Fig. 1.16 shows the simulated power-frequency plots of DDR IMPATTs based on conventional (Si, GaAs, InP) and WBG semiconductors (4H-SiC, Wz-GaN). The available experimental results are also shown in the figure (as small rectangular areas for SI DDRs and dots for GaAs and InP DDRs) for the sake of comparison. The experimental reports show that DDR SI IMPATT device delivers output power of 600 and 300 mW at 94 and 140 GHz which agree very well with the simulation results (Fig. 1.16). Available experimental results show that GaAs DDR device delivers 1.24 W at 60 GHz, 0.27 W at 95 GHz, and 0.10 W at 144 GHz [34,40,67] which are also in close agreement with the simulation results, shown as circular dots on the theoretical curve (Fig. 1.16). In case of DDR InP DDR IMPATTs experimental report, marked as dots on Fig. 1.16, shows that these devices provide 55 mW power at 84.8 GHz [68] which again agree well with the simulated value. It may be noted that while the simulated results for GaAs DDR IMPATTs are in close agreement with the experimental results at 60 GHz but above this frequency a little departure from the experimental value is observed. Similar feature is observed for DDR InP IMPATT devices at W-band. The possible reasons for obtaining lower power from the experimental devices are (i) immature device fabrication process technology and (ii) nonavailability of accurate device design. The experimental reports of fabrication and characterization of 4H-SiC and Wz-GaN DDR IMPATT devices at higher mm-wave and THz frequency band are not available in the literature and therefore simulated results on the RF power output could not be compared with the experimental data.

MM-WAVE AND THz IMPATTS BASED ON SOME WIDE BANDGAP SEMICONDUCTORS

Apart from experimental reports on fabrication and characterization of Si SDR and DDR IMPATTs, some reports of fabrication of IMPATTS made of GaAs, InP, and 4H-SiC are available in the literature. The favorable material properties of WBG semiconductors like Wurtzite-GaN (Wz-GaN) and type-IIb diamond can be utilized to use these materials as base semiconductors of DDR IMPATT devices for obtaining high power at THz frequencies. In this section, the potentiality of DDR IMPATTs based on WBG semiconductors will be explored as high power-high efficiency sources at THz frequency bands. The simulation study based on avalanche response approach reveals that the upper cut-off frequency of diamond IMPATTs is 1.50 THz, while the same for Si IMPATTs is much smaller, i.e., 0.50 THz. The reported simulation results show that DDR IMPATTs based on type-IIb diamond excel those based on Si as regard high power and high efficiency at THz frequency regime.

The high-frequency performance of DDR devices based on GaAs, InP, and Si are also compared with those of based on Wz-GaN. The results show that the performance of Wz-GaN DDR IMPATTs is significantly better than that of GaAs, InP, and Si DDR IMPATTs at both mm-wave and THz frequencies.

DDR IMPATTs Based on Diamond

Diamond, being a WBG semiconductor, has a lot of promise for THz IMPATTs. The n, p-layer widths (W_n, W_p) and donor, acceptor impurity density of n, p, and n + p $^+$layers (N_D, N_A, and N_{n+}, N_{p+}) are designed from TT consideration [50] to obtain optimum RF performance of DDR IMPATTs based on diamond and silicon at different mm-wave and THz frequencies. The values of W_n, W_p, N_D, and N_A for diamond and Si IMPATTs are given in Table 1.4 for where the serial numbers correspond to different design frequencies, f_d, as indicated in Table 1.3.

The doping concentrations of n^+- and p^+-layers (N_{n+} and N_{p+}) are usually taken to be 5×10^{25} m^{-3}. The diameters of mesa-etched circular junction, D_j, and corresponding junction areas of the device are obtained at different frequencies for both diamond and Si DDRs from thermal analysis so that the junction temperature is limited below 500 K [64,65]. The calculated values of D_j are given in Table 1.4. It is observed that the junction diameters (D_j) of DDR diamond IMPATTs are 35 and 2.5 μm at 94 GHz and 1.5 THz, respectively.

DC parameters of diamond and silicon DDR IMPATTs: a comparative study

The DC parameters of diamond and silicon DDR devices can be extracted from the large-signal parameters by computing their average values over the time period of a full oscillation cycle. Table 1.5 shows the DC parameters such as (i) peak electric field (ξ_P), (ii) breakdown voltage (V_B), (iii) avalanche voltage (V_A), (iv) ratio of drift zone voltage to breakdown voltage (V_D/V_B) where $V_D = V_B - V_A$, (v) avalanche layer width (x_A) where $x_A = |x_{A1}| + x_{A2}$, and (vi) ratio of avalanche layer width to total drift layer width (x_A/W; where $W = W_n + W_p$). The variations of ξ_P, V_B, and V_A with operating frequency are shown in Fig. 1.17 for both diamond and Si IMPATTs. Using Fig. 1.17 and Table 1.5, the DC properties of DDR diamond and Si devices can be compared at different design frequencies. Table 1.5 shows that with increasing frequency, the peak electric field (ξ_P) increases, while the breakdown voltage (V_B), avalanche zone voltage (V_A), and avalanche layer width (x_A) of the device decrease. The magnitude of junction field (ξ_p) at a fixed design frequency is higher in DDR diamond devices than in DDR Si devices. It may be noted that with the increase of frequency from 94 GHz to 1.5 THz, the junction field in DDR diamond IMPATTs increase from 9.10×10^7 to 1.46×10^8 V m^{-1} and that in DDR Si IMPATTs increase from $6.04 \times 10^7 - 1.23 \times 10^8$ V m^{-1}. The peak field at the junction of DDR diamond devices (ξ_P) is lower, while the breakdown voltage is higher as compared with those in DDR Si devices at the design frequency of 0.5 THz. At a particular frequency, the lower peak field at the junction of DDR diamond device is due to its larger depletion layer width ($W = W_n + W_p$) as compared with DDR Si device. The voltage across the drift layer ($V_D = V_B - V_A$) of diamond IMPATTs at different frequencies is calculated from the difference of breakdown voltage (V_B) and avalanche zone voltage (V_A). It is observed from Table 1.5 that with increasing frequency, DDR diamond IMPATTs have higher V_D/V_B ratio than DDR Si IMPATTs. For example, this ratio is 0. 4771 and 0.3346 at 94 GHz and 0.4897 and 0.1615 at 0.5 THz for DDR diamond and Si devices, respectively. The rate of decrease of V_D/V_B ratio at THz frequency is slightly sharper in DDR Si IMPATTs than in DDR diamond IMPATTs. The conversion efficiency is proportional to V_D/V_B ratio [66] and therefore the efficiency of DDR Si devices decreases a bit sharply as compared with that of diamond devices.

With increasing frequency, the x_A/W ratio of DDR diamond IMPATTs remains almost constant, while that of DDR Si IMPATTs increases appreciably. Increase of $x_A/$

TABLE 1.4
Design Parameters.

Semiconductor	Serial Number	f_d (GHz)	W_n (μm)	W_p (μm)	N_D ($\times10^{23}$ m^{-3})	N_A ($\times10^{23}$ m^{-3})	N_{n+} ($\times10^{25}$ m^{-3})	N_{p+} ($\times10^{25}$ m^{-3})	D_j (μm)
Diamond	1	94	0.780	0.720	0.460	0.530	5.000	2.700	35.0
	2	140	0.530	0.530	0.810	0.870	5.000	2.700	25.0
	3	220	0.320	0.320	1.350	1.490	5.000	2.700	20.0
	4	300	0.220	0.220	2.050	2.220	5.000	2.700	15.0
	5	500	0.120	0.120	3.750	4.100	5.000	2.700	10.0
	6	1000	0.052	0.052	9.500	10.00	5.000	2.700	5.0
	7	1500	0.030	0.030	36.00	37.00	5.000	2.700	2.5
Si	1	94	0.400	0.380	1.200	1.250	5.000	2.700	35.0
	2	140	0.280	0.245	1.800	2.100	5.000	2.700	25.0
	3	220	0.180	0.160	3.950	4.590	5.000	2.700	20.0
	4	300	0.132	0.112	6.000	7.300	5.000	2.700	15.0
	5	500	0.072	0.072	15.00	16.20	5.000	2.700	10.0

TABLE 1.5
Simulated DC Properties of Diamond- and Si-Based DDR IMPATTs at Different Frequencies.

Semiconducting Material	Serial Number	J_0 ($\times 10^8$ Am^{-2})	ξ_P ($\times 10^7$ Vm^{-1})	V_B (V)	V_A (V)	V_D $/V_B$ (%)	x_A (μm)	x_A/W (%)
Diamond	1	4.00	9.11180	111.54	58.33	47.71	0.638	43.88
	2	7.50	9.98950	63.16	28.01	55.65	0.328	30.94
	3	13.0	10.5458	38.72	17.92	53.71	0.198	30.94
	4	17.0	11.0065	26.90	12.57	53.27	0.132	30.00
	5	25.0	11.6943	15.56	7.941	48.97	0.078	32.50
	6	39.0	12.8940	7.761	4.283	44.85	0.038	36.08
	7	48.0	14.6692	3.223	2.094	35.09	0.016	26.67
Si	1	3.40	6.03700	24.36	16.21	33.46	0.348	44.62
	2	5.80	6.68700	19.02	13.64	28.66	0.270	51.42
	3	14.5	8.18700	13.99	10.40	25.66	0.172	49.86
	4	24.5	9.33700	11.71	9.25	21.01	0.136	55.74
	5	55.0	12.3120	9.35	7.84	16.15	0.089	63.03

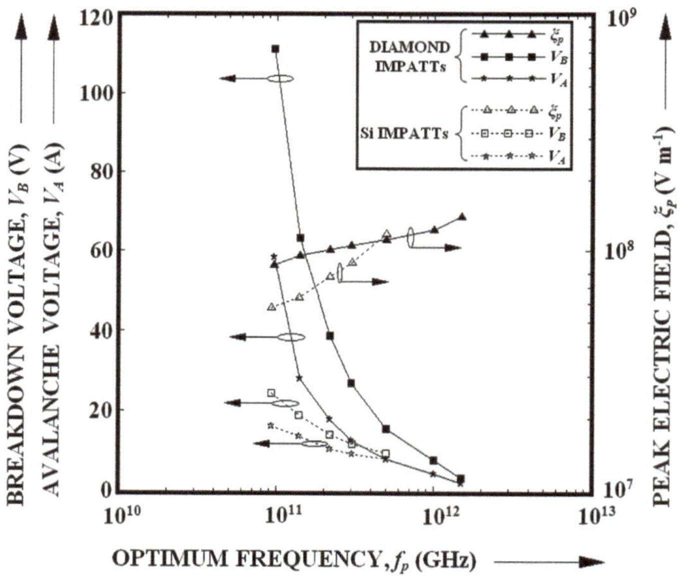

FIG. 1.17 Variations of breakdown voltage, avalanche zone voltage, and peak electric field with optimum frequency of double-drift region diamond and Si IMPATTs.

W ratio with increasing frequency indicates decrease of conversion efficiency due to decrease of V_D/V_B ratio [66]. Thus, the degradation of conversion efficiency at THz frequency will be more pronounced in DDR Si IMPATT devices than in DDR Si devices.

Large-signal properties of DDR diamond and Si IMPATTs at mm-wave and THz frequency bands

The simulated large-signal parameters of DDR diamond and Si IMPATTs are obtained at mm-wave and THz frequency bands for a voltage modulation of 50% and these are given in Table 1.6 for the sake of comparison. The parameters listed in the table are optimum frequency (f_p), avalanche resonance frequency (f_a), peak negative conductance (G_p), corresponding susceptance (B_p), quality factor (Q_p), negative resistance (Z_R), P_{RF}, and η_L. The admittance (G-B) plots for diamond- and Si-based DDR IMPATT devices at optimum frequencies of 94, 140, 220, and 300 GHz are shown in Fig. 1.18, while the G-B plots of diamond-based DDR IMPATTs at 0.5, 1.0, and 1.5 THz (solid lines) and Si-based DDR IMPATTs at 0.5 THz (dotted line) are shown in Fig. 1.19.

TABLE 1.6
Simulated High-Frequency Parameters of DDR IMPATT Devices Based on Diamond and Silicon.

Base Material	Serial Number	f_p (GHz)	f_a (GHz)	G_p ($\times 10^7$ S m^{-2})	B_p ($\times 10^7$ S m^{-2})	$Q_p = -(B_p/G_p)$	Z_R ($\times 10^{-10}$ Ω m^{-2})	P_{RF} (mW)	η_L (%)
Diamond	1	95.6	49.5	−0.3212	1.2541	2.40	−283.6800	7797.60	18.17
	2	140.0	99.0	−1.3181	2.9199	2.21	−128.4311	3226.40	13.88
	3	218.0	144.5	−2.9765	7.8421	2.63	−42.3141	1752.40	11.08
	4	301.0	192.1	−5.5742	16.0669	2.88	−19.2730	890.98	11.02
	5	502.0	283.9	−12.7406	52.1542	4.09	−4.4202	302.84	9.91
	6	1002.0	469.0	−37.7468	252.0855	6.68	−0.5809	55.79	9.39
	7	1501.0	704.4	−97.3996	660.1105	6.78	−0.2188	6.19	8.17
Si	1	93.0	52.0	−0.8815	3.6758	4.17	−61.6960	629.13	7.89
	2	139.5	70.9	−1.5069	8.5124	5.65	−20.1643	334.49	6.18
	3	218.5	111.5	−3.8668	19.5416	5.05	−9.7443	297.20	4.66
	4	301.5	141.3	−5.7154	40.5807	7.10	−3.4031	173.12	3.41
	5	501.5	196.7	−10.4471	121.2923	11.62	−0.7045	89.61	2.22

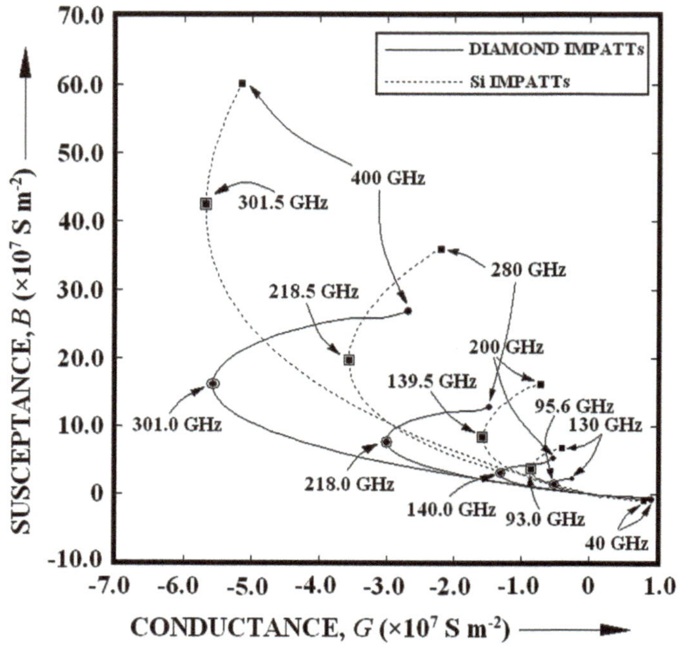

FIG. 1.18 Admittance (G-B) plots of diamond- and Si-based double-drift region IMPATT devices at optimum frequencies of 94, 140, 220, and 300 GHz.

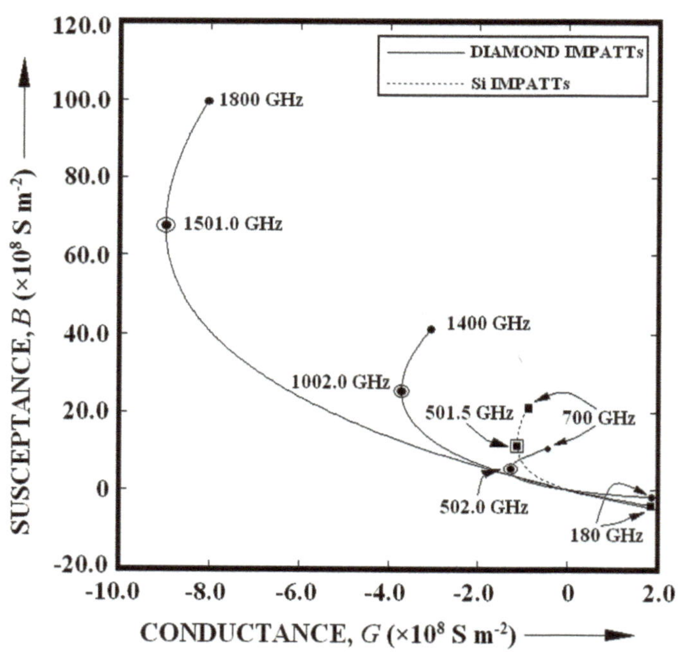

FIG. 1.19 Conductance-susceptance (G-B) plots of diamond-based double-drift region IMPATTs at 0.5, 1.0, and 1.5 THz (*solid lines*) and Si-based DDR IMPATTs at 0.5 THz (*dotted line*).

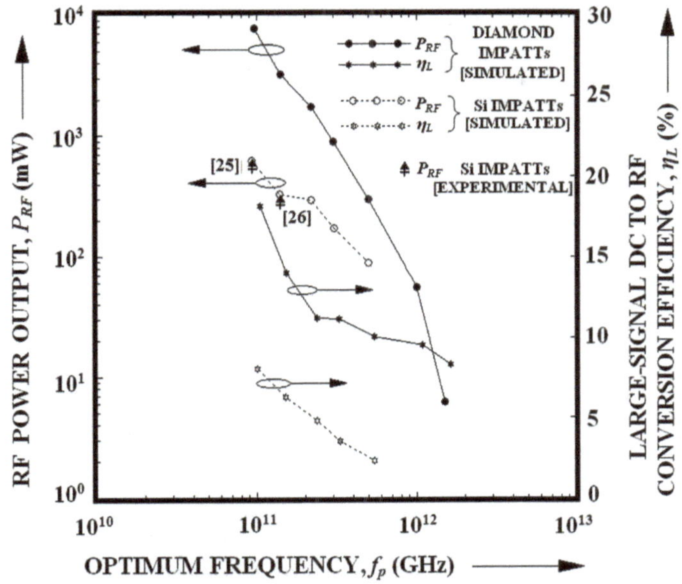

FIG. 1.20 Output power and large-signal efficiency versus optimum frequency for diamond- and Si-based DDRs.

The admittance (G-B) plots shown in Figs. 1.18 and1.19 provide the optimum frequencies (fp) at which the magnitudes of G and B attain the peak values as well as the avalanche resonance frequencies (f_a) at which the admittance curve intersects x-axis and the conductance changes from negative to positive values which means that oscillation will cease beyond this frequency. Table 1.6 shows that with increasing value of fp from 94 to 500 GHz, f_a increases from 49.5 to 283.9 GHz and 52.0–196.7 GHz in case of DDR diamond and Si devices, respectively. Thus, diamond DDR IMPATTs exhibit wider bandwidth of oscillation than its Si counterpart. The Quality factor at the optimum frequency, $Q_p = (-G_p/B_p)$, is a very good indicator of stability and growth rate of oscillation in IMPATT devices. The device design based on small-signal simulation should ensure that Q_p is nearly unity which means that the magnitude of conductance is almost same as that of susceptance at the optimum frequency. In this respect, quality factors of diamond DDR devices are better than corresponding Si DDR devices (Table 1.6) at all design frequencies under consideration. It is observed that the magnitude of negative resistance (Z_R) is higher in DDR diamond IMPATTs than in its silicon counterpart for five design frequencies up to 0.5 THz corresponding to serial numbers 1–5 (Table 1.6). This indicates higher power delivery from DDR diamond IMPATTs in comparison to DDR Si devices for the aforementioned five frequencies.

The large-signal power-frequency ($P_{RF}-\eta_L$) curves for diamond and Si DDRs are shown in Fig. 1.20 at a fixed voltage modulation of 50% and optimum frequencies of 94, 140, 220, and 300 GHz. It is observed from Fig. 1.20 and Table 1.6 that diamond IMPATTs provide higher output power with higher efficiency than Si IMPATTs at THz frequency band. It is observed that diamond-based DDRs provide large-signal peak output powers of 7.79 and 302.84 mW with 18.17% and 9.91% conversion efficiency at 94 GHz and 0.5 THz, respectively, for 50% voltage modulation (Table 1.6). On the other hand, Si-based DDRs provide large-signal peak powers of 629.13 and 89.61 mW with 7.89% and 2.22% efficiency at 94 and 500 GHz, respectively, for 50% voltage modulation. It is very important to note that at 1.5 THz frequency, diamond-based DDR devices can deliver significant large-signal power of about 6.19 mW with 8.17% conversion efficiency.

POSSIBLE FABRICATION STEPS OF (I) TYPE-IIB DIAMOND AND (II) Wz-GaN-BASED DDR IMPATT DEVICES

(i) Ion-implantation technique [69,70] can be used to fabricate DDR (n^+-n-p-p^+) IMPATT device based on diamond. Single crystal diamond can be grown successfully by chemical vapor deposition (CVD) techniques such as hot-filament CVD [71], microwave plasma-assisted CVD [72–77], DC arc plasma jet CVD [78], and other CVD methods [79–83]. The single crystal diamond is then doped either n-type or p-type to fabricate the junction of IMPATT device. Diffusion technique is not suitable for the junction growth since most of the impurities in diamond have low diffusivity. Reports of doping type-IIb diamond by ion-implantation [84,85] and CVD [86,87] process are available. Boron (B) can be successfully doped as acceptor type in diamond with an activation energy of 0.37 eV [88]. During the growth process of diamond by CVD, boron can be introduced in diamond in gaseous form as toxic diborane [89–91] or in solid form as either boron powder [92] or boron trioxide [87] or in liquid form as trimethyl borate [93] to obtain p-type epitaxial layer. But n-type doping of diamond is a tricky job. Nitrogen is used as n-type dopant in diamond [94]. The potential n-type dopants in diamond are lithium (Li), phosphorus (P), arsenic (As), and antimony (Sb). But the most promising n-type dopant in diamond is phosphorus. Koizumi et al. [95] successfully produced n-type diamond films with phosphorous by CVD process with an activation energy of 0.43 eV. Recently, several researchers have successfully doped diamond with phosphorus to make it n-type [96,97]. A p-n junction is successfully fabricated by implanting lithium [85] or arsenic [98] ions into p-type diamond crystals followed by high-temperature annealing.

Ta/Au and Ti/Au deposited on diamond [99–102] followed by annealing produce good ohmic contact. A specific contact resistance of $2 \times 10^{-5}\ \Omega\ \mathrm{cm}^2$ is reported from annealed Mo- and Ti-carbide contacts on highly doped diamond epitaxial films [103]. The specific contact resistance improves by two orders of magnitude if Mo-carbide is used in place of Ti-carbide as contact material with lightly doped type-IIb semiconducting diamonds [69].

(ii) Heteroepitaxial growth of Wz-GaN has been reported on sapphire [104,105], 6H-SiC [106], 4H-SiC [107,108], and AlN/Si [109] substrates by using techniques like hydride vapor phase epitaxy, metal-organic vapor phase epitaxy (MOVPE), low pressure metal-organic chemical vapor deposition (LP-MOCVD), plasma-assisted molecular beam epitaxy techniques (PA-MBE), etc. Homoepitaxial growth is preferred to heteroepitaxial growth since it provides better microelectronic and optoelectronic performance due to formation of low dislocation lines per unit area at the interface of substrate and epitaxy. Further homoepitaxial growth avoids the complex process steps like nitridation and nucleation. Homoepitaxial growth, i.e., GaN epilayer growth on GaN substrate has been reported using MBE [110], MOCVD [111], and MOVPE [112] techniques. Si and Mg have been used as donor and acceptor, respectively, to fabricate DDR n^+-n-p-p^+ structure [109]. Both donor and acceptor type doping in GaN wafer with impurity concentration exceeding $10^{25}\ \mathrm{m}^{-3}$ has been reported [104,105]. Deposition of Ni/Ag metal combination on highly doped n^+ and p^+ layers of Wz-GaN DDR structure followed by annealing has been reported [109] which provides nonrectifying ohmic contact.

The potentiality of DDR Wz-GaN IMPATT devices as regard their RF performance at mm-wave and THz frequency bands has been presented in this section. The comparative study on the high-frequency performance of DDR GaN IMPATTs with DDR GaAs, InP, and Si IMPATTs at sum-mm-wave and THz frequency bands presented in this section shows that DDR IMPATTs made of GaN is much superior to DDRs made of other semiconductors as regard high-power delivery with high efficiency.

QUANTUM DRIFT-DIFFUSION MODEL FOR THz IMPATTS

At THz frequency band, the depletion layer width of the device is very narrow less than 350 nm. The simulation technique based on drift-diffusion based classical model cannot accurately provide the RF performance of DDR IMPATTs at THz frequency band. Thus, quantum corrections should necessarily be incorporated in CLDD model to calculate the power and efficiency of the devices at THz regime. The quantum drift-diffusion (QDD) model uses quantum potentials or Bohm potentials [113,114]. The quantum theory of density gradient (DG) method [113–115] is used to simulate the device properties at THz frequency band.

In this section, large-signal high-frequency properties of DDR IMPATT devices made of different semiconductors, both conventional and WBG semiconductors, will be presented at THz frequency band where QDD model has been incorporated in the large-signal modeling. The validity of proposed QDD model can be easily tested by neglecting quantum corrections in the model and verifying whether the results are same as obtained from classical model.

Design and Material Parameters

The widths of the depletion layer (W_n, W_p), doping concentrations of n- and p-layers (N_D, N_A) and other structural parameters of DDR IMPATTs are appropriately chosen using TT consideration for operation at a particular design frequency (f_d) for a particular semiconductor at THz band. Sze and Ryder's formula [50] is helpful in this regard. The doping and structural parameters along with the bias current are optimized with respect to maximum large-signal efficiency at a particular THz frequency. The design parameters of the devices made of different materials are obtained at sub-mm-wave and THz frequency bands below the limiting frequency (f_u) above which IMPATT operation ceases [7,44]. The limiting frequencies of DDR devices made of both conventional semiconductors like Si and InP are reported as 0.5 and 1.0 THz, respectively, while those based on WBG semiconductors like 4H-Sic and Wz-GaN are reported as 1.0 and 5.0 THz, respectively [7,44]. Various design parameters obtained from simulation studies are shown in Table 1.7. The active layer of mesa-etched device has a diameter (D_j) and has been obtained from a thermal analysis, considering appropriate design of heat sink to prevent burn out failure of the device due to thermal runaway [64,65] and shown in the table.

The material parameters of the device are temperature dependent. Hence, the static and RF properties are also temperature dependent. Results show that with increasing junction temperature, both output power and efficiency of all DDRs increase. Optimum RF power is obtained with proper heat sink arrangement to keep the temperature of the device much more than the room temperature and much less than the burn out temperature of the semiconductor to avoid burn out problem of the device. The junction temperature of IMPATTs made of Si and InP is limited at 500 K to obtain optimum power from the device. The material parameters of Si and InP at a junction temperature of 500 K are taken from Ref. [46–49,116,117], while the available room temperature material parameters of 4H-SiC, Wz-GaN, and type-IIb diamond are obtained from Ref. [61–63,118–123].

QDD Model for THz IMPATT Devices

Microscopic and macroscopic theories have been used to explain the electron transport in solids. The microscopic theory deals with individual electrons, electron wave functions, density matrices, etc., while the macroscopic theory is based on electron population obtained from Fermi-Dirac distribution function and density of states function. The macroscopic theory involves DG theory which can be incorporated in QDD model subject to the existence of sufficient electron population whose average properties can be considered [115]. The DG theory can be used to explain the high-frequency properties of low-dimensional THz DDR IMPATTs where quantum confinement and tunneling play an important role.

CLDD model considers electron/hole gas density. On the other hand, DG theory considers not only the density of electron/hole gas but also their DG. In QDD model, the device equations of CLDD model are modified by incorporating quantum effects like quantum confinement and quantum tunneling. These quantum corrections can describe the transport phenomena in devices of low dimensions with sufficient accuracy.

The de Broglie wavelengths for electrons and holes are given by $\lambda_{n,p} = h\Big/\left(m^*_{n,p}\, v_{sn,sp}\right)$ where h is the Planck's constant. The classical limiting lengths below which quantum corrections are essential in THz IMPATT devices are given by $L^{QDD}_{CL(n,p)} = \sqrt{\hbar^2\Big/6m^*_{n,p}k_B T_j}$ where k_B is the Boltzmann constant and $\hbar = h/2\pi$ is the normalized Planck's constant [124]. These classical limiting lengths are calculated by using electron and hole effective mass values [48] and saturated drift velocities of carriers (v_{sn}, v_{sp}) [46,62,63,117,122,123] and given in Table 1.8. Table 1.8 shows that both de Broglie wavelength and classical limiting length of DDR IMPATT devices are much smaller than the active region dimensions of the devices at mm-wave frequency bands. With increasing frequency of operation (f_d), the dimension of the active region of the device ($W = W_n + W_p$) decreases which can be determined from $W_{n,p} = 0.37\, v_{sn,sp}/f_d$ [50]. The influence of quantum effect on the DC and RF properties of DDR IMPATTs based on different semiconductors depends on the operating frequency.

The static and large-signal parameters of the device made of different semiconductors are obtained at higher frequencies in mm-wave and THz band from both QDD and CLDD models. The purpose is to determine the frequency exceeding which the quantum effect is more or less appreciable.

The physical phenomena take place in semiconductor bulk along the symmetry axis of the device. Thus, one-dimensional (1D) model of reverse biased n^+-n-p-p^+ structure shown in Fig. 1.21 is used for the large-signal simulation of DDR IMPATTs. The snapshots of electric field, carrier current density, and carrier concentrations at different time intervals of a full oscillation cycle can be obtained from simultaneous numerical solution of device equations subject to appropriate

TABLE 1.7
Design Parameters.

Base Material	f_d (GHz)	J_0 ($\times 10^8$ Am^{-2})	W_n (μm)	W_p (μm)	N_D ($\times 10^{23}$ m^{-3})	N_A ($\times 10^{23}$ m^{-3})	N_{n+} ($\times 10^{25}$ m^{-3})	N_{p+} ($\times 10^{25}$ m^{-3})	D_j (μm)
Wz-GaN	94	1.050	1.5800	1.5800	0.590	0.600	5.000	2.700	35.00
	140	2.250	1.0500	1.0500	0.690	0.710	5.000	2.700	25.00
	220	4.275	0.7350	0.7350	1.050	1.100	5.000	2.700	20.00
	300	8.700	0.5350	0.5350	1.550	1.600	5.000	2.700	15.00
	500	18.375	0.3300	0.3300	2.860	2.900	5.000	2.700	10.00
	1000	45.000	0.1850	0.1850	6.840	7.200	5.000	2.700	5.00
	1500	55.500	0.1300	0.1300	9.800	10.50	5.000	2.700	2.50
	2000	72.000	0.1020	0.1020	13.500	14.500	5.000	2.700	1.20
	5000	88.500	0.0520	0.0520	35.500	36.500	5.000	2.700	0.70
InP	94	4.500	0.3200	0.3200	1.900	1.900	5.000	2.700	35.00
	140	7.700	0.2100	0.2100	3.400	3.400	5.000	2.700	25.00
	220	12.000	0.1300	0.1300	5.200	5.200	5.000	2.700	20.00
	300	20.000	0.1000	0.1010	7.200	7.200	5.000	2.700	15.00
	500	47.000	0.0650	0.0650	13.500	13.500	5.000	2.700	10.00
	1000	60.000	0.0285	0.0285	28.000	28.000	5.000	2.700	5.00
Type-IIb diamond (C)	94	4.000	0.7800	0.7200	0.460	0.530	5.000	2.700	35.00
	140	7.500	0.5300	0.5300	0.810	0.870	5.000	2.700	25.00
	220	13.000	0.3200	0.3200	1.350	1.490	5.000	2.700	20.00
	300	17.000	0.2200	0.2200	2.050	2.220	5.000	2.700	15.00
	500	25.000	0.1200	0.1200	3.750	4.100	5.000	2.700	10.00
	1000	39.000	0.0520	0.0520	9.500	10.000	5.000	2.700	5.00
	1500	48.000	0.0300	0.0300	36.000	37.000	5.000	2.700	2.50
4H-SiC	94	2.100	0.5800	0.5800	2.800	2.900	5.000	2.700	35.00
	140	4.300	0.4000	0.4000	4.900	5.000	5.000	2.700	25.00
	220	9.300	0.3000	0.3000	6.900	7.000	5.000	2.700	20.00
	300	16.600	0.2500	0.2500	9.500	10.500	5.000	2.700	15.00
	500	60.000	0.1600	0.1600	14.500	16.500	5.000	2.700	10.00
	1000	210.000	0.0900	0.0900	37.000	43.000	5.000	2.700	5.00
i	94	3.400	0.4000	0.3800	1.200	1.250	5.000	2.700	35.00
	140	5.800	0.2800	0.2450	1.800	2.100	5.000	2.700	25.00
	220	14.500	0.1800	0.1600	3.950	4.590	5.000	2.700	20.00
	300	24.500	0.1320	0.1120	6.000	7.300	5.000	2.700	15.00
	500	55.000	0.0720	0.0720	15.000	16.200	5.000	2.700	10.00

TABLE 1.8
The De Broglie Wavelengths and Classical Limiting Lengths for Electrons and Holes for Different Base Materials.

Semiconductor Material	T_j (K)	λ_n (nm)	λ_p (nm)	$L^{QDD}_{CL(n)}$ (nm)	$L^{QDD}_{CL(p)}$ (nm)
Wz-GaN	300	12.12	12.12	1.57	0.78
InP	500	43.33	21.35	1.03	0.70
C	300	3.46	2.93	0.59	0.48
4H-SiC	300	11.83	8.75	1.30	0.79
Si	500	31.46	14.18	1.21	1.81

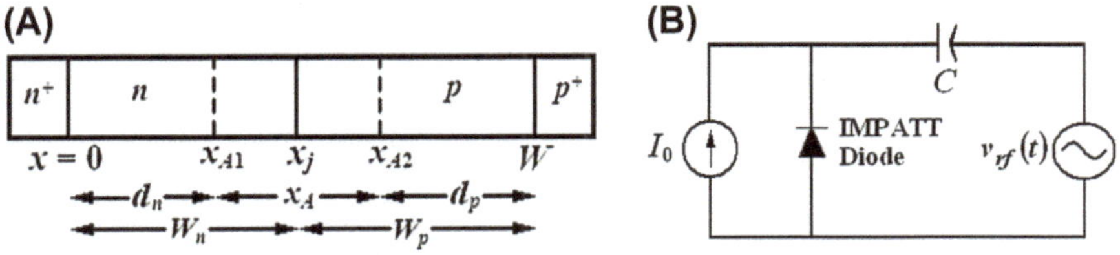

FIG. 1.21 **(A)** One-dimensional double-drift region IMPATT structure. **(B)** Equivalent circuit for analysis.

boundary conditions. 1D finite difference method [125] can be used for numerical solution of the necessary device equations which are both time and space dependent. The time- and space-dependent Poisson's equation, continuity equations, and current density equations are given in Eqs. (1.6)−(1.8).

$$D_x^2 V(x,t) = -(q/\varepsilon_s)[N_D(x) - N_A(x) + p(x,t) - n(x,t)], \quad (1.6)$$

$$D_t(p,n(x,t)) = \mp(1/q)D_x J_{p,n}(x,t) + G_{Ap,n}(x,t) + G_{Tp,n}(x,t), \quad (1.7)$$

$$J_{p,n}(x,t) = -q\mu_{p,n}\left[p,n(x,t)D_x(V(x,t) + Q_{p,n}(x,t)) \pm (k_B T_j/q)D_x(p,n(x,t))\right], \quad (1.8)$$

where $V(x,t)$ is the electric potential, $p(x,t)/n(x,t)$ are the hole/electron concentrations, $J_n(x,t)/J_p(x,t)$ are the electron/hole current density, and $G_{An}(x,t)/G_{Ap}(x,t)$ are the electron/hole generation rates. The avalanche generation rate of carrier is given by $G_{Ap}(x,t) = G_{An}(x,t) = \alpha_p(x,t)v_p(x,t)p(x,t) + \alpha_n(x,t)v_n(x,t)n(x,t)$, where $\alpha_p(x,t)$, $\alpha_n(x,t)$ are ionization rates and $v_p(x,t)$, $v_n(x,t)$ are saturated drift velocities of electrons and holes. The tunneling generation rates of carriers $G_{Tp}(x,t)$ and $G_{Tn}(x,t)$ are obtained from Ref. [126,127]. The above parameters in Eqs. (1.6)−(1.8) are both space and time dependent. The operators D_x and D_t in Eqs. (1.6)−(1.8) correspond to $\partial/\partial x$ and $\partial/\partial t$, respectively. $N_A(x)$ and $N_D(x)$ are the doping densities in p- and n-layer of DDR structure, respectively, at a position x in the depletion layer. The hole and electron mobilities are μ_p and μ_n, respectively, semiconductor permittivity is ε_s, electronic charge is q, and junction temperature is T_j. The electric field at the space point x at the instant of time t can be obtained from the space derivative of the electric potential, i.e., $\xi(x,t) = -D_x V(x,t)$.

DG theory considers that the electron gas is energetically sensitive with respect to its DG. DG model considers the quantum mechanical nonlocal effect by considering only the lowest order of $\hbar^2$ [113,114]. However, quantum corrections to the expressions of current density in classical model are considered up to third-order derivative terms. The quantum corrections $Q_p(x,t)$ and $Q_n(x,t)$ to the electric potential $V(x,t)$ at the space point x at the instant of time t are known as Bohm potentials [113] or quantum potentials given by

$$Q_{p,n}(x,t) = \left(2s_{p,n}/\sqrt{p,n(x,t)}\right)D_x^2\left(\sqrt{p,n(x,t)}\right), \quad (1.9)$$

where the coefficients s_p and s_n signify the DG strength of carrier gas and these are functions of material parameters of the base semiconductor and given by $s_{p,n} = (\hbar^2/4qm_{p,n}{}^* r_{p,n})$. In the expression of $s_{p,n}$, r_p, and r_n are dimensionless empirical parameters which take into account the statistical effect of DG model

[113,114,128,129]. At low temperature, the values of both these parameters in most of the semiconductors are nearly three [128].

Eqs. (1.6)–(1.8) can be solved numerically subject to the boundary conditions for electric field, ξ (x,t), and normalized current density, $P(x,t)$, at the edges of depletion layer. The expression for $P(x,t)$ is given by

$$P(x,t) = [J_p(x,t) - J_n(x,t)]/[J_p(x,t) + J_n(x,t)]$$
$$= [J_p(x,t) - J_n(x,t)]/J_t(t)$$

The boundary conditions for electric field are

$$\xi(x=0,t) = \xi(x=W,t) = 0$$

The boundary conditions for normalized current density are

$$P(x=0,t) = [(2J_p(x=0,t)\,/\,J_t(t)) - 1] \text{ and}$$
$$P(x=W,t) = [1 - (2J_n(x=W,t)\,/\,J_t(t))]$$

Here, $J_t(t) = \int_W (J_p(x,t) + J_n(x,t))dx$ is the total time-varying particle current density.

Large-Signal Simulation Technique Based on QDD Model

The equivalent circuit (Fig. 1.21B) for large-signal modeling and simulation considers IMPATT diode as voltage-driven oscillator where the RF voltage waveform is nonsinusoidal and given by

$$v_{rf}(t) = V_B \sum_{p=1}^{n} (m_x)^p \sin(p\omega t), \qquad (1.10)$$

The voltage waveform consists of $(n-1)$ harmonics whose fundamental frequency is $f = \omega/2\pi$. The device is connected across a coupling capacitor, C. The DC bias current is $I_0 = J_0 \times A_j$ where J_0 is the bias current density and A_j is the junction area of the device. Voltage-driven oscillator gives a current response at the output which is obtained from large-signal analysis and computer simulation. The parameter m_x is the ratio of amplitude of RF voltage to DC breakdown voltage called voltage modulation factor. The time-dependent diode voltage, $V_t(t)$, and voltage across the avalanche zone voltage $V_a(t)$ are integral of time-dependent field over the corresponding region. These voltages are evaluated through numerical integration of field over the depletion and avalanche layers, respectively. The DC parameters such as peak field at the junction, ξ_P, reverse voltage at breakdown, V_B, and the voltage across the avalanche layer, V_A, can be obtained from the corresponding time-dependent parameters, extracted from large-signal simulation program, by calculating their average values over a complete oscillation cycle. The voltage across the drift zone can then be calculated from $V_D = V_B - V_A$.

The large-signal program is run at different phase angles corresponding to the limit of one complete cycle (i.e., $0 \le \omega t \le 2\pi$). The simulation is repeated at consecutive cycles to confirm the stability of oscillation. The large-signal negative conductance, $G(f)$, and susceptance, $B(f)$, as functions of the fundamental angular frequency ($\omega = 2\pi f$) of the voltage source are both normalized with respect to junction area A_j of the device by assuming circular cross-sectional area of the device. Thus, $A_j = \pi(D_j/2)^2$ where D_j is the device effective junction diameter. The terminal current and voltage waveforms are obtained by carrying out detailed Fourier analysis. The quality factor of the device is calculated from $Q_p = -B_p/G_p$ where G_p and B_p are, respectively, the large-signal peak values of conductance and susceptance. The large-signal power delivered by the device at the optimum frequency is calculated from $P_{RF} = (1/2)(V_{RF})^2|G_p|A_j$, where V_{RF} is the RF voltage amplitude, and $|G_p|$ is the normalized magnitude of large-signal conductance with respect to junction area at the optimum frequency. The conversion efficiency of the device is calculated from the expression $\eta_L = (P_{RF}/P_{DC})$, where $P_{DC} = J_0 V_B A_j$ is the DC power input, J_0 is the sum of electron and hole current density, and P_{RF} is the RF power output.

Simulation Results

The fundamental large-signal device Eqs. (1.6)–(1.8) based on QDD model lead to respective DC equations by taking the voltage modulation factor, m_x = zero. Then numerical solution of DC equations is carried out subject to appropriate boundary conditions to obtain the respective DC parameters. The simulation results based on QDD model are shown in plots of V_B and V_A against optimum frequency for DDR IMPATT devices made of Wz-GaN, cubic, and 4H-SiC (Fig. 1.22). The same plots are also shown in Fig. 1.22 by neglecting the quantum corrections leading to the results of CLDD model. The percentage deviations of parameters, $\Delta X = (X)_{CLDD} - (X)_{QDD})/(X)_{CLDD}$ (%), where $X \equiv V_B$, V_A and V_D/V_B are obtained from CLDD and QDD models and shown as bar graphs in the insets of Fig. 1.22 for Wz-GaN, cubic, and 4H-SiC DDR IMPATTs. Fig. 1.23 shows the plots of V_B and V_A against optimum frequency and ΔX as bar graphs in the inset of the figure for DDR IMPATT devices made of InP and Si. Figs. 1.22 and 1.23 show that the quantum effect incorporated in CLDD model leads to appreciable increase of the magnitudes of V_B and V_A and

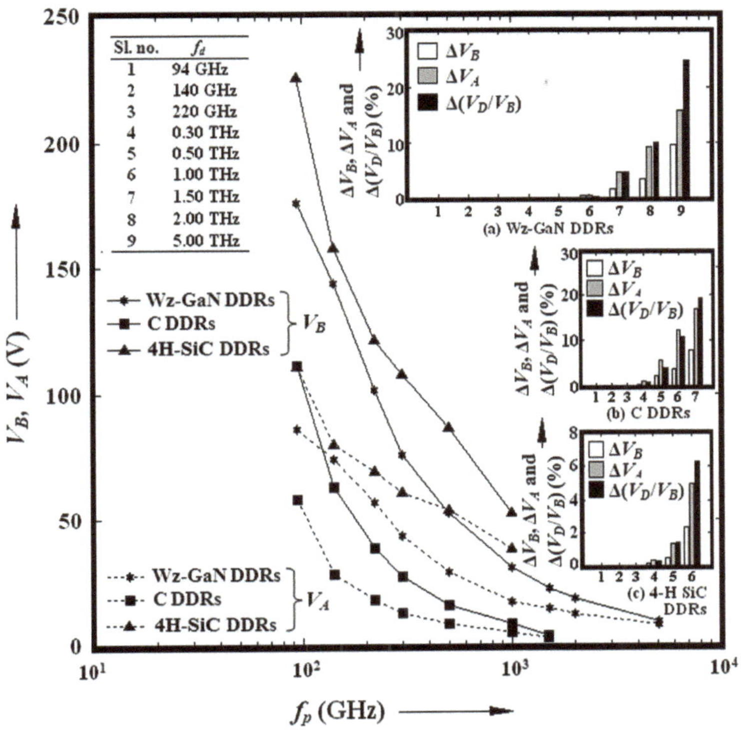

FIG. 1.22 Plots of V_B and V_A against optimum frequency for double-drift region (DDR) IMPATT devices made of Wz-GaN, cubic, and 4H-SiC based on quantum drift-diffusion model at $T_j = 300$ K. The percentage changes of parameters, ΔX for V_B, V_A, and V_D/V_B are shown as insets **(A–C)**, respectively, in the figure.

decrease of V_D/V_B of respective DDR IMPATTs particularly at THz band. It is further observed that significant changes of the DC parameters are observed at optimum frequencies of 1.50, 0.36, 0.50, 1.00 THz, and 267.10 GHz, respectively, and corresponding active layer widths, W, in the range 180–340 nm due to inclusion of quantum effect in the CLDD model for DDR IMPATTs made of Wz-GaN, InP, C, 4H-SiC, and Si. The percentage changes in DC parameters of all DDR devices due to quantum effect are found to be significant at frequencies higher than 1.0 THz.

The large-signal parameters such as avalanche resonance frequency (f_a), optimum frequency (f_p), peak negative conductance (G_p), susceptance (B_p), output power (P_{RF}), and conversion efficiency (η_L) of all DDR devices are obtained from CLDD and QDD models by taking $m_x = 0.5$. Table 1.9 shows the values of f_a and f_p obtained from CLDD and QDD models for all five DDR devices under consideration. Similarly, the percentage deviations of f_a and f_p, $\Delta Y = [(Y)_{CLDD}-(Y)_{QDD})/(Y)_{CLDD})$ (%), where $Y = f_a$ or f_p] are shown as bar graphs in Fig. 1.24A–E for five DDR devices made of different materials. Fig. 1.24A–E as well as Table 1.9 show that the quantum effect leads to an increase of both f_a and f_p for DDR IMPATTs based on five materials at higher mm-wave or THz frequencies and corresponding active layer thickness in the range of 180–340 nm.

The bar graphs in Fig. 1.25A–E show the simulated values of large-signal peak negative conductance ($|G_p|$) based on QDD and CLDD models for all five DDR devices under consideration. Significant decrease of $|G_p|$ for DDRs based on Wz-GaN, InP, C, 4H-SiC, and Si occurs above the frequencies 1.50, 0.36, 0.50, 1.00, and 0.267 THz, respectively. The magnitudes of G_p obtained from QDD and CLDD models are almost the same at frequencies below 250 GHz when the active layer dimension of the devices exceeds 0.34 μm.

Fig. 1.26 shows the plots of large-signal output power (P_{RF}) versus frequency of three DDR devices based on Wz-GaN, C, and 4H-SiC following CLDD and QDD models. The bar graphs in the inset of Fig. 1.26 marked as (a) and (b) show the percentage deviation in the simulated values of power output and conversion efficiency of the three DDRs with respect to QDD and CLDD models is given by $\Delta Z = [(Z)_{CLDD}-(Z)_{QDD})/(Z)_{CLDD})$ (%), where $Z = P_{RF}$ or η_L]. The figures show a decrease of magnitudes of both P_{RF}

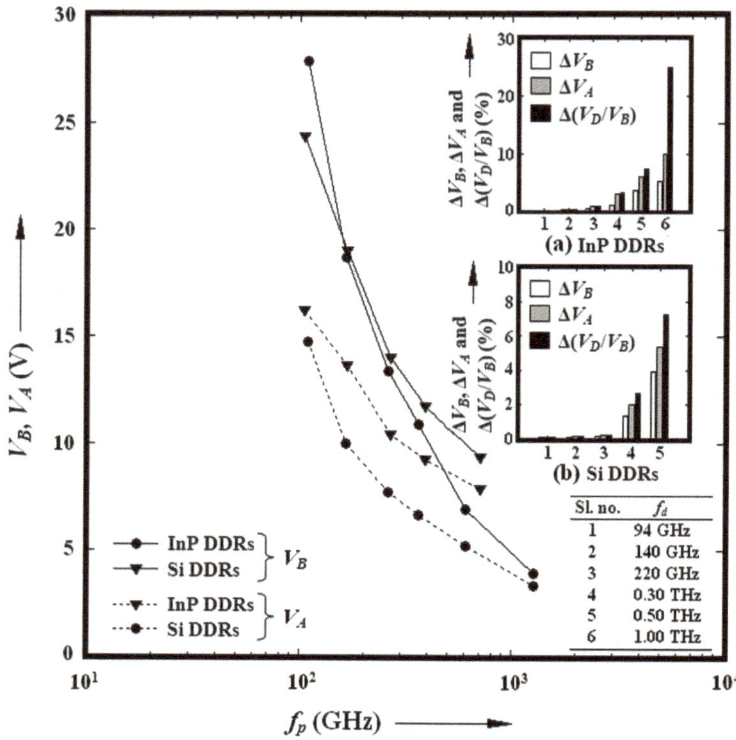

FIG. 1.23 Plots of V_B and V_A against optimum frequency for double-drift region (DDR) IMPATT devices made of InP and Si at $T_j = 500$ K following quantum drift-diffusion model. The percentage changes of parameters, ΔX of all these devices for V_B, V_A, and V_D/V_B, respectively, are shown as insets **(A–C)** in the figure.

and η_L of all DDR IMPATT devices at frequencies in THz band when quantum corrections are incorporated in the CLDD model. The quantum corrections made in CLDD model cause decrease of RF power output by approximately 14%–24% and decrease of efficiency by about 16%–30% for DDR Wz-GaN, cubic, and 4H-SiC IMPATTs at the optimum frequencies of 5.0, 1.5, and 1.0 THz, respectively. On the other hand, the quantum effect causes reductions of output power and efficiency of DDR Si and InP IMPATTs by around 20%–22% and 23%–25% at the optimum frequencies of 0.5 and 1.0 THz, respectively. Inclusion of quantum effect in CLDD model causes decrease in the value of $|G_p|$ which leads to decrease of RF power output at THz frequencies.

At THz frequency bands, it is observed that both output power and efficiency of DDR IMPATT devices are slightly degraded when QDD model is applied in the simulation. However, the quantum corrections to CLDD model lead to more accurate device design providing more precise magnitudes of RF output power and conversion efficiency of THz IMPATTs.

Thus, the design parameters of THz DDR IMPATTs based on QDD model and NSVE large-signal simulation presented in this chapter will be extremely useful for fabrication of THz solid-state sources using IMPATT devices.

Fig. 1.27 shows the variations of total depletion width (W) of Wz-GaN, InP, C, 4H-SiC, and Si DDRs with optimum frequency. The bar graphs in the inset of Fig. 1.27 clearly show the variations of the classical limiting frequencies (f_{CLLT}) of the aforementioned devices.

The active layer widths corresponding to the classical limiting frequencies of DDR IMPATTs based on Wz-GaN, InP, C, 4H-SiC, and Si are found to be 260, 201, 180, 240, and 340 nm, respectively. It is observed from Fig. 1.27 that quantum effect causes modulation of RF properties of IMPATT devices based on different semiconductors when the active layer widths shrink below the range of 180–340 nm depending on the base semiconductor. In spite of the fact that the active layer width of DDR type-IIb diamond (C) IMPATTs operating at 0.50 THz is very narrow, the RF properties

TABLE 1.9
Simulated Values of

		(A) WZ-GAN DDRS ($T_J = 300$ K)		(B) INP DDRS ($T_J = 500$ K)		(C) C DDRS ($T_J = 300$ K)		(D) 4H-SIC DDRS ($T_J = 300$ K)		(E) SI DDRS ($T_J = 500$ K)	
DD Model	**Sl. No.**	f_a (GHz)	f_p (GHz)	f_a (GHz)	f_p (GHz)	f_a (GHz)	f_p (GHz)	f_a (GHz)	f_p (GHz)	f_a (GHz)	f_p (GHz)
CLDD	1	67.70	95.10	69.39	108.30	49.50	95.60	52.35	95.20	69.50	104.90
	2	97.90	140.80	107.30	165.31	99.00	140.00	86.59	142.21	91.90	166.60
	3	139.80	220.30	149.79	263.53	144.50	218.00	120.04	221.11	170.80	267.10
	4	196.51	300.31	205.19	366.11	192.11	301.10	167.69	300.60	225.60	386.90
	5	290.82	506.32	368.11	611.00	283.92	502.00	283.01	502.31	342.80	695.90
	6	433.01	1004.41	516.09	1283.90	469.01	1002.00	399.42	1004.40	—	—
	7	788.83	1505.81	—	—	704.40	1501.00	—	—	—	—
	8	1446.90	2008.91	—	—	—	—	—	—	—	—
	9	3060.00	5030.10	—	—	—	—	—	—	—	—
QDD	1	67.70	95.10	69.39	108.30	49.50	95.60	52.35	95.20	69.50	104.91
	2	97.90	140.80	107.30	165.31	99.00	140.00	86.59	142.21	91.92	166.65
	3	139.80	220.30	149.84	263.63	144.50	218.00	120.04	221.11	170.94	267.36
	4	196.51	300.31	205.89	368.30	192.13	301.10	167.71	300.70	226.39	390.02
	5	290.84	506.32	369.86	617.35	284.45	503.72	282.11	502.72	345.82	707.59
	6	433.20	1005.10	521.76	1307.98	471.32	1009.02	401.50	1013.24	—	—
	7	791.00	1512.92	—	—	710.14	1520.90	—	—	—	—
	8	1454.80	2025.40	—	—	—	—	—	—	—	—
	9	3090.71	5106.70	—	—	—	—	—	—	—	—

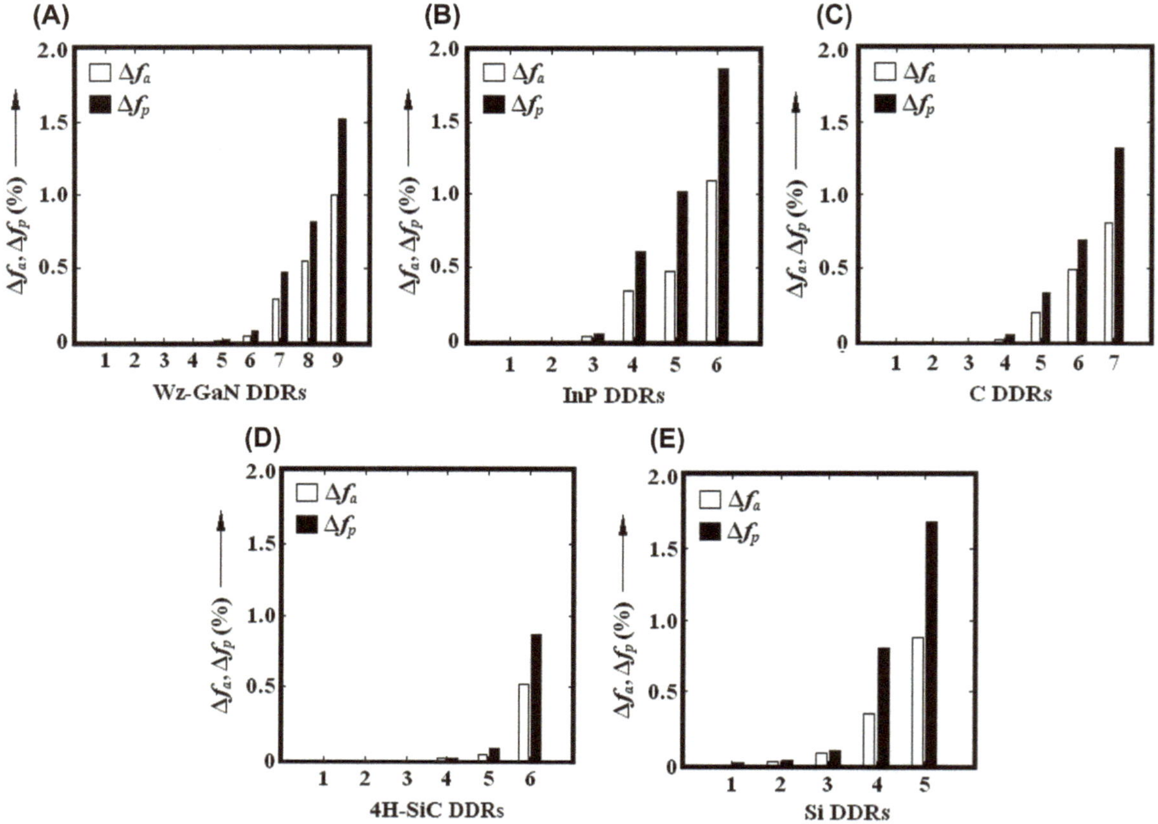

FIG. 1.24 Bar graphs showing the percentage deviations of f_a and f_p due to quantum effect inclusion: **(A)** Wz-GaN (*Tj* = 300 K), **(B)** InP (*Tj* = 500 K), **(C)** C (*Tj* = 300 K), **(D)** 4H-SiC (*Tj* = 300 K), and **(E)** Si (*Tj* = 500 K) double-drift region (DDR) IMPATTs (serial numbers 1, 2, 3, ..., 9 in the horizontal axes of the figures **(A–E)** correspond to different frequencies shown in Table 9.3).

of the device is not significantly affected by quantum confinement and quantum tunneling phenomena. On the other hand, the RF properties of DDR Si IMPATTs are appreciably affected due to quantum effect at much lower frequency of 267.10 GHz when the active layer width of the device is 340 nm. The quantum effect becomes more pronounced when the active width of DDR Si devices shrinks further below 340 nm.

CONCLUSION

In this chapter, the potentiality of IMPATT devices based on different semiconductors particularly the WBG ones has been presented for operation at THz frequency band. The suitability of IMPATTs based on both normal bandgap and WBG semiconductors as potential THz sources has been studied by ART analysis. The design, modeling, and simulation of DDR and SDR IMPATTs based on various semiconductors as well as the DC and RF properties of these devices at millimeter wave and THz frequency bands have been reviewed. The possibility of IMPATTs operating at THz frequency band depends on the base semiconductor used for IMPATT fabrication as revealed from ART analysis which determines the upper cut-off frequency. InP IMPATTs are capable of delivering power up to 1 THz frequency which is its cut-off frequency. The avalanche resonance limited frequencies of GaAs and Si IMPATTs are, however, lower than InP IMPATTs. It has been observed that DDR IMPATTs based on WBG semiconductors like 4H-SiC and Wz-GaN are potential candidates for THz operation since these devices are capable of delivering high power with high conversion efficiency at THz frequencies. The results indicate that IMPATT devices based on Wz-GaN are without any competition above 1 THz as regard delivering high power with high conversion efficiency.

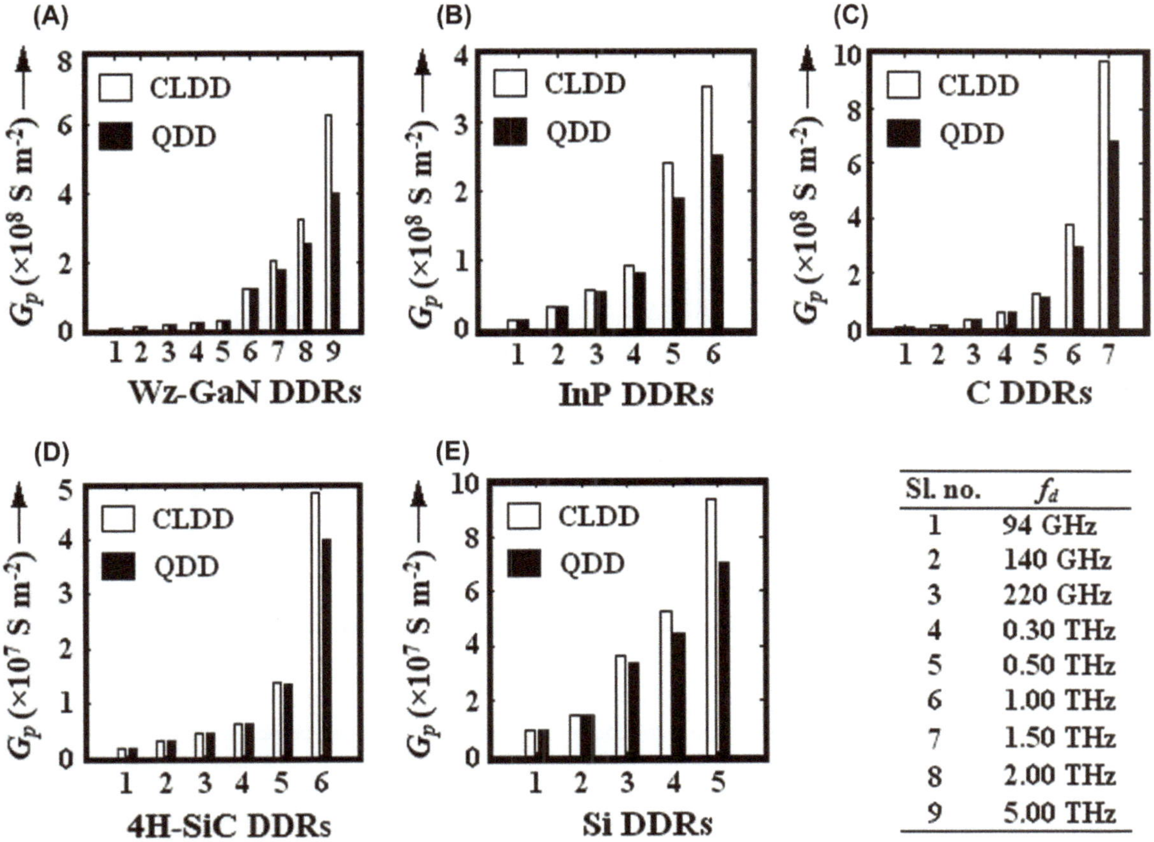

Sl. no.	f_d
1	94 GHz
2	140 GHz
3	220 GHz
4	0.30 THz
5	0.50 THz
6	1.00 THz
7	1.50 THz
8	2.00 THz
9	5.00 THz

FIG. 1.25 Bar graphs showing the magnitudes of large-signal peak negative conductance ($|G_p|$) based on QDD and CLDD models for double-drift region (DDR) devices based on **(A)** Wz-GaN ($T_j = 300$ K), **(B)** InP ($T_j = 500$ K), **(C)** C ($T_j = 300$ K), **(D)** 4H-SiC ($T_j = 300$ K), and **(E)** Si ($T_j = 500$ K) (serial numbers 1, 2, 3, ..., 9 in the horizontal axes of the figures **(A–E)** correspond to different frequencies shown in Table 9.3).

The avalanche resonance limited frequencies of DDR IMPATTs based on GaN, diamond, and Si IMPATTs are found to be 1.00, 1.50, and 0.50 THz, respectively. The results show that diamond IMPATTs deliver much higher RF power with significantly higher conversion efficiency at both mm-wave and THz frequencies as compared with their Si counterparts. Thus, DDR diamond IMPATTs can also be used as potential sources for generating THz oscillation up to 1.5 THz due to their faster avalanche response. The effect of tunneling on the millimeter wave and THz performance of DDR diamond IMPATTS is practically negligible. The simulation results are encouraging and the design results presented in this chapter are useful input data for fabrication of mm-wave and THz DDR diamond IMPATTs by using ion-implantation or suitable CVD techniques.

In this chapter, a QDD model has been presented for large-signal simulation of DDR IMPATT devices based on conventional and WBG semiconductors operating at higher mm-wave and lower THz frequencies. It is observed that the mm-wave and THz performance of DDR IMPATTs based on Wz-GaN, InP, C, 4H-SiC, and Si are affected by quantum phenomena such as quantum confinement, quantum tunneling, etc., arising at certain limiting frequency (f_{CLLT}). The simulation provides the avalanche resonance limited frequencies of DDR IMPATTs which is highest for Wz-GaN in THz band. The quantum effect on the large-signal properties will not be appreciable if the dimension of the active layer of the device is larger than the de Broglie wavelength of electrons or holes at the design frequencies in mm-wave and THz bands. However, more accurate prediction of large-signal power and conversion efficiency of the device can be made due to incorporation of quantum corrections in the drift-diffusion model.

The design parameters of Si, GaAs, InP, 4-H SiC, Wz-GaN, and type-IIb diamond DDR IMPATTs, presented in this chapter, will be useful to select the

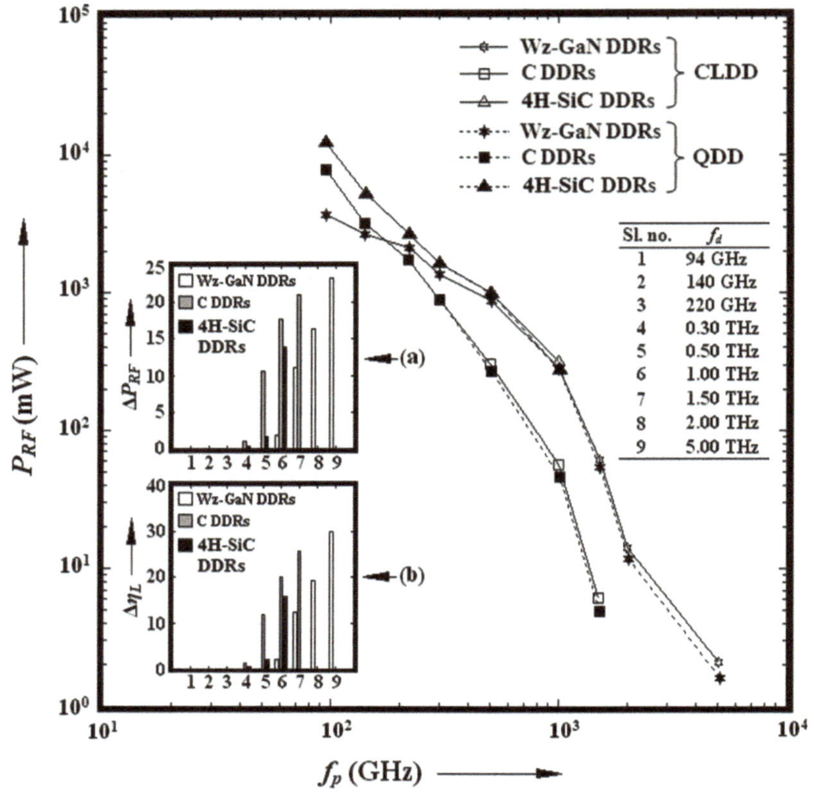

FIG. 1.26 Plots of power versus frequency for double-drift region (DDR) devices based on Wz-GaN, C, and 4H-SiC based on CLDD and QDD models. Insets in the figure show bar graphs of percentage deviation of power and efficiency.

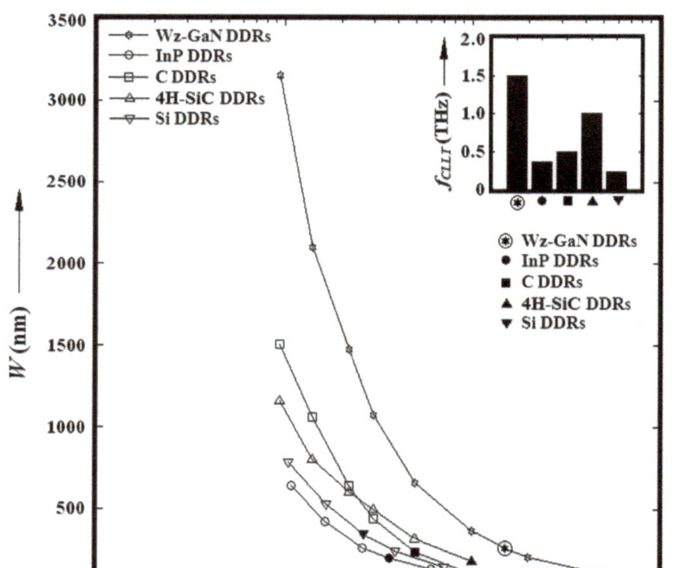

FIG. 1.27 Variations of total depletion width of Wz-GaN, InP, C, 4H-SiC, and Si double-drift regions (DDRs) with optimum frequency; classical limiting frequencies of respective devices are shown as bar graphs in inset of the figure.

proper base materials for IMPATTs for operation at THz frequency band. The results presented in this chapter will be very much useful to the experimentalist for fabrication and characterization of THz DDR IMPATTs.

In conclusion, the great potential of Wz-GaN and type-IIb diamond as base materials of DDR IMPATTs can be explored to experimentally realize these devices for THz operation.

AUTHOR DETAILS

Dr. Suranjana Banerjee received B.Sc. (Hons.) in Electronics and B.Tech and M.Tech degrees in Radio Physics and Electronics from the University of Calcutta. She was awarded a PhD (Engineering) degree from Indian Institute of Engineering, Science and Technology (IIEST), Shibpur. She joined the Department of Electronics and Telecommunication Engineering, IIEST, Shibpur, as an Assistant Professor in 2016 and she is presently working as Assistant Professor in the Department of Electronics of Dum Dum Motijheel College under West Bengal State University (WBSU). She is the principal author of about 30 research papers in referred technical and scientific journals. Her present area of research is Design and Simulation of Avalanche Transit Time (ATT) Devices based on wide bandgap semiconductors for Terahertz application.

REFERENCES

[1] W. Feng, J.C. Cao, Theoretical study of THz current oscillations in $GaAs_{1-x} N_x$, Journal of Applied Physics 104 (2008) 013111, https://doi.org/10.1063/1.2952017.

[2] M. Wollitzer, J. Buchler, F. Schafflr, J.F. Luy, D-band Si-IMPATT diodes with 300 mW CW output power at 140 GHz, Electronics Letters 32 (1996) 122–123.

[3] C. Dalle, P. Rolland, G. Lieti, Flat doping profile double-drift silicon IMPATT for reliable CW high power high-efficiency generation in the 94-GHz window, IEEE Transactions on Electron Devices 37 (1990) 227–236.

[4] M. Mukherjee, N. Mazumder, S.K. Roy, Prospects of 4H-SiC double drift region IMPATT device as a photo-sensitive high-power source at 0.7 terahertz frequency regime, Active and Passive Electronic Components 2009 (2009) 1–9.

[5] A.K. Panda, D. Pavlidis, E. Alekseev, DC and high-frequency characteristics of GaN-based IMPATTs, IEEE Transactions on Electron Devices 48 (2001) 820–823.

[6] S. Banerjee, M. Mukherjee, J.P. Banerjee, Bias current optimization of Wurtzite-GaN DDR IMPATT diode for high power operation at THz frequencies, International Journal of Advanced Science and Technology 16 (2010) 12–20.

[7] A. Acharyya, J.P. Banerjee, Prospects of IMPATT devices based on wide bandgap semiconductors as potential terahertz sources, Applied Nanoscience (November 2012), https://doi.org/10.1007/s13204-012-0172-y. Published online.

[8] L. Yuan, A. James, J.A. Cooper, M.R. Melloch, K.J. Webb, Experimental demonstration of a silicon carbide IMPATT oscillator, IEEE Electron Device Letters 22 (2001) 266–268.

[9] R.J. Trew, J.B. Yan, P.M. Mock, The potentiality of diamond and SiC electronic devices for microwave and millimeter-wave power applications, Proceedings of the IEEE 79 (5) (1991) 598–620.

[10] P.M. Mock, R.J. Trew, RF performance characteristics of double-drift MM-wave diamond IMPATT diodes, in: Proc. of IEEE/Cornell Conf. Advanced Concepts in High-Speed Semiconductor Devices and Circuits, 1989, pp. 383–389.

[11] W. Shockley, Negative resistance arising from transit time in semiconductor diodes, Bell Labs Technical Journal 33 (1954) 799–826.

[12] W.T. Read, A proposed high frequency negative resistance diode, Bell Labs Technical Journal 37 (1958) 401.

[13] R.L. Johnson, B.C. DeLoach, B.G. Cohen, A silicon diode microwave oscillator, Bell Labs Technical Journal 44 (1965) 369–372.

[14] T. Misawa, The negative resistance in *p-n* junctions under avalanche breakdown conditions Part-1, IEEE Transactions on Electron Devices ED-13 (1966) 137–151.

[15] M. Mukherjee, N. Majumder, Optically illuminated 4H-SiC terahertz IMPATT device, Egyptian Journal of Solids 30 (1) (2007) 87–101.

[16] M. Mukherjee, N. Majumder, S.K. Roy, Prospects of 4H-SiC double drift region IMPATT device as a photo-sensitive high power source at 0.7 terahertz frequency regime, Active and Passive Electronic Components 2008 (2008) 1–9.

[17] T.A. Midford, R.L. Bernick, Millimeter wave CW impatt diodes and oscillators, IEEE Transactions on Microwave Theory and Techniques MTT.27 (1979) 483.

[18] T. Ishibashi, M. Ohmori, 200 GHz 50 mW CW oscillation with Si DDR Impatts, IEEE Transactions on Microwave Theory and Techniques MTT-24 (1976) 858.

[19] J.J. Berenz, F.B. Fank, T.L. Hierl, Ion-implanted p-n junction indium-phosphide IMPATT diodes, Electronics Letters 14 (21) (1978) 683–684.

[20] K.V. Vassilevski, A.V. Zorenko, K. Zekentes, Experimental observation of microwave oscillations produced by pulsed Silicon Carbide IMPATT diode, Electronics Letters 37 (2001) 466.

[21] D.L. Scharfetter, W.J. Evans, H.L. Johnson, Double drift region p+pnn+ avalanche diode oscillators, Proceedings of the IEEE 50 (1970) 1131.

[22] T.E. Seidel, R.E. Davis, D.E. Jglesias, DDR ion-implanted (p+pnn+) mm-wave IMPATT diodes, Inst. Electron Devices Meeting, Washington DC, USA, 28–30th October 1970, n.d., pp.52.

[23] J.C. De Jaeger, R. Kozlowski, G. Salmer, High efficiency GaInAs/InP heterojunction impatt diodes, IEEE Transactions on Electron Devices ED 30 (1983) 790.

[24] G.N. Dash, S.P. Pati, Computer aided studies on the microwave characteristics of InP/GaInAs and GaAs/GaInAs heterostructure single drift region impact avalanche transit didoes, Journal of Physics D Applied Physics 27 (1994) 1719.

[25] J.K. Mishra, A.K. Panda, G.N. Dash, An extremely low-noise heterojunction IMPATT, IEEE Transactions on Electron Devices ED-44 (12) (1997) 2143–2148.

[26] N. S Dogan, J.,R. East, M. Elta, G.I. Haddad, Millimeter wave heterojunction MITATT diodes, IEEE Transactions on Microwave Theory and Techniques MTT 35 (1987) 1304.

[27] M.J. Bailey, Hetrojunction IMPATT diodes, IEEE Transactions on Electron Devices 39 (1992) 1829.

[28] Y. Takanashi, Y. Horikoshi, InGaAsP/InP avalanche photodiode, Japanese Journal of Applied Physics 17 (1978) 2065.

[29] Y. Takanashi, Y. Horikoshi, Ioniozation coefficient of InGaAsP/InP APD, Japanese Journal of Applied Physics 18 (1979) 2173.

[30] J.F. Luy, A. Casel, W. Behr, E. Kasper, A 90-GHz double-drift IMPATT diode made with Si MBE, IEEE Transactions on Electron Devices 34 (1987) 1084–1089.

[31] H.C. Huang, A modified GaAs IMPATT structure for high-efficiency operation, IEEE Transactions on Electron Devices 20 (5) (1973) 482–486.

[32] R.E. Goldwasser, F.E. Rosztoczy, High efficiency GaAs low-hig-low IMPATTs, Applied Physics Letters 25 (1974) 92.

[33] C.O. Bozler, J.P. Donelly, R.A. Murphy, R.W. Laton, R.N. Sudhury, W.T. Lindley, High efficiency ion implanted Lo-hi-lo GaAs IMPATT diodes, Applied Physics Letters 29 (1976) 123.

[34] H. Eisele, Selective etching technology for 94 GHz, GaAs IMPATT diodes on diamond heat sinks, Solid-State Electronics 32 (3) (1989) 253–257.

[35] H. Eisele, GaAs W-band IMPATT diode for very low noise oscillations, Electronics Letters 26 (2) (1990) 109–110.

[36] H. Eisele, G.I. Hadded, GaAs single-drift flat profile IMPATT diodes for CW operation at D band, Electronics Letters 28 (23) (1992) 2176–2177.

[37] M.J. Kearney, N.R. Couch, J.S. Stephens, R.S. Smith, Low noise, high efficiency GaAs IMPATT diodes at 30GHz, Electronics Letters 28 (8) (1992) 706–708.

[38] M. Curow, Proposed GaAs IMPATT device structure for D-band applications, Electronics Letters 30 (19) (1994) 1629–1631.

[39] M. Tschernitz, J. Freyer, H. Grothe, GaAs read-type IMPATT diodes for D-band, Electronics Letters 30 (13) (1994) 1070–1071.

[40] M. Tschernitz, J. Freyer, 140 GHz GaAs double-Read IMPATT diodes, Electronics Letters 31 (7) (1995) 582–583.

[41] J.P. Banerjee, S.P. Pati, S.K. Roy, High frequency characterization of double drift region InP and GaAs diode, Applied Physics A 48 (1984) 437–443.

[42] M. Mukherjee, S. Banerjee, J.P. Banerjee, Dynamic characteristics of III-V and IV-IV semiconductor based transit time devices in the terahertz regime: a comparative analysis, Terahertz Science and Technology 3 (2010) 98–109.

[43] M. Mukherjee, N. Mazumder, S.K. Roy, K. Goswami, Terahertz frequency performance of double drift IMPATT diode based on opto-sensitive semiconductor, in: Proc. of Asia-Pacific Microwave Conference, 2007, pp. 1–4.

[44] A. Acharyya, S. Banerjee, J.P. Banerjee, Calculation of avalanche response time for determining the high frequency performance limitations of IMPATT devices, Journal of Electron Devices 12 (2012) 756–760.

[45] K.V. Vassilevski, A.V. Zorenko, K. Zekentes, K. Tsagaraki, E. Bano, C. Banc, A. Lebedev, 4H-SiC IMPATT diode fabrication and testing, in: Technical Digest of International Conference on SiC and Related Materials, Tsukuba, Japan, 2001, pp. 713–714.

[46] C. Canali, G. Ottaviani, A.A. Quaranta, Drift velocity of electrons and holes and associated anisotropic effects in silicon, Journal of Physics and Chemistry of Solids 32 (1971) 1707–1720.

[47] W.N. Grant, Electron and hole ionization rates in epitaxial Silicon, Solid-State Electronics 16 (1973) 1189–1203.

[48] C. Canali, G. Ottaviani, A.A. Quaranta, Electronic Archive: New Semiconductor Materials, Characteristics and Properties. Available from: http://www.ioffe.ru/SVA/NSM/Semicond/index.html. (Accessed June 2014).

[49] B.V. Zeghbroeck, Principles of Semiconductor Devices, Colorado Press, USA, 2011.

[50] S.M. Sze, R.M. Ryder, Microwave avalanche diodes, Proceedings of IEEE, Special Issue on Microwave Semiconductor Devices 59 (1971) 1140–1154.

[51] S.K. Roy, J.P. Banerjee, S.P. Pati, A Computer analysis of the distribution of high frequency negative resistance in the depletion layer of IMPATT diodes, in: Proc. 4th Conf. on Num. Anal. of Semiconductor Devices (NASECODE IV) (Dublin), Ireland, 1985, pp. 494–500.

[52] H.K. Gummel, J.L. Blue, A small-signal theory of avalanche noise in IMPATT diodes, IEEE Transactions on Electron Devices 14 (1967) 569–580.

[53] J.P. Banerjee, J.F. Luy, F. Schaffler, Comparison of theoretical and experimental 60 GHz Silicon IMPATT diode performance, Electronics Letters 27 (1991) 1049–1050.

[54] Y. Takayama, Effect of temperature on devices admittance of GaAs and Si IMPATT diodes, IEEE Transactions on Microwave Theory and Techniques MTT 23 (1975) 673.

[55] Y. Hirachi, H. Nishi, M. Shireda, Y. Fukakawa, Millimeter wave IMPATT diodes with improved efficiency by using ion-implanted ohmic contact, Proceeding of the IEEE Letters 63 (1975), 1367-1367.

[56] M.S. Gupta, A simple approximate method to estimate the effect of carrier diffusion in Impatt diodes, Solid-State Electronics 18 (1975) 327.
[57] M. Chive, E. Constant, M. Lefebvre, J.P. Ribetich, Effect of tunneling on high efficiency impatt avalanche diode, Proceedings of the IEEE 63 (1975) 824–826.
[58] K.B. Winterbon, Ion Implantation Range and Energy Deposition Distributions, vol. 2, IFI/Plenum Press, New York, 1975.
[59] I. Doumitria, G. Salmer, E. Constant, High frequency limitation of silicon IMPATT diode velocity modulation, Journal of Applied Physics 46 (1975) 1831.
[60] C.P. Wan, Y.S. Chang, E.J. Denoglar, Multilayer epitaxially grown silicon IMPATT diodes at millimeter wave frequencies, Journal of Electronic Materials 4 (1) (1975) 119–129.
[61] E.A. Konorova, Y.A. Kuznetsov, V.F. Sergienko, S.D. Tkachenko, A.K. Tsikunov, A.V. Spitsyn, Y.Z. Danyushevski, Impact ionization in semiconductor structures made of ion-implanted diamond, Soviet Physics - Semiconductors 17 (1983) 146.
[62] D.K. Ferry, High-field transport in wide-bandgap semiconductors, Physical Review B: Condensed Matter 12 (1975) 2361.
[63] C. Canali, E. Gatti, S.F. Kozlov, P.F. Manfredi, C. Manfredotti, F. Nava, A. Quirini, Electrical properties and performances of neutral diamond nuclear radiation detectors, Nuclear Instruments and Methods 160 (1979) 73.
[64] A. Acharyya, J. Mukherjee, M. Mukherjee, J.P. Banerjee, Heat sink design for IMPATT diode sources with different base materials operating at 94 GHz, Archives of Physics Research 2 (1) (2011) 107–126.
[65] A. Acharyya, B. Pal, J.P. Banerjee, Temperature distribution inside semi-infinite heat sinks for IMPATT sources, International Journal of Engineering Science and Technology 2 (10) (2010) 5142–5149.
[66] D.L. Scharfetter, H.K. Gummel, Large-signal analysis of a silicon Read diode oscillator, IEEE Transactions on Electron Devices 6 (1) (1969) 64–77.
[67] M.G. Adlerstein, S.L.G. Chu, GaAs IMPATT diodes for 60 GHz, IEEE Electron Device Letters 5 (1984), 97-97.
[68] H. Eisele, C.C. Chen, G.O. Munns, G.I. Haddad, The potential of InP IMPATT diodes as high-power millimetre-wave sources: first experimental results, in: IEEE MTT-S International Microwave Symposium Digest 2, 1996, pp. 529–532.
[69] C.A. Hewett, J.R. Zeidler, Issues in diamond device fabrication, Diamond and Related Materials 1 (1992) 688–691.
[70] Takeuchi, et al., Diamond PN Junction Diode and Method for the Fabrication, United States Patent, patent no. US 6,727,171 B2, Apr. 27, 2004.
[71] M. Kamo, Y. Sato, S. Matsumoto, N. Setaka, Journal of Crystal Growth 62 (1983) 642.
[72] P. Post, The business and technical outlook for CVD diamond and diamond-like carbon, in: Proc 2nd Gorham Advanced Materials Conf, Monterey, CA, 1993.
[73] M. Füner, C. Wild, P. Koidl, Novel microwave plasma reactor for diamond synthesis, Applied Physics Letters 72 (1998) 1149–1150.
[74] Q. Liang, C.Y. Chin, J. Lai, C.S. Yan, Y. Meng, H. Mao, R.J. Hemley, Enhanced growth of high quality single crystal diamond by microwave plasma assisted chemical vapor deposition at high gas pressure, Applied Physics Letters 94 (2009) 024103–024104.
[75] P.K. Tyagi, A. Mishra, K.N. Narayanan, P. Rai, M.K. Sing, U. Palnikar, D.S. Misra, F.L. Normand, Step growth in single crystal diamond growth by microwave plasma chemical vapor deposition, Diamond and Related Materials 15 (2–3) (2005) 304–308.
[76] R.J. Hemley, Y.-C. Chen, C.-S. Yan, Growing diamond crystals by chemical vapor deposition, Elements 1 (2005) 105–108.
[77] K. Fabisiak, E. Staryga, CVD diamond: from growth to application, Journal of Achievements in Materials and Manufacturing Engineering 37 (2) (2009) 264–269.
[78] K. Kurihara, K. Sasaki, M. Kawarada, N. Koshino, High rate synthesis of diamond by DC plasma jet chemical vapor deposition, Applied Physics Letters 52 (437–438) (1988).
[79] A. Hiraki, H. Kawarada, J. Wei, J.I. Suzuki, Preparation and characterization of wide area, high quality diamond film using magnetoactive plasma chemical vapor deposition, Surface and Coatings Technology 43/44 (1990) 10.
[80] T. Yara, M. Yuasa, M. Shimizu, H. Makia, A. Hatta, J. Suzuki, T. Ito, A. Hiraki, Fabrication of diamond films at low pressure and low-temperature by magneto-active microwave plasma chemical vapor deposition, Japanese Journal of Applied Physics 33 (1994) 4404.
[81] T.D. Mantei, Z. Ring, M. Schweizer, S. Tlali, H.E. Jackson, Low temperature synthesis of diamond films with electron cyclotron resonance plasma chemical vapor deposition, Japanese Journal of Applied Physics 35 (1996) 2516.
[82] Y. Matsui, A. Yuuki, M. Sahara, Y. Hirose, Flame structure and diamond growth mechanism of acetylene torch, Japanese Journal of Applied Physics 28 (1989) 1718.
[83] C. Pan, J.C. Withers, C.H. Stoessei, R.O. Loutfy, Chemical vapor deposition of diamond using fullerenes for diamond nucleation and growth precursors, in: Proc. of 4th Internal Symp on Diamond Mater, 1995, p. 130.
[84] V.S. Vavilov, M.A. Gukasya, M.I. Guseva, T.A. Karatygia, E.A. Konorova, Conductivity of diamond doped by implantation of phosphorus ions, Soviet Physics: Semiconductors 9 (1976) 962–964.
[85] V.S. Vavilov, E.A. Konorova, E.B. Stepanova, E.M. Trukhan, Infrared photoconductivity of diamond doped by implanting lithium ions, Soviet Physics: Semiconductors 13 (1979) 604–606.
[86] N. Fujimori, T. Imai, A. Doi, Characterization of conductining diamond films, Vacuum 36 (1–3) (1986) 99–102.

[87] K. Okhano, H. Naruki, Y. Akiba, T. Kurosu, M. Iida, Y. Hirose, Synthesis of diamond thin films having semiconductor properties, Japanese Journal of Applied Physics 27 (1988) L173–L175.
[88] G.H. Glover, Solid-State Electronics 16 (1973) 973.
[89] J. Mort, D. Kuhman, M. Machonkin, M. Moragan, F. Jansen, K. Okumura, Y.M. Legrice, R.J. Nemanich, Boron doping of diamond thin films, Applied Physics Letters 55 (1989) 1121–1122.
[90] H. Shiomi, H. Nakahata, T. Imai, Y. Nishibayashi, N. Fujimori, Electrical characteristics of metal contacts to boron-doped diamond epitaxial films, Japanese Journal of Applied Physics 28 (1989) 758.
[91] K. Miyata, K. Kumagai, K. Nishimura, K. Kobashi, Morphology of heavily B doped diamond films, Journal of Materials Research 8 (1993) 2845.
[92] S.A. Grot, C.W. Hatfield, G.S. Gildenblat, A.R. Badzian, T. Badzian, Electrical properties of selectively grown homoepitaxial diamond films, Applied Physics Letters 58 (1991) 1542–1543.
[93] R. Locher, J. Wagner, F. Fuchs, C. Wild, P. Hiesinger, P. Gonon, P. Koidl, Boron doped diamond films: electrical and optical characterization and the effect of compensating nitrogen, Materials Science and Engineering B 29 (1995) 211.
[94] S. Kajihara, A. Antonelli, J. Bernholc, in: Proc Fall 1989 MRS Meeting, Boston, MA, vol. 162, 1989, p. 315.
[95] S. Koizumi, T. Murakami, T. Inuzuka, K. Suzuki, Growth and characterization of phosphorous doped (111) homoepitaxial diamond thin films, Applied Physics Letters 71 (1997) 1065–1066.
[96] H. Kato, T. Makino, S. Yamasaki, H. Okusi, *n*-type diamond growth by phosphorus doping on (001) oriented surface, Journal of Physics D Applied Physics 43 (2010) 374017.
[97] J. Chevallier, M.A. Pinault, J. Barion, T. Kociniewski, F. Jomard, C. Saguy, R. Kalish, Different approaches for the *n*-type doping of diamond, in: International Workshop on Physics of Semiconductor Devices, 2007, pp. 813–818.
[98] J. Chevallier, M.A. Pinault, J. Barion, T. Kociniewski, F. Jomard, C. Saguy, R. Kalish, Electrical properties of diamond doped by implantation of lithium ion, Soviet Physics: Semiconductors 13 (1979) 635–638.
[99] C. Zhen, Y. Wang, S. He, Q. Guo, Z. Yan, P. Yuejiao, Ohmic contacts to boron-doped diamond, Optical Materials 23 (2003) 117–121.
[100] C.A. Hewett, M.J. Taylor, J.F.L. Zeidler, M.W. Geis, Specific contact resistance measurements of ohmic contacts to semiconducting diamond, Journal of Applied Physics 77 (2) (1995) 755–760.
[101] M.S. Alexander, M.N. Latto, P.W. May, D.J. Riley, G.P. Moreno, A simple route to ohmic contacts on low boron-doped CVD diamond, Diamond and Related Materials 12 (2003) 1460–1462.
[102] J. Wan, R.Q. Zhang, H.F. Cheung, Energetics of Ti atom diffusion into diamond film, Computational Materials Science 23 (2003) 73–79.
[103] C.A. Hewett, J.R Zeidler, M.J. Taylor, C.R. Zeiss, K.L. Moazcd. Specific contact resistance measurements of ohmic contacts to diamond, Proceedings of the 2nd International Conference on the New Diamond Science and Technology, Washington D.C., September 23 27, 1990.
[104] S.K. Noh, C.R. Lee, S.E. Park, Doping characteristics of Si-doped n-GaN epilayers grown by low-pressure metal-organic chemical vapor deposition, Journal of the Korean Physical Society 32 (1998) 2851–2856.
[105] A. Usikov, O. Kovalenkov, V. Soukhoveev, V. Ivantsov, A. Syrkin, V. Dmitriev, A.Y. Nikiforov, S.G. Sundaresan, S.J. Jeliazkov, A.V. Davydov, Electrical and optical properties of thick highly doped p-type GaN layers grown by HVPE, Physica Status Solidi 5 (2008) 1829–1831.
[106] K. Jeganathan, M. Shimizu, H. Okumura, Growth of strain free GaN layers on 6H-SiC (0001) by plasma-assisted molecular beam epitaxy, Physica Status Solidi 0 (2002) 143–147.
[107] J.K. Jeong, J.H. Choi, H.J. Kim, H.C. Seo, E. Yoon, C.S. Hwang, Buffer-layer-free growth of high-quality epitaxial GaN films on 4H-SiC substrate by metal-organic chemical vapor deposition, Journal of Crystal Growth 276 (2005) 407–414.
[108] S. Bose, S.K. Mazumder, Fabrication and characterization of a GaN/(4H)SiC vertical pn power diode using direct and interfaced epitaxial-growth approaches, Journal of Semiconductors 34 (2013) 044001–044004.
[109] M.Z. Mohd Yusoff, A. Baharin, Z. Hassan, H.A. Hassan, M.J. Abdullah, MBE growth of GaN pn-junction photodetector on AlN/Si(111) substrate with Ni/Ag as ohmic contact, Superlattices and Microstructures 56 (2013) 35–44.
[110] E.R. Glaser, M. Murthy, J.A. Freitas, D.F. Storm, L. Zhou, D.J. Smith, Optical and magnetic resonance studies of Mg-doped GaN homoepitaxial layers grown by molecular beam epitaxy, Physica B: Condensed Matter 401–402 (2007) 327–330.
[111] J.L. Weyher, P.D. Brown, A.R.A. Zauner, S. MuKller, C.B. Boothroyd, D.T. Foord, P.R. Hageman, C.J. Humphreys, P.K. Larsen, I. Grzegory, S. Porowski, Morphological and structural characteristics of homoepitaxial GaN grown by metalorganic chemical vapour deposition (MOCVD), Journal of Crystal Growth 204 (4) (1999) 419–428. https://doi.org/10.1016/S0022-0248(99)00217-1.
[112] C. Kirchner, V. Schwegler, F. Eberhard, M. Kamp, K.J. Ebeliig, MOVPE homoepitaxy of high-quality GaN: crystal growth and devices, Progress in Crystal Growth and Characterization of Materials 41 (2000) 57–83.
[113] M.G. Ancona, H.F. Tiersten, Macroscopic physics of the silicon inversion layer, Physical Review B: Condensed Matter 35 (1987) 7959–7965.
[114] M.G. Ancona, Z. Yu, R.W. Dutton, P.J.V. Voorde, M. Cao, D. Vook, Density-gradient analysis of MOS tunnelling,

IEEE Transactions on Electron Devices 47 (12) (2000) 2310–2319.

[115] M.G. Ancona, Density-gradient theory: a macroscopic approach to quantum confinement and tunneling in semiconductor devices, Journal of Computational Electronics 10 (2011) 65–97.

[116] I. Umebu, A.N.M.M. Chowdhury, P.N. Robson, Ionization coefficients measured in abrupt InP junction, Applied Physics Letters 36 (1980) 302–303.

[117] B. Kramer, A. Micrea, Determination of saturated electron velocity in GaAs, Applied Physics Letters 26 (1975) 623–624.

[118] K. Kunihiro, K. Kasahara, Y. Takahashi, Y. Ohno, Experimental evaluation of impact ionization coefficients in GaN, IEEE Electron Device Letters 20 (12) (1999) 608–610.

[119] A.O. Konstantinov, Q. Wahab, N. Nordell, U. Lindefelt, Ionization rates and critical fields in 4H-silicon carbide, Applied Physics Letters 71 (1997) 90–92.

[120] M. Ito, S. Kagawa, T. Kaneda, T. Yamaoka, Ionization rates for electrons and holes in GaAs, Journal of Applied Physics 49 (1978) 4607.

[121] C.W. Kao, C.R. Crowell, Impact ionization by electrons and holes in InP, Solid-State Electronics 23 (1980) 881–891.

[122] S.C. Shiyu, G. Wang, High-field properties of carrier transport in bulk wurtzite GaN: Monte Carlo perspective, Journal of Applied Physics 103 (2008) 703–708.

[123] K.V. Vassilevski, K. Zekentes, A.V. Zorenko, L.P. Romanov, Experimental determination of electron drift velocity in 4H-SiC p^{+}-n-n^{+} avalanche diodes, IEEE Electron Device Letters 21 (2000) 485–487.

[124] C.D. Falco, E. Gatti, A.L. Lacaita, R. Sacco, Quantum-corrected drift-diffusion models for transport in semiconductor devices, Journal of Computational Physics 204 (2) (2005) 533–561.

[125] J. Douglas, Y. Yuan, Finite Difference Methods for the Transient Behavior of a Semiconductor Device, IMA Preprint Series#286, Institute for Mathematics and Its Applications, University of Minnesota, Minnesota, 1987.

[126] M.E. Elta, The Effect of Mixed Tunneling and Avalanche Breakdown on Microwave Transit-Time Diodes (Ph.D. dissertation), Electron Physics Lab., Univ. of Mich., Ann Arbor, MI, 1978. Tech. Rep.

[127] E.O. Kane, Theory of tunneling, Journal of Applied Physics 32 (1961) 83–91.

[128] M.G. Ancona, Macroscopic description of quantum-mechanical tunnelling, Physical Review B: Condensed Matter 42 (1990) 1222–1223.

[129] M.G. Ancona, Density-gradient analysis of field emission from metals, Physical Review B: Condensed Matter 46 (1992) 4874–4883.

CHAPTER 2

Terahertz Sources Based on Difference-Frequency Generation for Spectroscopy and Biomaterial Analysis

SRINIVASA RAO RAGAM, PHD • PU ZHAO, PHD • YUTAKA OYAMA, PHD

INTRODUCTION

This book chapter mainly focused on terahertz (THz) radiation, design and development of the THz sources based on nonlinear optical (NLO) method, and potential applications of THz radiation for spectroscopy and biomaterial analysis. The THz spectrum spans the frequency range between 100 GHz and 10 THz. This region bridges the gap between the electronics and photonics [1]. The generation and detection of radiation in the frequency range of 100 GHz−10 THz is difficult; scaling and extrapolating known concepts of the microwave or infrared ranges is not possible. Upscaling of microwave devices suffers from the transit time limitation of classical devices. Downscaling of photonic concepts conflicts with the fact that the energy of a THz photon is substantially smaller than the thermal energy. However, the THz region has attracted a lot of importance in last decade as a variety of applications with a potentially great impact have been identified, especially in the area of chemical sensing, biomedical imaging, and spectroscopy [2,3].

Historically, the fields of chemistry and astronomy have been an inspiration for developing THz sources and detectors as the molecular rotational and vibrational resonances play an important role. With increased number of many research teams and their constant efforts, recently this THz gap is filled and has a potential to fulfill real-world applications [3].

Spectral transparency through various materials is one of the most interesting properties of THz radiation, thus making it possible to "see" through a variety of materials such as paper, plastic, fabric, ceramic, wood, and so on. This special property enables the way to nondestructive and noninvasive inspection of packages of many kinds from mail envelope in post offices to luggage and personal belongings in airports. It is important to know that various organic molecules exhibit strong absorption and dispersion due to rotational and intermolecular vibrations in the THz frequency range. These transitions will specify the targets. This enables chemical identification and brings out spectroscopic detection, testing, and analysis technique. These superior properties such as penetration and chemical identification make up the unique feature of the THz radiation, not to be found in any other part of the EM spectrum [4].

Also, THz radiation promises some advantages over X-ray imaging, such as highly reduced risk of irradiation and increased image contrast to differentiate between various soft materials and possibility of chemical identification. The THz photon (whose energy is in order of meV) is weaker than X-ray photon by about a million times, and hence it is safer to use on the human body. Therefore, THz wave technology has potential application in biomedical engineering, in the fields such as protein analysis, detection of skin cancer, tooth decay, etc. [3,4]. However, THz waves are strongly absorbed by water and reflected with metals. The water concentration contained in the biosamples are strongly absorbed THz radiation. In addition, the scattering of THz waves by biosamples makes the detection and identification of bioagents difficult. However, when bioparticles become airborne, the THz waves could still be used to fingerprint the airborne bioparticles. In contrast, this feature is becoming advantageous in the case of reflection spectroscopic measurements. Since almost all aerosol particles have diameters $\leq 10\ \mu m$, scattering of the THz waves by the bioaerosol particles suspended in the air is negligible. Also, due to the presence of atmospheric windows (mainly due to absorption dips of the water vapor), THz waves could eventually be used for probing as well as imaging for distances of 100m−10 km.

Terahertz Biomedical and Healthcare Technologies. https://doi.org/10.1016/B978-0-12-818556-8.00002-1

It is well known that infrared radiation (IR) is also used for chemical identification. But, a very few materials are transparent to infrared compared with THz waves. In addition to this, scattering by target is much stronger for infrared waves, which prevents their use in many noninvasive applications. Millimeter waves and microwaves are generally not chemically sensitive and also have poor image resolution compared to THz waves. IR spectrum is rather intended to specify the localized vibrations in molecules, whereas the THz wave spectrum is characterized in the weak intermolecular vibrations between molecules [5]. Therefore, THz sources have very important applications, especially in spectroscopy and imaging. Using THz spectroscopy, it should be possible to detect explosives or drugs/biological agents even if they are concealed. Hence, this technology is very useful for homeland security and biomedical applications for identification of dangerous chemicals and standoff security screening. It is important to develop portable THz sources, and the output frequency can be tuned in the entire THz domain for fulfilling the practical applications. The concept is based on NLO effect by utilizing the NLO crystals such as GaP, GaAs, $LiNbO_3$, GaSe, and DAST [2,4].

THz sources based on quantum cascaded laser and photomixer have made tremendous advances [6,7]. However, they both have disadvantages that have not been well improved. Although the THz source based on parametric processes and difference-frequency generation (DFG) has the intrinsic feature of low quantum efficiency, it is still among one of the approaches that has highest potential to achieve truly portable THz source [8,9]. In addition, the DFG technology can be built on the solid-state laser industry that is already a mature field. There are various laser mediums and laser systems that can function as the pump source for this THz source [10]. For example, we achieved a portable THz source at 1.64 THz (182 μm) by optically mixing dual wavelengths generated from a neodymium: yttrium lithium fluoride (Nd:YLF) laser [11]. THz frequency tuning and high output power (mW range) are necessary for enabling practical applications in THz domain.

DEVELOPMENT OF A COMPACT MONOCHROMATIC TERAHERTZ SOURCE BY PUMPING WITH ND:YLF LASER

For THz generation using NLO method, NLO crystals such as GaP, $ZnGeP_2$, and GaSe are widely used [12]. Phase matching is the key for achieving the coherent THz output signal. Nd:YLF crystal has two well-known transitions at 1047 nm (286.5 THz, π-polarization) and 1053 nm (284.9 THz, σ-polarization), respectively [11]. By utilizing one Nd:YLF crystal, up to 1 μW THz average power at 182.42 μm (1.643 THz) was generated inside a GaSe crystal (thickness 15 mm). However, it is important for us to note that the two laser transitions share the same upper level inside the laser gain medium, which means that they constitute a competitive relation in consuming the population inversion. Thus, when the output power of one wavelength grows at a higher rate, the power of the other wavelength will grow at a lower rate or even become saturated. This property actually inhibits the power scaling of the THz DFG power and also reduces the stability of the THz DF. Besides, this THz source can only rely on the laser medium that has dual-wavelength transitions, which include a quite limited choices, such as Nd:YLF (1047 nm and 1053 nm) [13], Nd:YAG (1319 nm and 1338 nm) [14], and $Nd:GdVO_4$ (1063 nm and 1065 nm) [10]. As a result, the THz wavelength will be fixed and cannot be tuned.

A prototype of incorporated resonator for solid-state laser which is used as the pump source for portable THz device was proposed. The output powers of the solid-state laser are dramatically improved. Correspondingly, the THz output power scaling with a factor of 2.5 times was achieved. This is made possible by using two diodes pumping scheme as well as the introduction of another Nd:YLF crystal. It is noted that the compactness of the whole system is not much influenced by the newly optimized configuration. Moreover, this laser cavity is not uniquely limited by implementing laser with laser mediums possessing dual-frequency transitions, like Nd: YLF. It is possible that laser medium with single frequency transition would also be added into the choices of laser mediums with output coupler. As a result, we could achieve THz source with different wavelengths as an output.

Experimental Method

The schematic laser design of the incorporated resonator is shown in Fig. 2.1. The cavity for 1053 nm consists of mirror 1, polarizer, and output, and the cavity for 1047 nm consists of mirror 2, polarizer, and output coupler. The cavity design is similar with our previous work at the first glance [11]. However, this new cavity configuration is completely different. In our previous work, the Nd:YLF crystal was placed at the shared arm of the 1047 and 1053 nm cavities. As a result, both the radiation of 1047 and 1053 nm transitions would access the same population inversion within only a single Nd:YLF crystal pumped by the same diode laser.

A polarizer is placed inside the cavity to separate the orthogonal and parallel laser beams at 1047 and 1053 nm. This new method of placing the intracavity polarizer introduces gain competition between the two radiations inside the laser crystal. Due to this gain competition, it was observed that power fluctuates between the 1047 nm and 1053n nm beams. In our new approach, another Nd:YLF with the same parameters was introduced, see Fig. 2.1. In the new configuration, the intracavity polarizer divides the two laser crystals. This solves the issue of gain competition as the two gain mediums are separately accessible by 1047 and 1053 nm laser transitions. A Q-switch (acousto-optic) is employed in the shared cavity for modulating the laser beams in the pulsed mode. A shared output coupler with transmittance of T = 25% (reflectivity = 75%) at both 1047 and 1053 nm is another modification from our previous work. Moreover, the spatial overlap of the two beams is automatically satisfied in this approach. To do frequency mixing, we can simply place the frequency converter after the laser output. Therefore, the whole system could be truly compact.

The two Nd:YLF crystals were separately pumped by two diode lasers at 808 nm through pigtail fibers. The two pump beams were then collimated and focused onto the Nd:YLF crystals through a couple of convex lenses, respectively. It is worth noting that the pumping power illuminated on both laser crystals could be tuned separately. This property is very important for the pulses synchronization of the dual-frequency beams when the lasers are operated at pulsed mode. To ensure the pulse synchronization, the pulse buildup times of the two lasers have to be exactly the same. According to the fundamentals of Q-switched laser, the laser pulse is not generated instantly after the acoustic-optic becomes highly transparent. When the acoustic-optic Q-switch is instantly open, the time taken to generate a laser pulse depends on the pulse buildup time. This depends on many parameters such as coefficient of output coupler, laser medium, losses inside cavity, pump laser power, and the stimulated emission cross section of laser medium. Once the cavity is tuned and well aligned, then the only thing that can change the pulse buildup time is the pumping level. Indeed, in this incorporated resonator, we can flexibly change the pumping level of the two lasers separately simply by varying the driving currents of the two diode lasers.

The relation between Q-switched laser output power and the pump powers at 1047 and 1053 nm was studied at a pulse repetition rate of 3.8 kHz, see Fig. 2.2. It is observed that output powers at both the wavelengths of 1047 and 1053 nm increased linearly, without having any gain competition problem. In this configuration, the laser output powers obtained were 2.3 and 1.5 W for 1047 and 1053 nm, respectively, with conversion efficiency 24% and 16%.

This is a very good improvement as the output power increased twice from our previous results. In addition, the average power ratio of 1047–1053 nm is 1.52. This value is quite close to the stimulated cross sectional ratio 1.5, which is $1.8 \times 10^{-19}\ cm^{-2}$ at 1047 nm versus $1.2 \times 10^{-19}\ cm^{-2}$ at 1053 nm [11]. The dependence of pulse width on laser pump power is plotted as shown in Fig. 2.3. It is observed that the laser pulse width at 1047 and 1053 nm reduced at almost the same rate with respect to the pump power increment. This is evident from the characteristics of actively Q-switched laser [13].

The laser pulse widths at 1047 and 1053 nm were measured to be 13 and 11 ns, respectively, with a pump power of 9.5 W, and the pulse profiles are shown in the inset of Fig. 2.3. From the figure, it is observed that there is a very good synchronization between the two laser pulses.

THz DFG was carried out by using a 15 mm long GaSe crystal. Experimental setup is shown in Fig. 2.4. Convex lens, L1 (focal length = 15 cm), works as a beam collimating component. In the dashed line circled part, the two beams are split by cubic beam splitter BS1 and recombined by BS2.

This is especially designed for type II DFG in which the power flux of interacted o and e lights will separate

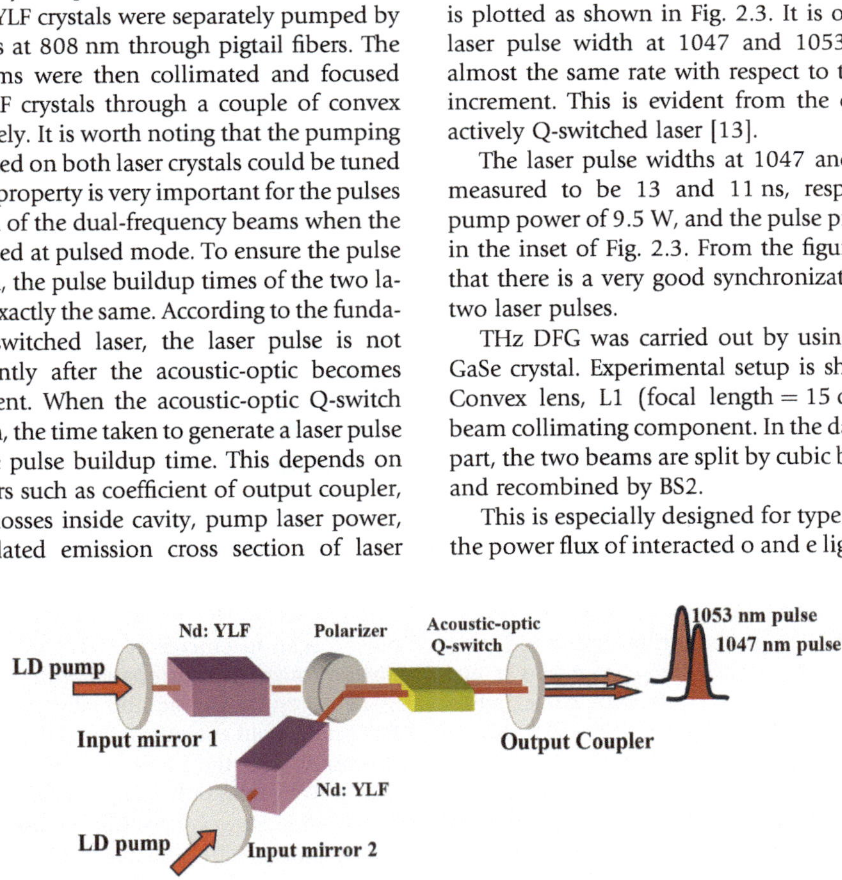

FIG. 2.1 Experimental setup for the incorporated resonator.

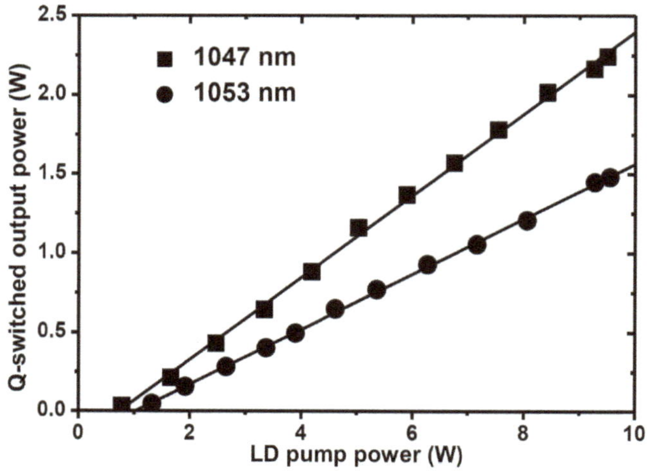

FIG. 2.2 Q-switched output power versus pump power at two different wavelengths. Dots and squares correspond to data points; straight lines correspond to linear fits to data points.

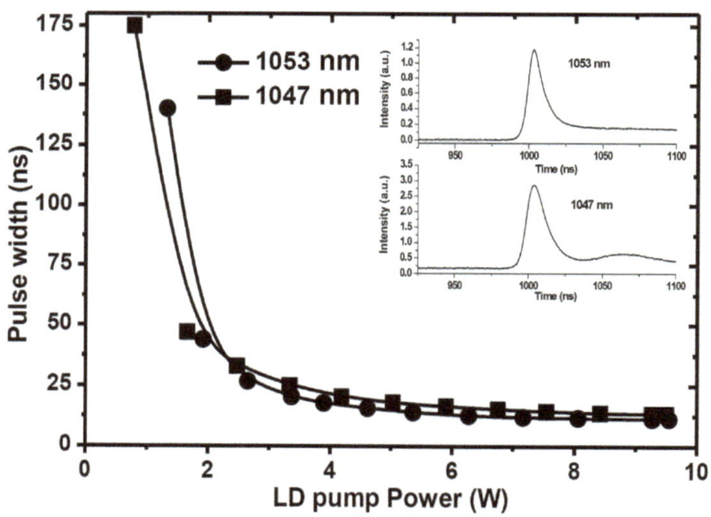

FIG. 2.3 Pulse widths versus the LD pump power.

from each other inside birefringent crystal. Indeed, in the circled part, the introduction of mirrors M1 and M2 will make it quite flexible for the beams overlapping inside GaSe crystal. Correspondingly, the conversion efficiency of DFG can be further optimized. It is worth noting that the dashed line circled part is not necessary for the DFG in crystals with cubic lattice structure, like GaP [15]. We measured the THz power dependence on the 1047 and 1053 nm summed power, as shown in Fig. 2.5. At the highest incident power, we achieved 2.356 μW THz radiation at 1.64 THz (182.4 μm), corresponding to a conversion efficiency of $0.633 \times 10^{-4}\%$. The solid line corresponds to the quadric fitting. When the laser power is more than about 3 W, the THz power began to increase linearly. This is due to the reason that a tailed pulse began to emerge at 1047 nm, which has a 1.5 times stronger gain compared with 1053 nm.

As a result, any additionally increased power of 1047 nm would enter the tailed pulse, which is not synchronized with the pulse at 1053 nm. Therefore, the THz power would only increase linearly with the power of 1053 nm. However, we still achieved the THz output power scaling with a factor of 2.5 times. Considering

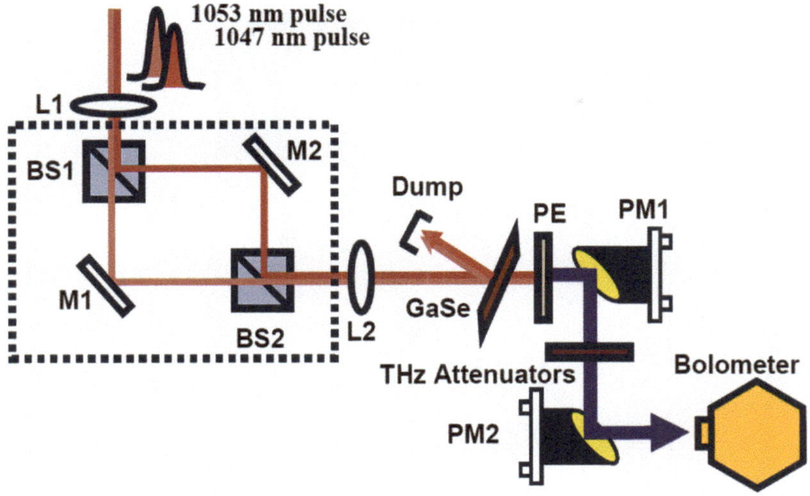

FIG. 2.4 Experimental setup for THz DFG generation: L1, collimating convex lens; L1, focusing convex lens; BS1–BS2, beam splitter; M1–M2, high reflection mirrors; PE, high-density white polyethene filter; PM1–PM2, parabolic mirrors.

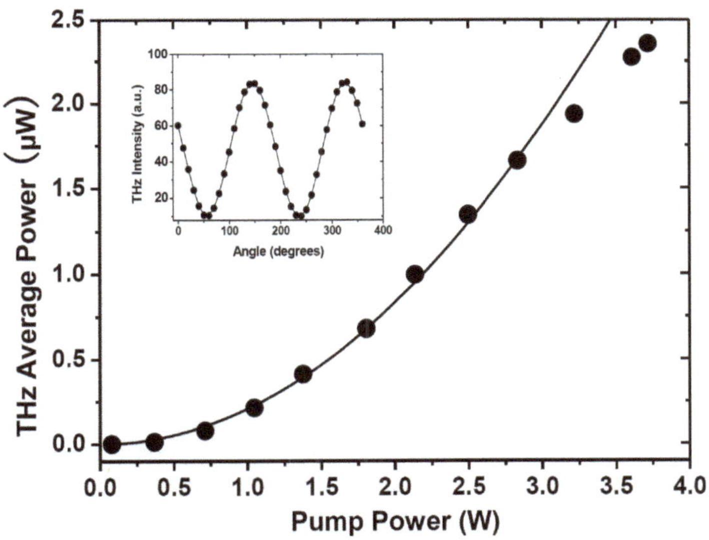

FIG. 2.5 Terahertz intensity versus 1047 and 1053 nm summed power.

the power improvements of the pump power at 1047 and 1053 nm, this scaling-up factor could be 4.7. It is expected that we can further improve the THz output power by optimizing the resonator and solving the problem of tailing pulse. In addition, we have measured the polarization of the THz radiation as a function of the azimuthal angle of a THz polarizer, shown in inset of Fig. 2.5. It is obvious that the power dependence shows a perfect trigonometric function.

TERAHERTZ GENERATION BASED ON STACKED GAP CAVITY MIRROR WITH INTRACAVITY CONFIGURATION

To achieve high efficiency frequency conversion, intracavity scheme is an important approach in which a high-power fundamental wave undergones a standing wave pattern inside the laser cavity. For efficient THz wave generation, it was reported that the intracavity parametric process [16] and intracavity DFG schemes

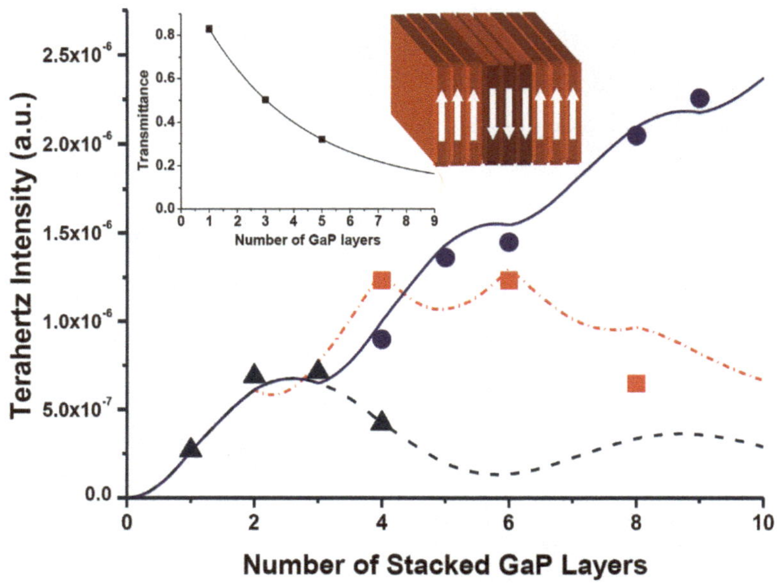

FIG. 2.6 THz intensity generated from GaP stacks in terms of different stacking configurations. Triangle, every one-layer reversed; rectangular, every two-layer reversed; round, every three-layer reversed. Inset, transmittance of laser beam through GaP stacks.

are very promising [17]. It must be noted that surface emitting scheme is very suitable in the both methods as THz wave propagates with wide angle in the direction of pump beams. This method will take care the issue of high absorption at THz frequencies in most of NLO crystals. However, the cavity alignment and THz detection are difficult in this method, and hence, a collinear approach is proposed. It should be noted that the NLO crystals must be highly transparent for both THz and infrared frequencies. It was demonstrated using an NLO crystal of GaAs inside OPO at the wavelength of 2 μm [18]. The wavelength of THz can be tuned by selecting two different laser crystals [19,20]. It is well known that from literature, there are hundreds of Nd-doped crystals or ceramics available with lasing wavelengths from 1.03 to 1.1 μm [19]. Two-photon absorption (TPA) is very dominant around 1 μm for GaAs crystal, and hence GaAs is not a suitable candidate for THz intracavity generation.

It is well known that GaP crystal exhibits a low TPA coefficient around 1 μm. Our group has successfully demonstrated an efficient THz pulse using GaP crystal with pump laser pulses at 1 μm [21,22]. Moreover, the GaP crystal can be employed for cavity-enhanced DFG scheme [23]. This shows that GaP is a potential NLO crystal for intracavity laser applications. In our experiments, we have used the industry-grade GaP plates, which were cut along the [110] direction and are highly polished. The GaP plates diameter and the thickness are measured as 48 mm and 660 μm, respectively. We have used a total of nine GaP plates for stacking, and this is employed as an output coupler. This gives a sufficient reflection coefficient that is required for the output coupler. The reflectivity of the stacked GaP plates were tested by using a solid-state Nd:YLF. The results are shown in the inset of Fig. 2.6, which gives the transmittance of laser beam through GaP stacks with different number of layers. From Fig. 2.6, it is evident that the transmittance reduces with an increase in the number of GaP stacked plates and transmittance reaches 20% with 9 plates. Our group successfully generated efficient THz signal at 1.64 THz by mixing two wavelengths at near-IR using a Nd:YLF laser as a pump source [20]. The two wavelengths at 1047 and 1053 nm in the near-IR have orthogonal polarization directions. It is very important to maintain the phase-matching condition in DFG scheme to achieve the efficient THz output signal, hence the polarization of these near-IR wavelengths should be parallel to [1$\bar{1}$0] and [001] onto the GaP crystal.

Three stacking configurations were explored in order to determine the optimized orientation direction. Efficient THz pulses were generated by pumping the near-IR beams at 1047 and 1053 nm on the GaP stacks in the intracavity configuration. In this experimental method, we have used different combinations of GaP plates as an output coupler. Eventually, the generated THz intensity is depicted in Fig. 2.6. Also, the theoretical

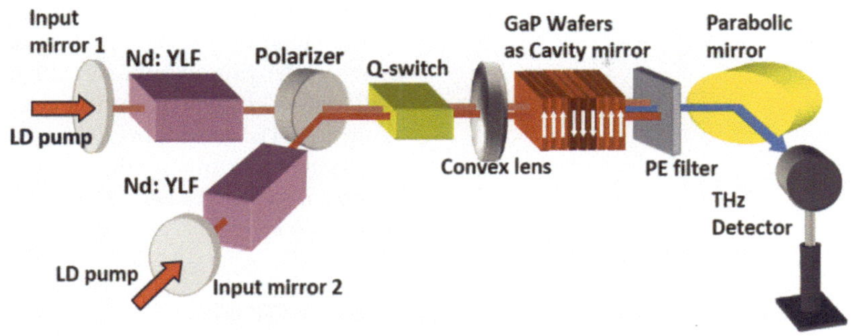

FIG. 2.7 The experimental setup for the configuration of intracavity DFG. PE filter, high-density white polyethylene filter.

modeling for THz outpower dependence with GaP plates for coherence length about 2 mm was shown in Fig. 2.6. It is obvious to note that our experimental results well agree with the theoretical modeling. The multiple reflections in the GaP wafers give rise to get high reflection coefficient. It is observed that the intracavity output power gradually reduces with the number of GaP plates. This shows that the intracavity intensity is much higher than the intensity finally emitted from the laser. In our configuration, the GaP are stacked by air so that orientation of the each plate is still can be varied, which is different from diffusion bonding scheme [24]. Thus, to achieve the highly efficient THz wave generation in the quasi phase–matched configuration, it is very important to align the GaP plate orientation for different coherence lengths at different output frequencies in THz domain.

We have successfully demonstrated the THz generation with GaP crystal in the intracavity scheme using Q-switched dual-frequency solid-state laser at 1 μm. Fig. 2.7 shows the experimental setup for THz intracavity configuration. Compared with the external cavity scheme, the THz power generated in the intracavity mode is greatly enhanced. We have used several stacked GaP wafers (plates), which can be employed as an output coupler for the dual-wavelength laser, see Fig. 2.7. Note that this configuration is little different from the experimental setup shown in Ref. [20]. It is due to the fact that we utilize GaP stacked plates as output coupler and make it portable. The laser cavity for wavelength at 1053 nm consists of input mirror 1, polarizer, convex lens, and GaP stack, and the laser cavity for wavelength at 1047 nm consists of input mirror 2, polarizer, convex lens, and GaP stack.

An intracavity polarizer is employed to combine the dual wavelengths that are having different polarizations. Here, the laser crystals are a-cut Nd:YLF (Nd doped at 1.0% and $4 \times 4 \times 10\ mm^3$), which are placed at separate cavities but combined by intracavity polarizer. For pulsed mode operation of the laser, we placed an acoustic-optic Q-switch inside the laser cavity. A focusing lens (biconvex lens) with focus length of $f = 10$ cm was employed inside cavity to achieve a focused beam on the GaP stack. By satisfying the phase-matching condition, DFG process will occur for efficient THz pulse generation. For signal processing, white polyethylene (PE) filter was used to block the near-IR beams. THz radiation is guided by a parabolic mirror, and room temperature–operated THz detector such as Golay cell measures the output signal.

A fiber coupled 808 nm diode lasers were used as pump lasers for Nd:YLF crystals. The Q-switch pulse repetition rate is around 4 kHz. In our experiments, the output powers of the Nd:YLF laser at 1047 and 1053 nm were 42 and 56 mW and the laser pulse widths are 280 and 170 ns, respectively. Hence, the THz average power was measured to be 200 nW. Fig. 2.8 shows the THz output power dependence on near-IR laser pump power.

THz power fluctuations were observed as we moved the stack not vertically or horizontally but perpendicularly to the direction of laser beams. This may be due the change of reflection coefficient induced by the air gaps among GaP plates. We have calculated the reflection coefficient of GaP from the theory of transmission matrix approach dealing with nonperiodic dielectric stack [24]. To see the performance of our new approach of GaP stack intracavity method, we compared the output performance with that of the external cavity THz configuration. An output coupler with a coupling efficiency of 5% was replaced with GaP plates. With this configuration, the output laser power was 902 mW at 1047 nm and 510 mW at 1053 nm, respectively, and the average THz power was measured to be

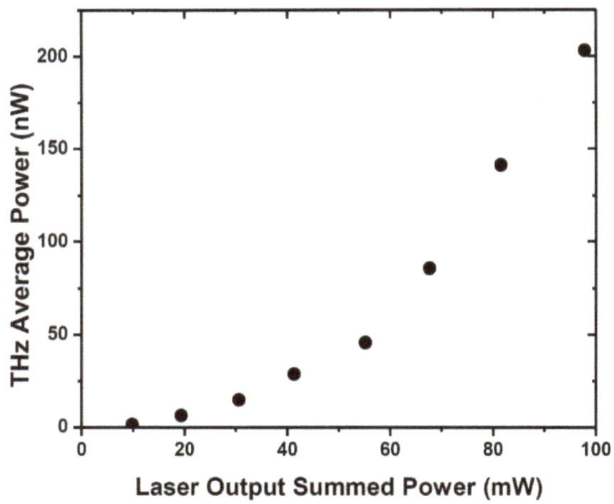

FIG. 2.8 THz power dependence versus corresponding laser powers emitted from the GaP stack.

2 nW. Obviously, this very lower value compared with the THz power obtained in the intracavity scheme. It is very important to mention that THz power stability is a concern in intracavity nonlinear process. Hence, the stability of THz output power was measured and shown in Fig. 2.9.

The THz power stability is within ±6%, for 10 min duration, which is important for practical of applications. In addition, THz beam wavelength was also measured by using a Si etalon. The experimental value of measured wavelength is 186 μm, which is very close to the value of 182.4 μm, obtained from two pump laser wavelengths. In our new configuration, the stacked GaP wafers employ as output coupler and NLO medium for THz generation. This new design makes the THz system not only portable but also a simple configuration for ease of operation based on dual-frequency solid-state laser.

APPLICATIONS

High-Resolution THz Spectrometer Using GaP Crystal and Pumping with CW Diode Lasers

We constructed a THz transmission spectroscopy system using GaP crystal and pumping with compact diode lasers, namely distributed feedback laser (DFB) and external cavity laser diode (ECLD). Fig. 2.10.1 shows the schematic diagram of an automatic measurement system for THz transmission spectroscopy. For efficient DFG signal generation, phase-matching condition has to be satisfied and it is automatically fulfilled by using a rotating and linearly translating stage controller with a polarizer. The DFB laser wavelength can be tuned from 1055 to 1062 nm with a line width of 4 MHz by software. The ECLD wavelength can be tuned from 1040 to 1075 nm with a line width of

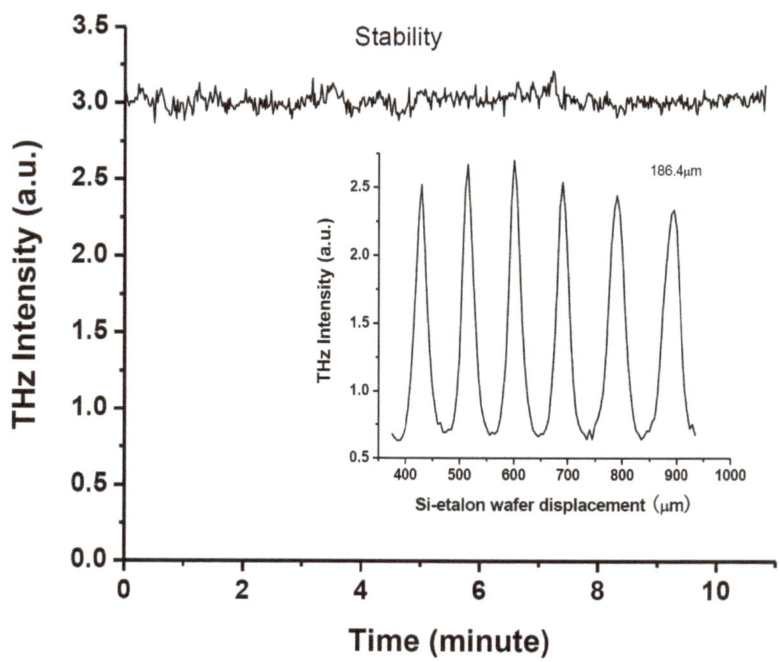

FIG. 2.9 Temporal stability of THz intensity. Inset, THz power being transmitted through a Si etalon as a function of the displacement between two Si wafers.

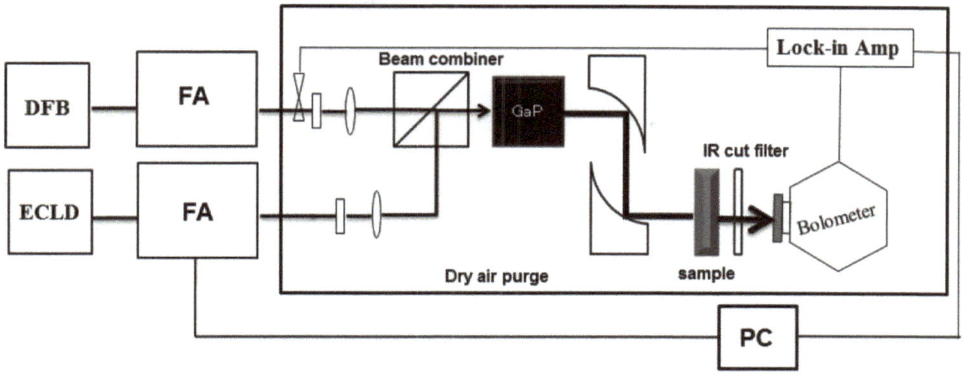

FIG. 2.10.1 Schematic diagram of THz spectrometer using GaP.

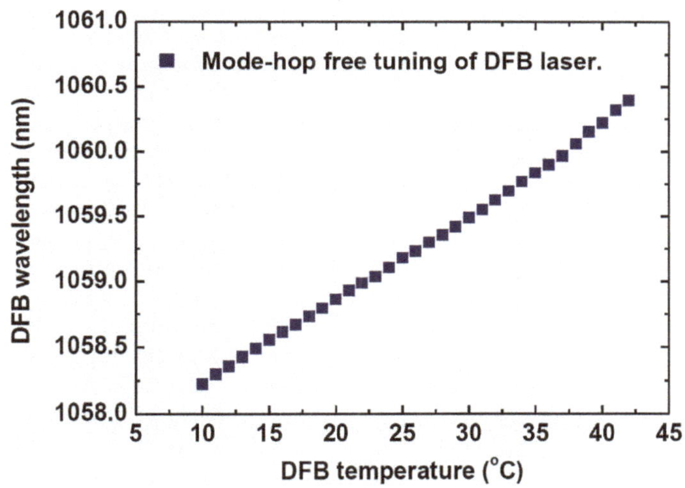

FIG. 2.10.2A The calibration graph for DFB laser temperature and its wavelength.

4 MHz. Since, the output power of the laser diodes is in the order of mW, two Yb doped fiber amplifiers were employed to amplify the intensity of the laser diodes up to 3 W. We have selected a 10 mm-long GaP as NLO crystal for our experiment. Both the input and output faces of GaP crystal are transparent for near-IR and THz frequencies, and hence GaP crystal was coated with Al_2O_3.

The polarizations laser diodes were maintained in the <001> and <110> directions. The line width of ECLD laser was measured as 2.15 MHz using a Fabry–Perot etalon. The THz signals are detected with 4 K Si bolometer.

Study of Water Vapor Transmittance Spectra

Using our simple and effective method, the transmission spectra of water vapor from 1.55 to 2.95 THz were measured at room temperature and atmospheric pressure conditions by tuning the DFB laser wavelength. Fig. 2.10.2A shows the calibration graph for DFB laser temperature and its wavelength. It is seen that the temperature–wavelength relation is linear with slope = (10 °C/0.661 nm). By automatically tuning the wavelength of DFB, a mode hope free tuning of THz wave obtained is about 600 GHz. Fig. 2.10.2B shows the THz frequency relation with its output power.

Figs. 2.10.3A–C show the water vapor absorption spectra of THz waves in the frequency range 1.5-3 THz at atmospheric pressure and room temperature conditions. It is observed that the FWHM of absorption lines are in several GHz order.

The scan rate is 310 MHz/step for 1.5 THz to 2.5 THz and 160 MHz/step for 2.5 THz–3 THz frequency range. The red lines/arrows indicate the data from NASA database [25–27]. It is observed that every single line of

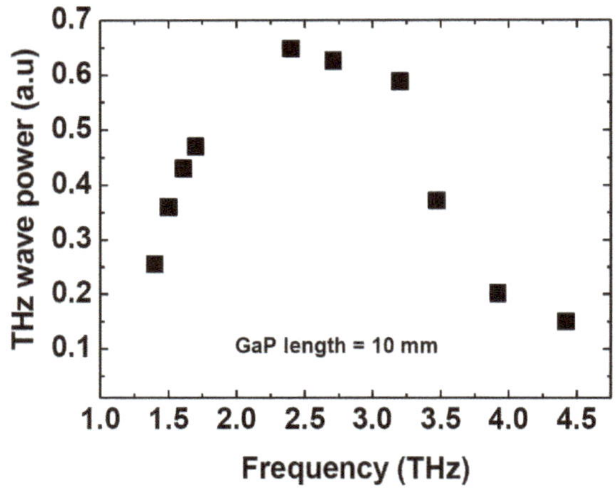

FIG. 2.10.2B The THz frequency relation with its output power.

water vapor absorption can be identified. It is well known that the line width of the water vapor absorption lines decreases with decrease of the pressure. We placed a 50 mm-long chamber in the THz beam line. The air inside the chamber is vacuumed by a turbo molecular pump.

In this experimental arrangement, THz beam travels 10 cm in the atmosphere and 5 cm inside the chamber before it is detected by the bolometer, which is placed very close to the outer face of the chamber. Fig. 2.10.3D depicts the THz water vapor absorption spectrum at room temperature and pressure of 1 mTorr inside the chamber. The scan rate is 15 MHz/step. It is seen that the absorption line at 1.61172 THz is narrowed when THz wave is passed through the chamber with high vacuum. The FWHM of the absorption line at 1.61169 THz is measured to be 168 MHz. Redline shows the spectrum data from NASA database.

Study of White Polyethylene THz Spectra

In PE, the low-frequency lattice vibrations arise from weak H—H atom interactions forming a PE crystal lattice. Absorption peak at 2.2 THz (73 cm^{-1}) in PE crystal is attributed to B_{1u} translational lattice vibration mode. We have investigated the very fine frequency shift of B_{1u} translation vibration modes of PE samples. We set up a purge bag in the THz wave path using the PE bag to cancel water vapor absorption of THz waves. The dry air is supplied to the bag by air dryer machine.

We did experiments to check the reduction of water vapor absorption with purging time. Also, we checked the stability of the THz wave and back ground noise of the bolometer when there is no THz wave generation. DFB laser wavelength is tuning from 1058 to 1060 nm automatically. ECLD laser wavelength is 1050.83 nm. The difference frequency is tuned from 2.002 to 2.477 THz. Fig. 2.10.4A and 2.10.4B depicts the transmission and absorption spectra of white PE in the frequency from 1.97 to 2.45 THz. It is worth to mention that the line width of the THz wave source is estimated to be < 8 MHz. By using CW THz spectroscopic system, more accurate measurement of absorption spectra of many chemicals is possible, compared with that of pulsed THz spectroscopic systems.

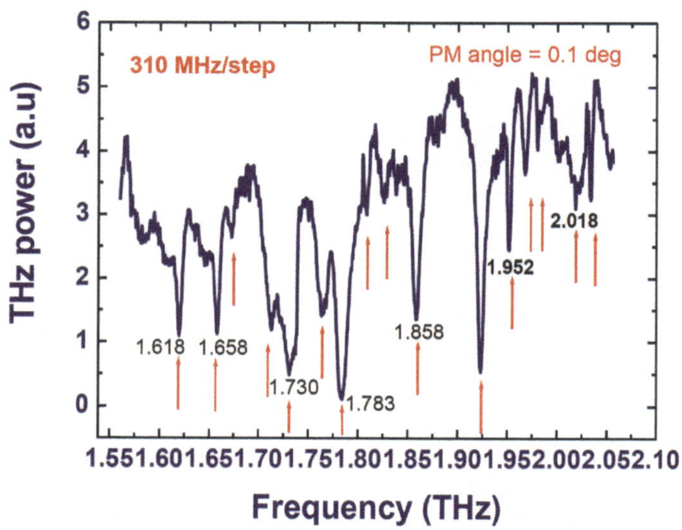

FIG. 2.10.3A The water vapor absorption spectra of THz waves in the frequency range 1.5–2 THz at atmospheric pressure and room temperature conditions. The redlines indicate the data of NASA database.

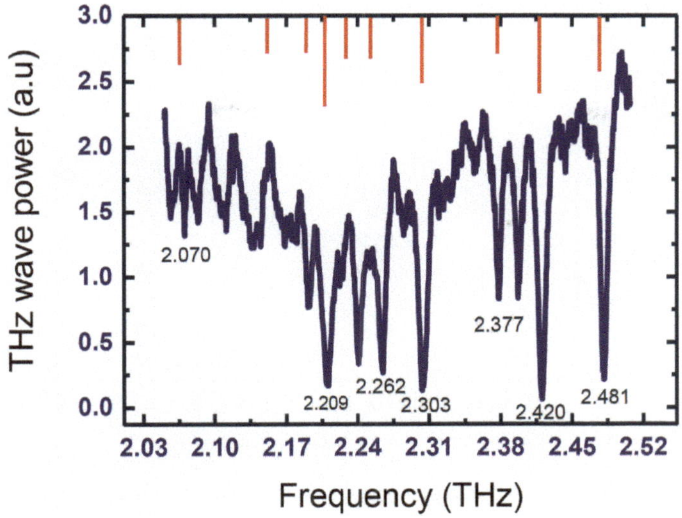

FIG. 2.10.3B The water vapor absorption spectra of THz waves in the frequency range 2–2.5 THz at atmospheric pressure and room temperature conditions. The redlines indicate the data of NASA database.

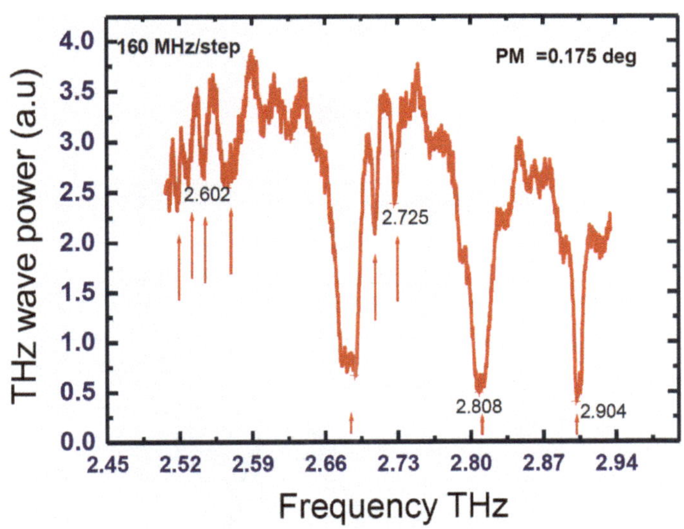

FIG. 2.10.3C The water vapor absorption spectra of THz waves in the frequency range 2.5–3 THz at atmospheric pressure and room temperature conditions. The redlines indicate the data of NASA database.

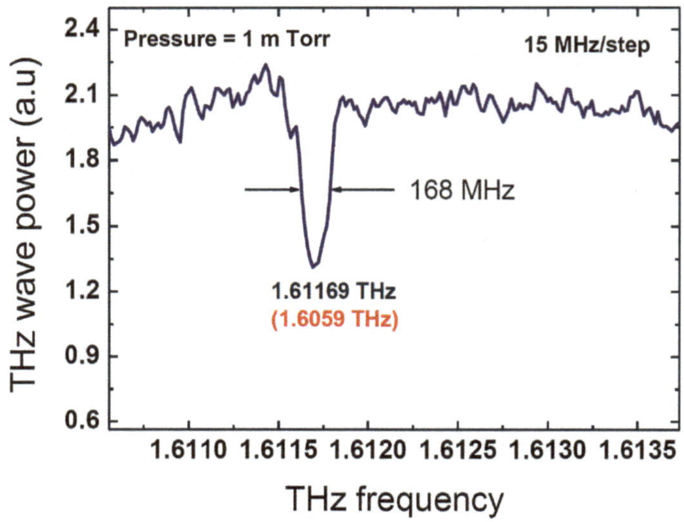

FIG. 2.10.3D The THz spectrum of the water vapor absorption at room temperature and pressure of 1 mTorr inside the chamber.

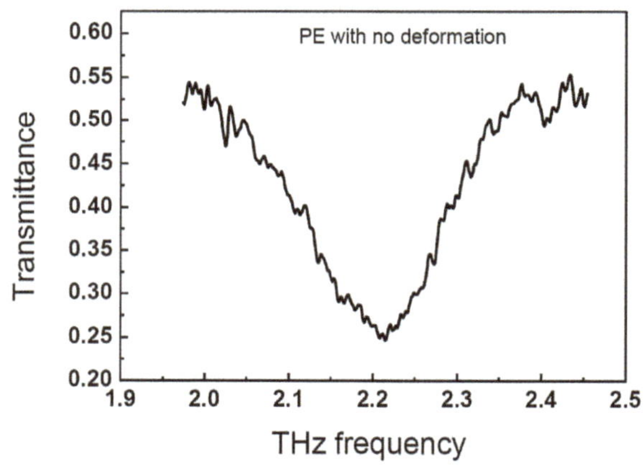

FIG. 2.10.4A Transmission spectrum of white PE.

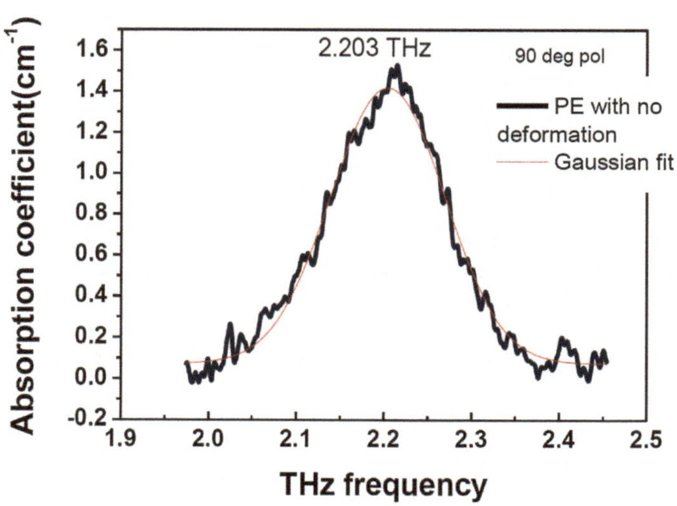

FIG. 2.10.4B Absorption spectrum of white PE.

CONCLUSION

For implementing THz wave technology in practical applications, a high-power and portable THz sources are desirable. In order to get THz power scaling, the effects of pump laser beam divergence, the effective interaction length in noncollinear mixing, and also the absorption in the NLO crystal must be considered. With this motivation, a THz spectroscopy system uses laser diodes as pump and GaP crystal as NLO medium on the basis of DFG method. The THz absorption spectra of white PE and water vapor were studied from 1.5 to 3 THz. The THz spectroscopy system has potential applications in biomedical engineering such as protein analysis, pharmaceutical industry, and nondestructive analysis of materials in high-resolution THz spectroscopy.

REFERENCES

[1] M.A. Piestrup, R.N. Fleming, R.H. Pantell, Continuously tunable submillimeter wave source: Applied Physics Letters 26 (1975) 418–421.

[2] Y.J. Ding, W. Shi, Widely tunable, monochromatic, and high-power THz sources and their applications, Journal of Nonlinear Optical Physics and Materials 12 (2003) 557–585.

[3] M. Tonouchi, Cutting-edge terahertz technology, Nature Photonics 1 (2007) 97–105.

[4] K. Kawase, Y. Ogawa, Y. Watanabe, H. Inoue, Nondestructive terahertz imaging of illicit drugs using spectral fingerprints, Optics Express 11 (2003) 2549–2554.

[5] B. Ferguson, X.- C Zhang, Materials for terahertz science and technology, Nature Materials 1 (2002) 26–33.

[6] S. Kumar, B.S. Williams, S. Kohen, Q. Hu, J.L. Reno, Applied Physics Letters 84 (2004) 2494–2496.

[7] S. Verghese, K.A. McIntosh, E.R. Brown, Applied Physics Letters 71 (1997) 2743–2745.

[8] K. Kawase, J. Shikata, K. Imai, H. Ito, Applied Physics Letters 78 (2001) 2819–2821.

[9] W. Shi, Y.J. Ding, N. Fernelius, K. Vodopyanov, Optics Letters 27 (2002) 1454–1456.

[10] B. Wu, P.P. Jiang, D.Z. Yang, T. Chen, J. Kong, Y.H. Shen, Optics Express 17 (2009) 6004–6009.

[11] P. Zhao, S. Ragam, Y.J. Ding, I.B. Zotova, Optics Letters 35 (2010) 3979–3981.

[12] W. Shi, Y.J. Ding, Applied Physics Letters 83 (2003) 848.

[13] W. Shi, Y.J. Ding, Optics Letters 27 (2002) 1454.

[14] T.M. Pollak, W.F. Wing, R.J. Grasso, E.P. Chicklis, H.P. Jenssen, IEEE Journal of Quantum Electronics 18 (2) (1982) 159–163.

[15] W. Koechner, M. Bass, Solid-State Lasers, Springer, New York, 2003.

[16] W. Shi, Y.J. Ding, Optics Letters 30 (2005) 1030–1032.

[17] D.J.M. Stothard, T.J. Edwards, D. Walsh, C.L. Thomson, C.F. Rae, M.H. Dunn, P.G. Browne, Line-narrowed, compact, and coherent source of widely tunable terahertz radiation, Applied Physics Letters 92 (2008) 141105.

[18] M. Scheller, J.M. Yarborough, J.V. Moloney, M. Fallahi, M. Koch, S.W. Koch, Room temperature continuous wave milliwatt terahertz source, Optics Express 18 (2010) 27112–27117.

[19] J.E. Schaar, K.L. Vodopyanov, M.M. Fejer, Intracavity terahertz-wave generation in a synchronously pumped optical parametric oscillator using quasi-phase-matched GaAs, Optics Letters 32 (2007) 1284–1286.

[20] F. Trager, Handbook of Lasers and Optics, Springer, New York, 2007.

[21] P. Zhao, S. Ragam, Y.J.J. Ding, I.B. Zotova, Power scalability and frequency agility of compact terahertz source based on frequency mixing from solid-state lasers, Applied Physics Letters 98 (2011) 131106.

[22] Y. Jiang, Y.J. Ding, I.B. Zotova, Power scaling of widely-tunable monochromatic terahertz radiation by stacking high-resistivity GaP plates, Applied Physics Letters 96 (2010) 031101.

[23] Y. Jiang, D. Li, Y.J.J. Ding, I.B. Zotova, Terahertz generation based on parametric conversion: from saturation of conversion efficiency to back conversion, Optics Letters 36 (2011) 1608–1610.

[24] E.B. Petersen, W. Shi, A. Chavez-Pirson, N. Peyghambarian, A.T. Cooney, Efficient parametric terahertz generation in quasi-phase-matched GaP through cavity enhanced difference-frequency generation, Applied Physics Letters 98 (2011) 121119.

[25] L.A. Coldren, S.W. Corzine, Diode Lasers and Photonic Integrated Circuits, John Wiley & Sons, New York, 1995.

[26] http://www.jpl.nasa.gov/.

[27] F.C. De Lucia, Optics and Photonics News 14 (2003) 44.

CHAPTER 3

Advanced Materials and Structures for Terahertz Engineering

NILESH MUKHERJEE, PHD • NURNIHAR BEGUM, PHD • P. SONI REDDY, PHD • RAHUL MONDAL, PHD • SUSHANTA SARKAR, PHD • PARTHA PRATIM SARKAR, PHD

The terahertz (THz) waves being intermediate to the microwave and the visible light spectrum exhibit partial property of both the microwave and the visible spectrum. However, microwaves have penetration property for many nonmetallic substances, but the microwaves tend to differentiate between materials with less precision in terms of penetration, absorption, and reflection. Hence, materials generally do not show any specific signature property when incident with microwaves. In case of visible spectrum, light waves when incident on a material show specific reflection, absorption, and penetration property for the material, which shall be the specific signature of the material with respect to the light waves being incident. However, most of the materials available are opaque to the light waves, i.e., the visible light waves cannot penetrate through them, thus limiting the parameters. In case of THz waves, it penetrates most of the material though its absorption is high. But, this acts as a helpful property as the absorption is very specific for different materials, thus giving the signature touch to the waves. Hence, all the physical aspects, i.e., transmission, reflection, and absorption, of the THz waves with respect to a material can be studied to analyze a material.

In any THz system, apart from the THz source and detectors, the system components form the major bulk of the system. In THz system, the components mainly include the following:

1. THz lenses
2. THz polarizers
3. THz prisms
4. THz windows
5. THz mirrors
6. THz waveguides

All the above components are passive in nature but they determine the end application of the THz system. As with other system, the material to be used for the components depends on how the material interacts with physical phenomenon it has to deal. For example, in case of electric system, the material used for transmission has to be a good conductor to electricity and the material used to prevent unwanted exposure should be a bad conductor to electricity. For optical system, the material used for transmission has to be transparent to optical spectrum; the material used for preventing the optical transmission from optical interferences should be opaque to optical spectrum. Similarly, the material for use in the fabrication of THz components should satisfy the properties in THz range as required by the function of the component.

For electromagnetic radiation, the most vital part being the transmission line, the following are the categories of material that can be used as waveguide in THz frequency range:

1. Free space
2. Hollow metallic waveguide
3. Dielectric
4. Parallel plate waveguide
5. Photonic crystal fiber (PCF)
6. Coaxial waveguide
7. Metal wire waveguide

TERAHERTZ GAP

Research on THz technology is immature till date and it has tremendous potential. There are a number of THz radiation sources like cosmic background radiation, blackbody radiation, etc. Most of these

Terahertz Biomedical and Healthcare Technologies. https://doi.org/10.1016/B978-0-12-818556-8.00003-3

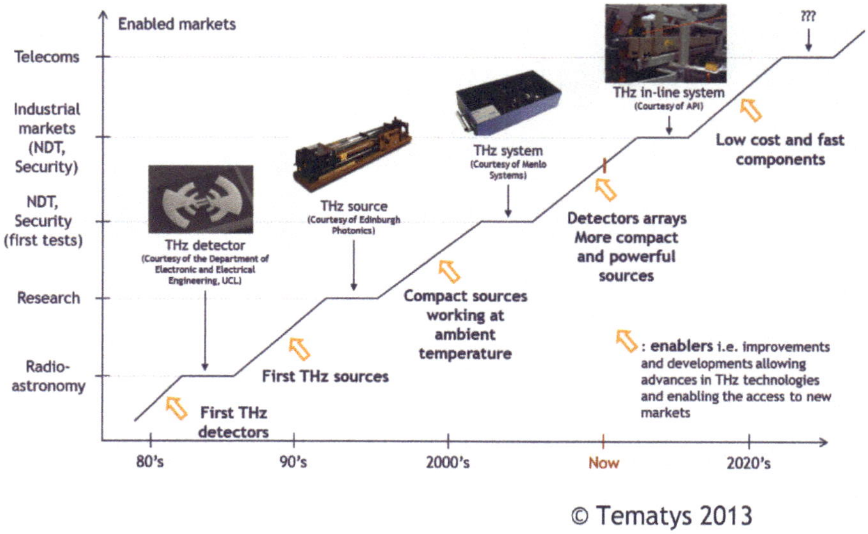

FIG. 3.1 Market trends in terahertz (THz) technology [11].

sources are incoherent in nature. As a result, utilization is rare. If generation and detection of THz radiation are compared with those of other frequency ranges, there is no doubt that THz wave generation and detection are not still well established. It is very difficult to handle this technology by conventional semiconductor technology. As the photon energy of THz wave is much smaller than that of near infrared of visible light, it is also very difficult to control this THz wave with existing photonic technology. Researchers may find tremendous potential in this field.

Vacuum tube generators like backward wave oscillators (BWOs) and Free Electron Lasers (FELs) can generate high power THz wave using microwave concept. Low power THz waves may be generated by multiplying semiconductor oscillator frequency. Semiconductor lasers can also generate THz radiation.

Recently, semiconductor manufacturing technology has been advanced very shortly. This helps THz systems and applications to be more feasible. Also with the advancement of photonics and microwave technology, THz technology is also being advanced.

A new approach of research like designing of THz antennas has also been started. Presently, in the universe, microwave spectrum is highly populated for communication system. Now, high capacity communication system requires wider bandwidth than existing microwave spectrum. As a solution, possible frequency range can be found in THz frequency ranges.

BASICS OF TERAHERTZ TECHNOLOGY

THz is indicated between the millimeter and infrared regions of electromagnetic spectrum. The range of THz is 300 GHz−10 THz. THz is not harmful as X-ray for medical imaging. Also in spectroscopy, THz detects more information about hidden objects than other electromagnetic waves [1−3]. Due to its transmission properties in light, THz technique is appropriate for checking the material inside the envelope without opening the wrapper [4]. Development of THz is mainly included in research field for imaging, tomography, or spectroscopy which consists of source, components, and detectors [5−8]. Total evaluation of THz technology is given in Fig. 3.1 [4,9,10,11].

As per a review of MIT, THz technology is going to be one of the most emerging technologies which may cause a drastic change in the field of technology. In near future, development of THz technology may usher in a new era enabling implementation of online industrial inspection systems. It is predicted that within 2021 THz technology may grow more than 5 times than that of the year 2016 in valuation. Fig. 3.1 shows the market trends in THz technology [11,12].

TERAHERTZ SPECTROSCOPY

There are three main parts of the THz spectroscopy, i.e., source, component, and detector. THz radiation is generated and manipulated by source and components, respectively. Radiated THz is detected by detector [8].

Now in brief THz sources, components, and detectors are being described.

TERAHERTZ SOURCES

There are different types of sources which are responsible for THz radiation [4,8]. These are shown in Table 3.1 below. The various types of sources are thermal [13–15], electronic (vacuum and solid state) [16,17], laser [18,19], laser pumped (continuous and pulsed) [20], and mechanical excitation (peeling tape and surface information) [21,22]. Thermal sources are included cosmic background radiation [13], Globar [14,15], and mercury lamp [23]. Extended interaction klystron, traveling-wave tube, gyrotron, FEL, etc., are falling in the vacuum electronic THz source [24–28]. Different solid-state electronic THz sources are Gunn diodes [17], transistors, frequency multiplication, and superconductor [29–31]. Laser type sources are gas, semiconductor, and quantum cascade [18,32–35].

If an incident electromagnetic wave is incident on a nonlinear device or medium, nonlinear frequency conversion takes place. As a result, THz radiation is generated. This way of generation of THz radiation is explained in Fig. 3.2A [62]. When two optical photons of frequencies w_1 and w_2 interact with a new linear crystal, a THz photon is generated with $W_T = w_1 - w_2$. This is called difference frequency generation method. Broadband THz (B.W. = 10 THz) can be generated by femtosecond laser pulser.

Harmonics of microwave signal by utilizing diodes having strong nonlinear I-V characteristics can also be used as process of generation of THz signal.

Radiation of electromagnetic wave takes place due to time-varying currents or by accelerating charges. It is shown in Fig. 3.2B [62]. Likewise, if laser beams excite a biased photoconductive (PC) antenna, it can generate THz radiation. The basic formation of metal antenna is a semiconductor substrate with two metal electrodes deposited on it. If the gap between the two electrodes is excited by an optical beam, photocarriers are generated and these free carriers are accelerated by a static bias field. Thus, photocurrent generated is time varying corresponding to intensity. Consequently, femtosecond laser pulses generate THz radiation with broadband.

Both of BWO and FEL generate THz radiation. There is a remarkable difference in size. First one is laboratory size equipment. But the second one is a large equipment. However, they are similar in mechanism of THz radiation generator. A periodic structure undulates an electron beam in both the cases. However, periodic structure for BWO is a metal grating and that for FEL is a magnetic array. Here, basically periodic accelerating electron beam generates CW THz radiation.

TABLE 3.1
List of Terahertz sources.

Source type	Representative references
Thermal	
Cosmic background radiation	[13]
Globar	[14, 15, 36]
Mercury lamp	[23]
Vacuum electronic	[16]
Backward-wave oscillator	[37– 39]
Extended-interaction klystron	[24]
Traveling-wave tube	[25]
Gyrotrons	[26, 27]
Free-electron lasers	[28, 40]
Synchrotrons	[41]
Solid-state electronic	
Gunn diodes	[17]
Transistors	[29]
Frequency multiplication	[30]
Superconductor	[31]
Lasers	
Gas	[18]
Semiconductor	[32, 33]
Quantum cascade	[34, 35]
Sources pumped by lasers	
Continuous	
Photomixer	[20]
Mechanical resonance	[42]
Pulsed	
Photoconductive switches	[43, 44]
Air	[45, 46]
Magnetic dipoles	[47]
Terahertz parametric oscillator	[48]
Optical rectification	[49]
Bulk	[50, 51]
Surface	[52, 53]
Transient currents	[54, 55]
Diffusion/ Drift	[56-61]
Mechanical excitation	
Peeling tape	[21]
Surface formation	[22]

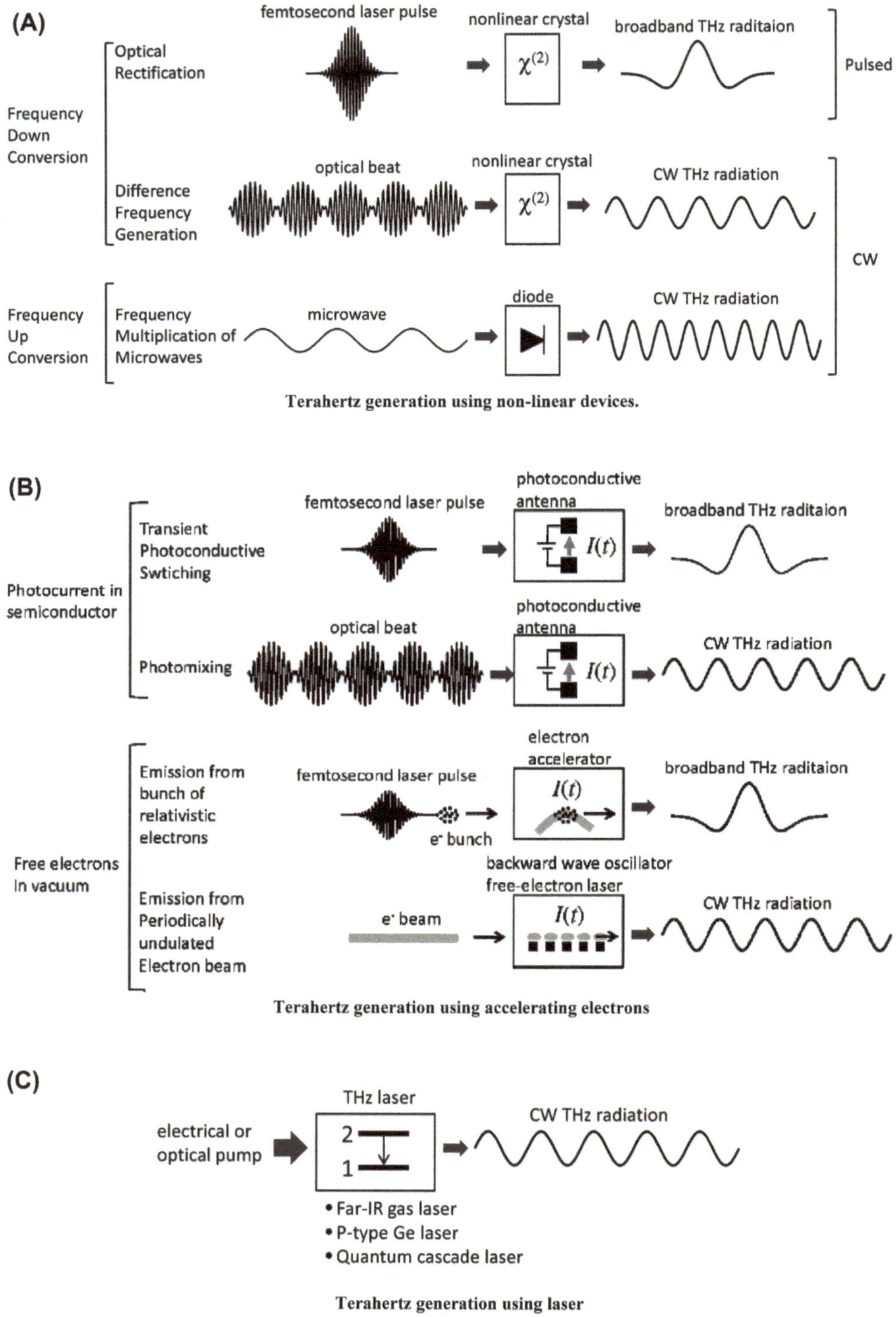

FIG. 3.2 Terahertz (THz) Sources. **(A)** THz generation using nonlinear devices. **(B)** THz generation using accelerating electrons. **(C)** THz generation using laser.

In Fig. 3.2C [62], it is shown that the basic requirement of laser action is a two-level quantum system with population inversion. One of the electrically pumped solid-state lasers is a P-type germanium laser. One of the semiconductor heterostructure lasers is a quantum cascade laser (QCL). This type of heterostructure laser is formed by periodically alternating layers of dissimilar semiconductors. THz photons are involved in transitions between subbands of these semiconductors. When electron undergoes successive intersubband transitions in a QCL, coherent THz radiation is generated.

TERAHERTZ COMPONENTS

Different THz components are listed below in Table 3.2 [4,8].Usually THz mirror components have been formed by metal. Nowadays doped and undoped GaAs [63], high-resistivity silicon and hybrid of polypropylene [64], and photonic crystal have been applied for THz components [65–68]. Conventionally lenses are made of plastics. These THz lenses are manufactured by molding process [67], thin and light weight Fresnel zone plates [68], and paper [69].

TERAHERTZ DETECTORS

Initially, THz detectors performed on the basis of thermometric property which means change in size or electrical resistance with temperature of a material. A tuned metamaterial absorber and a biomaterial related with microelectromechanical systems are other THz detectors [74–76]. Various thermal THz detectors are thermocouple, thermopile, pyroelectric, thermomechanical, bolometer (most sensitive detector), etc. [4,8]. Optical sampling is one of the processes to detect the THz pulses. To detect the THz, different sampling techniques are related such as free-space electro-optic (EO) sampling, antenna detection, synchronous, and asynchronous optical sampling [77].

Some detectors of THz radiation are listed in Table 3.3.

THz detection is basically of two types: (i) coherent detection and (ii) noncoherent detection. In coherent detection, both amplitude and phase of the field are measured. In noncoherent detection, only the field intensity is measured.

Commonly used coherent detection is illustrated in Fig. 3.3. Here, in time domain, actual electric field of broadband THz pulses is measured by EO sampling. In a nonliner optical crystal, birefringence is induced by THz field. This is proportional to the field amplitude. An optical probe can determine the entire waveform by measuring the induced birefringence as a function of relative time delay between THz and optical pulses.

In time domain, THz pulse may also be measured by sensing with a PC antenna. If photocarriers are injected

TABLE 3.2
List of Terahertz components.

Component	Representative references
Mirrors	
Semiconductor	[63]
Hybrid	[64]
Photonic crystal	[65]
Lenses	
Molded	[66]
Variable focal length	[67]
Fresnel zone plates	[68]
Plasmonic resonance	[70]
Paper	[69]
Polarizers	
Reconfigurable	[71]
Metamaterials	
Absorber	[72]
Modulator	[73]

TABLE 3.3
List of Terahertz detectors.

Detector type	Representative references
Thermal	
Thermocouple	[78]
Thermopile	[79]
Pyroelectric	[80]
Thermomechanical	[74,75]
Bolometer	[81]
Superconductor	[82]
Imaging arrays	[83]
Electro-optic	
Optical rectification	[84]
Electro-optical sampling	
Electronic	
Direct electronic	[85], [86]
Photoconductive gating	[87]

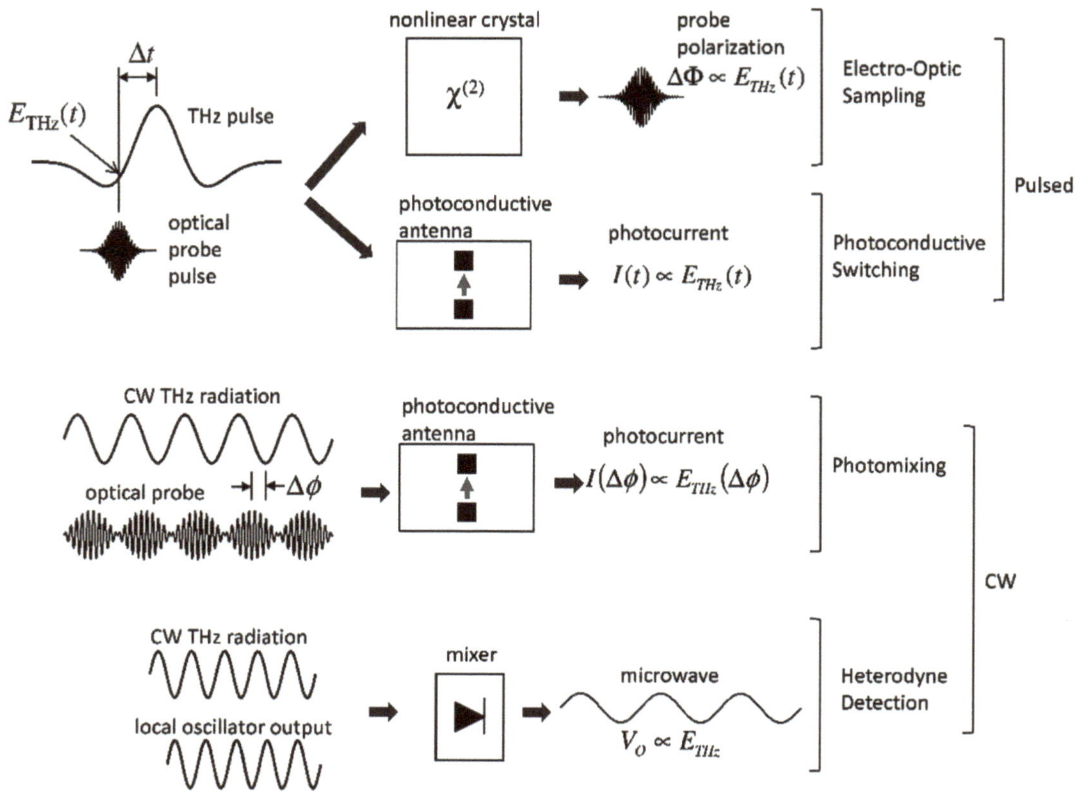

FIG. 3.3 Coherent detection of Terahertz (THz) radiation.

by optical probe pulse, a current in the PC gap is induced by THz field. THz field amplitude and photocurrent are proportional. By measuring the photocurrent, THz pulse can be mapped out.

CW THz radiation can also be measured by photomixing. This is done by exploiting PC switching. Relative phase between optical beat and THz radiation is dependent on photocurrent.

Heterodyne detection is done by a mixer which is a nonlinear device. Commonly used mixer may be a Schottky diode. In a mixer, the output signal is downconverted in frequency. The inputs to the mixer are a THz signal with frequency W_S, and the reference radiation with frequency W_{LO} is a fixed one. The output of the mixer is $W_D = W_S - W_{LO}$. The THz signal amplitude and the amplitude of the mixer output signal will be proportional.

Thermal sensors like bolometers, Golay cells, pyroelectric devices, etc., are some of the incoherent detectors. Generally, in such type of incoherent detectors a radiation absorber is attached to a new link. Temperature is increased in the absorber by radiation energy, and this temperature rise is measured by a thermometer. Specific scheme to measure the temperature rise is different for different thermal detectors. An electrical resistance thermometer is used in the bolometer. Heavily doped Si or Ge is used to make that electrical resistance thermometer. Operation of bolometer is done generally in cryogenic temperature. Pyroelectric material is employed in a pyroelectric detector. Spontaneous electric polarization takes place by temperature change in pyroelectric material. In a Golay cell, small volume of gas is formed from heat inside a sealed chamber behind the absorber. Membrane deformation caused by the pressure increase is detected by the optical reflectivity measurement. Response to radiation by the thermal detectors covers a broad spectral range.

RESEARCHES ON TERAHERTZ SOURCES, COMPONENTS, AND DETECTORS

In modern research field, THz technology is a very interesting topic. It is quiet immature topic in research. So there is a scope to develop the technology. Various research work related to THz technology is presented here.

Feng Liu et al. presented a high power THz source emerged on a PCF amplifier system. The femtosecond laser amplifier has been used as laser pump source due to its compact size, high stability, high reception rate, etc., for producing the ultrashort THz pulses. The compact system with THz output up to 150 μW and high efficiency has been obtained by applying shorter THz pulses which is generated by large mode area photonic crystal fiber (PCF) amplifier pulse sources [88].

Jianming Dai et al. described in their invited paper about the recent advancement of THz generator and detector related to laser-induced gas plasma. "THz wave air photonics" is the combination of THz source and detector in gaseous medium. It can detect THz wave in remote and indicated the hazardous materials. They achieved THz electric field above 1.5 MV cm^{-1} from gas plasma [89].

THz quantum well photodetector (QWP), which is sensitive in THz frequency range, is used as a detector for imaging system of a key in an envelope by T Zhou et al. in the year of 2012. In this letter, compositions of described THz QWP are 23 modules made of 22.1 nm GaAs wells and 95.1 nm $Al_{0.015}Ga_{0.985}As$ barriers. For imaging of the sample, they used a blackbody source as a background radiation. They demonstrated that THz QWP focal plane array may be created for possible real-time imaging [90].

Mary Lou P. Bailey et al. presented a water-based optical absorber with PMMA (plexiglass). They tuned effective refractive index to get maximum return loss by maintaining a glycerol layer on the water level. Return loss of the absorber lies between 230 and 250 GHz. Maximum return loss has been achieved at 240 GHz with PMMA thickness 1.72 mm. The absorber is suitable for eliminating unwanted beam in THz spectroscopy by precise tuning of resonating frequency and measurement of THz dielectric properties [91]. Jianming Dai et al. presented theoretical and experimental improvement regarding THz sources, detectors, and components in laser-induced gas plasma [92].

COMPARISON OF THZ AND MM WAVE SCANNING

Frequency of operation of millimeter wave is around 30 GHz which correspond to wavelength of 10 mm. Imaging technology in this frequency range [93] has been developed a lot. Through some barrier materials, wave in this frequency range penetrates better than THz wave. Still there are reasons to favor THz wave imaging. Resolution of THz imaging is 10 times better than millimeter wave imaging as its wavelength is around 10 times shorter than MM wave. So identification of any hidden object must be better by THz wave imaging than mm wave imaging [94]. Also concealed content and potential threats can be analyzed spectroscopically by THz wave for identification.

THZ SPECTRA

Non-polar and non-metallic solids are partially reflective and partially transparent in THz radiation in the frequency range of 0.2–5 THz. These types of materials may be plastics or ceramics. Generally, in THz radiation polar liquid like water is highly absorptive, whereas in this radiation nonpolar liquids are transparent. THz time-domain spectroscopy of organic molecules can be used to examine their vibrational characteristics. The same information can also be studied with the help of Fourier transform infrared (FTIR) analysis. Far-infrared spectral analysis through computer-based stimulation technique is another alternative method in this regard. They are associated with intermolecular hydrogen bond relative motions [95–97]. In the THz range, gases may have distinctive spectroscopic fingerprints [98].

SAMPLE PREPARATION

Spectroscopic testing requires preparation of samples, which can be done in various ways. For security-based applications, it is desired that the THz spectra are not dependent on the sample preparation method. However, it is found that in certain cases, the THz spectra are sensitive to impurities or fillers introduced during sample preparation and/or structural changes of the material. Due to this, in the above-mentioned cases, the sample preparation method has minor or significant effects on the THz spectra. RDX spectra in the range of THz may be dissimilar in nature [99–101]. This is due to the fact that multiple reflections take place inside the sample and also between the holder of the sample and itself. More than one reflection from the system may also take place [102].

A process of sample preparation refers to pelletizing the explosive powders/crystals to determine the inherent characteristic of the material [103]. Pressing samples into pellet form is a common practice in far-infrared THz transmission spectroscopy for ascertaining the THz transmission spectra. Sometimes, materials which are nonreactive to THz radiations are used as filler/binding materials to form pellets of the sample explosive/crystal powders. An alternative method involves grinding the sample explosive/crystals into fine powders of grain size almost equal to 300 μm, i.e., the THz wavelength. Thus, THz radiations can effectively interact with the finely grinded sample powders. An example of a filler material is polyethylene. The filler material, generally transparent in THz, permits dilute concentrations of the highly absorbing agent to be measured.

The matrix material and/or the pressed pellet are able to impact the measured THz spectra. As an example, reduction of the effect of dielectric mismatch leads to minimization of scattering, and the dielectric mismatch can be made smaller by using a matrix material having a refractive index value close to that of the refractive index of the powder. One dielectric material of a composite material is considered to be immersed in any other dielectric host and then the spectroscopic data of the composite material are examined. This is followed by Garnett theory [104]. The THz spectra are largely dependent on the effective dielectric of the composite material. The effective dielectric of the composite material is modified due to the interaction between the neighboring grains of powder, which occurs because of the proximity of the grains to each other [105]. In Ref. [101], it can be seen that there are many THz peaks in RDX. This happens as the powder is of crystalline nature. Also, long range oscillations occur in the crystal. An extensive THz spectral analysis of sample materials in the form of pellets should be conducted in order to obtain pure spectral characteristics of the test sample. Since the pellets are formed utilizing filler materials, various types and fractional combinations of such materials should be considered. This method would ensure the spectral characteristics to be independent of the filler material configurations used in sample preparation. Thereby, the spectral characteristics so obtained would truly reflect the test sample nature in presence of THz radiations.

While there are various preparation methods, several spectral characteristics of explosives are replicable, and not dependent on sample preparation. For example, though the sample preparation method causes a little deviation in the spectra of RDX and C4, different peaks may occur which are independent of whether RDX mixture (C4) or RDX powder is measured. A complete and useable practical explosive detection system based on THz sensing must be able to detect explosive or its constituent chemicals without fail. For example, ammonium nitrate (AN) in pure form or a complete C4 bomb system using explosives must be equally detectable by the system.

EXPLOSIVES

Table 3.4 displays an overview of materials with their reported absorbance peak positions. The phonon modes corresponding to the crystalline structure result in sharp absorption peaks, which is an important feature of the THz spectra [103]. This outcome results from intramolecule vibrations of RDX [101]. If the scattering from the structure is of the order of the wavelength of the THz signal, then that may cause the existence of broad features. This generally takes place in materials that have fibers or grains [111].

It must be noted that the range 0–55 THz includes various absorption features which can be used to distinctively detect the explosive/drug. Comparison between the THz spectra of C4 and RDX is shown in Fig. 3.4 [100,101]. In the dataset absorption features are seen of 0.8, 1.5, 2.0, 2.2, and 3 THz. When RDX combines with matrix material to form C4, it is observed that dominant absorption nature of RDX still exists. The spectral transmittance feature data presented in Ref. [101] are more detailed and present spectral feature of RDX at 1.1 THz which was otherwise invisible in the data from Ref. [100].

A sharp absorption peak in THz spectra of different crystalline explosives like RDX [101] and TNT [108] has been observed. With the help of density functional theory, a comparison has also been done between these THz spectral assignments of peaks with an SPARTAN ab initio molecular simulations [112] study. These simulation results show a good agreement with measured THz absorption when the molecular vibrational modes of TNT is greater than 5 THz.

The vibration modes of one single RDX molecule were also compared with the measured FTIR data beyond 600 cm^{-1} [112]. Absorption peak of most explosives is usually not observed below 1 THz. But RDX shows a different result as its absorption does not match to inherent molecular vibrational mode. Peak absorption of RDX at 0.8 THz is observed (Fig. 3.4). Molecular rotations of the nitro ($-NO_2$) group or RDX molecule, a weak hydrogen bond formation between two RDX molecules, etc., might be the probable causes of this THz absorption peak.

THz spectral characteristics of the first nine explosives in the frequency range of 0.1–3 THz are listed in Table 3.4. There are different techniques available for detection of THz fingerprint. But these techniques require a relatively high vapor pressure. THz spectroscopy offers a potentially useful detection technique for detection of those explosives which typically have low vapor pressure [103].

THz signal can detect amorphous explosives similar to explosives like RDX which are crystalline in nature. AN mixed with fuel oil (FO) is generally used in car/truck bomb as an improvised explosive device (IED). A uniformly increasing THz attenuation characteristic

TABLE 3.4
THz Frequency Positions for Maximum Absorbance of Some Explosives.Conversion to Units of Wave Numbers Requires Multiplication by 33

Material	Explosive	Semtex-H	PE4	RDX/C4	PETN	PETN	HMX	HMX	TNT	TNT	TNT	NH_4NO_3
Feature band center position frequency (THz)		0.72, 1.29, 1.73, 1.88, 2.15, 2.45, 2.57	0.72, 1.29, 1.73, 1.94, 2.48, 2.21, 2.69	0.72, 1.26, 1.73	1.73, 2.51	2.01	1.58, 1.91, 2.21, 2.57	1.84	1.44, 1.91	1.7	5.6, 8.2, 9.1, 9.9	4, 7
Reference		[99]	[99]	[72,101,107]	[99]	[103]	[99]	[103]	[99]	[103]	[107,108]	[103,109]

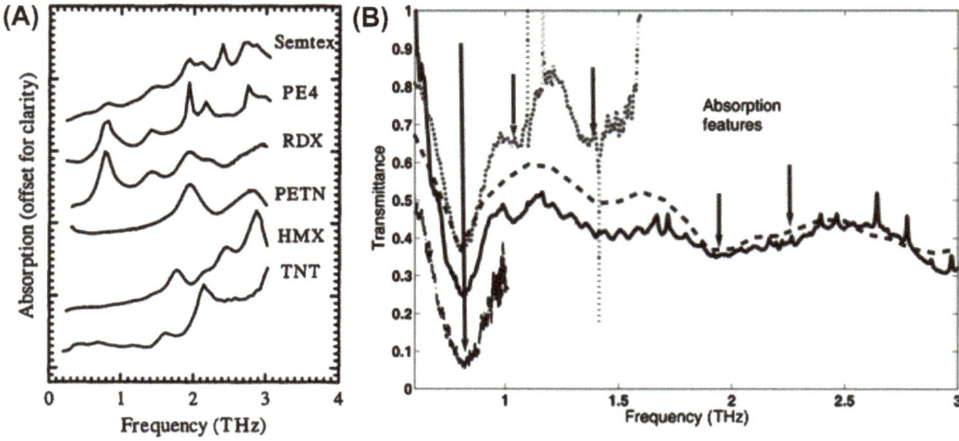

FIG. 3.4 **(A)** Absorption characteristics of few explosives [100]. **(B)** Comparison of transmittance characteristics of RDX obtained by different methods [100,101]. *Dotted line*: C4 using THz time-domain spectroscopy (TDS) [101], *dashed line*: RDX [100], *solid line*: RDX using Fourier transform infrared [101], and *bottom line*: RDX using THz-TDS [101]. The sharp rise or fall in the C4 curve is due to traces of water. It may be inferred that the absorption characteristics of RDX at 3, 2.2, 2.0, 1.5, and 0.8 THz are in confirmation with its transmittance characteristics at the same frequencies.

instead of sharp characteristics is found for the explosive material AN in the frequency range of 0–3 THz [103,109].

In Fig. 3.5, experimentally measured THz spectra of AN [109] are compared with the data of Ref. [103]. From this figure, we can see that, as the THz frequency increases up to 3 THz, the THz absorption (extinction coefficient) increases. Also, two subtle oscillations seem in the 3–7 THz range. (Due to multiple reflections in the 20 μm sample, ~70 cm^{-1} wide oscillations in the transmission from 10 to 20 THz are observed). Some distinct features are seen between RDX and AN. THz spectra of RDX show unique spectral features in the 0.2–3 THz range which may be helpful to identify RDX. However, such unique feature is not exhibited by AN.

Hence, some special consideration is required for the THz detection of AN, along with other "featureless" explosives. One alternative solution for these "featureless" explosives is to design a THz system that operates where the presence of fingerprint spectra might occur. Another option may be the detection of FO of ANFO explosives. As the slopes of THz absorption over frequency of different

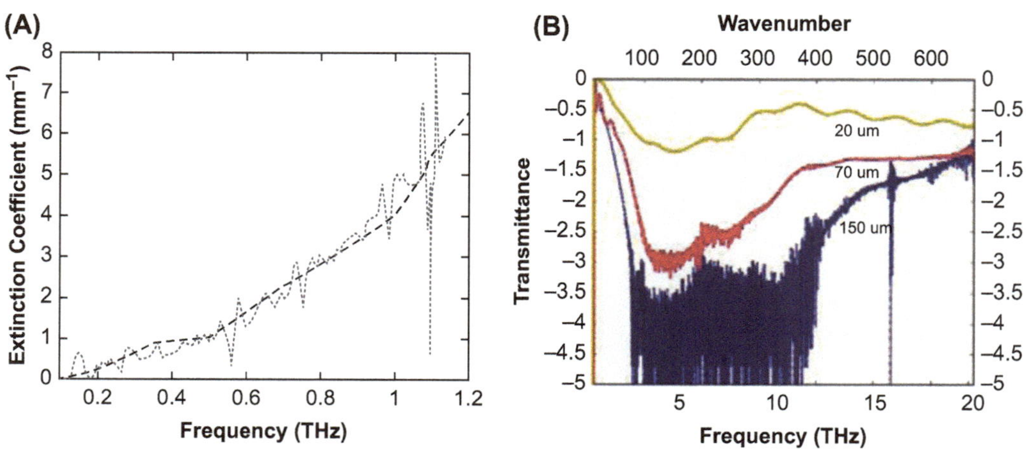

FIG. 3.5 **(A)** Terahertz (THz) characteristic of NH_4NO_3 (1 mm) as mentioned in Ref. [109] (*dotted line*) and as in Refs. [103] (*dashed line*). **(B)** THz spectrum characteristics of ammonium nitrate with nominal thickness [109].

explosives are not similar, thus the third method of identification of the explosives may be based on increasing order of slope of THz absorption in the 0.2–3 THz range. AN is basically transparent at lower frequency (0.2 THz), while it is opaque at the higher frequency (2.5 THz). This unique property of AN in presence of THz radiations enables the fourth detection method to provide a quick and efficient analysis of any explosive containing traces of AN.

ILLICIT DRUGS

THz spectroscopy of explosive materials is a vast area and quite extensively studied by the researchers over the years. Compared with this illegal drugs detection using THz spectroscopy is an area least explored so far. Although few research works have been reported in literature on the detection of illegal drugs using THz spectroscopy [100,110,113], the research in this area is quite limited. Different materials exhibit uniquely different characteristics in presence of THz radiations. Some materials like materials used for packaging appear completely transparent, while others appear opaque. Each chemical drug show unique spectral characteristics in presence of THz radiations. Thereby, compared with normal X-ray, millimeter wave, and infrared imaging, THz imaging not only allows one to easily "see" through the layers of "barrier" materials used to conceal a threat material but also allows one to clearly differentiate between illicit and legal drugs [110].

THz sources having discrete tunable characteristics were used by Kawase et al. [110] to image commonly used drugs like aspirin, MDMA (DL-3, 4-methylenedioxymethamphetamine), and methamphetamine. The findings of Kawase et al [110] related to these drugs are used as a reference and their THz absorption characteristics are displayed in Table 3.5 for the frequency range of 1.3–2 THz. The THz images of these drugs were taken by placing individual 20 mg of each drug inside polyethylene bags concealed in an envelope. Subsequently, at seven different THz frequencies, the THz images of each drug sample are taken and investigated by component spatial pattern analysis [114] method. The results obtained by the above analysis process inherently suffered from an error of 10%. The same author group has also confirmed that identification of the spatial patterns of various drugs can be successfully done even when they are placed in complex mixtures or aligned one above the other. This finding shows great promise to establish the use of THz imaging in security applications where any deliberate attempts to confuse the sensing system can be successfully handled. The authors have reported the THz spectral characteristics for some of the common drugs like D-amphetamine and drugs available over-the-counter like L-methamphetamine, acetaminophen (Tylenol), and caffeine in Ref. [110].

BARRIER MATERIALS

In realistic scenarios, materials like cloth, paper, etc., are commonly used to conceal the target threat material in a package. Such materials used to hide the threat material are known as "barrier" materials. In presence of a THz source, these "barrier" materials display their own transmission spectral characteristics. Thus, while performing THz imaging of the threat material, the THz transmission spectral characteristics of the "barrier" materials also need to be considered. For example, if a "barrier" material is found to absorb the THz radiation, the thickness of the "barrier" material needs to be fine tuned so that the THz image of the threat material can be properly generated without any hindrance. Alternatively, the "barrier" materials could possibly show similar THz transmission spectral characteristics as that of the targeted threat material. In such a scenario, the desired THz spectral characteristics of the threat material like explosives or illicit drugs get masked by that of the "barrier" material. Most of the "barrier" materials commonly used like cloth, paper, and plastic exhibit increasing THz spectral absorption characteristics with frequency, mostly under the 3 THz range [100,111,113,115].

Consideration of "barrier" materials in THz spectroscopic image detection [107,108] of landmines is different from the above-mentioned process. At present worldwide there are approximately 100 million landmines buried. Anti-personnel mines are very difficult to detect using conventional ground-penetrating radar systems. Owing to their small size and low metal content, they appear quite similar to rocks. Spatial resolutions of nearly ~1 mm can be achieved using THz technology which is approximately 10 times better than the conventional mine detection methods used so far.

The "barrier" materials in the process of detecting landmines are soil, sand, water, and rocks. Intuitively, these "barrier" materials will affect the ability to detect the non-metallic mines concealed underneath it significantly. Loss due to THz absorption in sand is found to be 8.2 dB cm^{-1}%, where % is the water weight percentage. A sample proof of concept of the ability to detect the nonmetallic mines hidden underneath soil using THz was tested. This was done by neoprene grommet imaging under dry sand of around 1.2 cm below

TABLE 3.5
THz Frequency Positions for Maximum Absorbance of Some Drugs. Conversion to Units of Wave Numbers.

Material	Drugs	Methamphetamine	MDMA	Lactose α-monohydrate	Icing Sugar	Co-Codamol	Aspirin, Soluble	Aspirin, Caplets	Acetaminophen	Terfenadine	Naproxen Sodium
Feature band center position frequency (THz)		1.2, 1.7–1.8	1.4, 1.8	0.54, 1.20, 1.38, 1.82, 2.54, 2.87, 3.29	1.44, 1.61, 1.82, 2.24, 2.57, 2.84, 3.44	1.85, 2.09, 2.93	1.38, 3.26	1.4, 2.24	6.5	3.2	5.2, 6.5
Reference		[110]	[110]	[99]	[99]	[99]	[99]	[99,110]	[111]	[111]	[111]

[108]. ID and OD of neoprene grommet were 12.7 and 25.4 mm. The image was extracted by scanning at an interval of 300 μm for 100×100 pixels. The targeted grommet was clearly visible in the extracted image.

ATMOSPHERE

The transmission characteristics of "barrier" materials in THz imaging is extremely important for detection of threat materials usually concealed within the vicinity of 3 m, i.e., close proximity or beyond 3 m, i.e., stand-off proximity. In the detection mechanism of remotely hidden threat materials (i.e., stand-off proximity) using THz radiations, the atmosphere plays the role of "barrier" material since the THz signals must propagate in the atmosphere over short distances (3–100 m). Discussions on the propagation of THz signals through the humid atmosphere have been presented by several research groups [95,98,116]. Water and oxygen dominates the absorption of THz signals in the atmosphere [98] at specific frequencies. Nevertheless, several transmission bands are also present across the THz frequency band as illustrated in Fig. 3.6 [95]. The attenuation of the THz signals in these transmission bands is purely frequency dependent. An approximate THz attenuation value of 50 dB km^{-1} is observed at 0.8 THz. In order to minimize the atmospheric attenuation of THz signals in a stand-off sensing system, the entire operating procedure should be tuned to these transmission bands. Other THz atmospheric absorption factors excluding water vapor and oxygen includes dust, smoke, fog, and rain which also have a significant effect on the THz transmission. It is assumed that the presence of water vapors or humidity or rain in the atmosphere would lead to greater attenuation of the THz signals transmitted through it. Size of typical micron-scale atmospheric particles like pollens, dust, smoke, etc., is much smaller than the wavelength of the THz signals. So, the presence of these types of atmospheric particles does not scatter the THz signals significantly [116]. However, the experimental validation of this assumption of low atmospheric scattering of THz signals by typical micron-scale atmospheric particles is yet to be made and presented in literature [116].

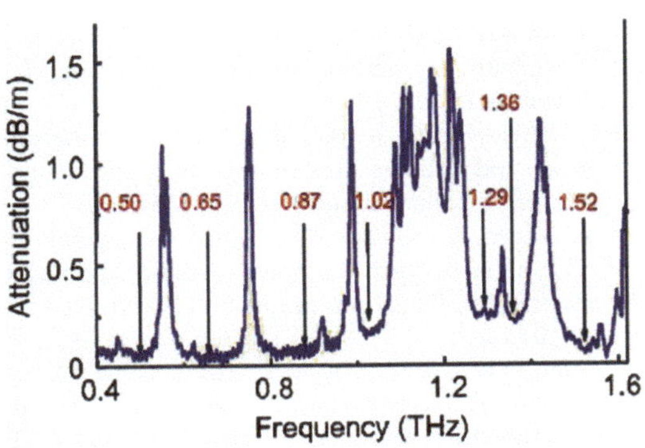

FIG. 3.6 Atmospheric Tx bands in the frequency range of terahertz (THz) [95].

CONCLUSION

Due to unique property to provide distinct material characteristics, THz wave finds application in different fields. From medical application to preventing illegal activities, from the study of biological objects to material analysis, the application potential is very vast. The economic and strategic importance of THz technology is immense if it is applied efficiently. The practical application is only possible when the components used/required could be readily produced and available in conformity with the tolerance, uncertainty, and flexibility of the end application. A scientific phenomenon can be applied to work only when the ancillary system components are available. The properties of the THz wave, no matter how beneficial it is, may be put to work only when right materials are used to make the necessary components. Given the research being done in the material science for use in THz region, the development of THz devices is imminent. As new materials are being researched and developed for use in THz region, new components with greater efficiency and reliability are becoming available. This is leading to the ever-increasing application of the THz wave.

REFERENCES

[1] W.H. Hayt, J.A. Buck, Engineering Electromagnetics, McGraw-Hill, 2001.

[2] E.J. Nichols, J.D. Tear, Joining the infrared and electric wave spectra, The Astrophysical Journal 61 (1925) 17–37.

[3] P. Kumar, S. Pratyush, R. Mishra, S. Behera, An Introduction to Terahertz Technology, its History, Properties and Application, Conference paper, 2015.

[4] R. Lewis, Materials for terahertz engineering, in: S. Kasap, P. Capper (Eds.), Springer Handbook of Electronic and Photonic Materials, Springer, Cham, 2017, pp. 1339–1350.

[5] D.M. Mittleman, R.H. Jacobsen, M.C. Nuss, T-ray imaging, IEEE Journal of Selected Topics in Quantum Electronics 2 (1996) 679–692.

[6] D.M. Mittleman, S. Hunsche, L. Boivin, M.C. Nuss, T-ray tomography, Optics Letters 22 (1997) 904–906.

[7] D.M. Mittleman, R.H. Jacobsen, R. Neelamani, R.G. Baraniuk, M.C. Nuss, Gas sensing using terahertztime-domain spectroscopy, Applied Physics B 67 (1998) 379–390.

[8] R.A. Lewis, A review of terahertz sources, Journal of Physics D: Applied Physics 47 (374001) (2014) 1–11.
[9] K. Sakai, Private Communication, 2014.
[10] K. Sakai, Pioneering studies and cutting-edge approaches in the terahertz-waves region, in: Proc. 34th Int. Conf. Infrared, Millimeter, and Terahertz Waves, IRMMW-THz 2009, 2009.
[11] T. Robin, C. Bouyé, J. Cochard, d'Humières B., Terahertz Components & Systems: Technology and Market Trends. www.photonics21.org.
[12] PreScouter Inc., Report 9 Disruptive Technologies Changing the World, 2015.
[13] C. Thacker, A. Cooray, J. Smidt, F. De Bernardis, K. Mitchell-Wynne, A. Amblard, R. Auld, M. Baes, D.L. Clements, A. Dariush, G. De Zotti, L. Dunne, S. Eales, R. Hopwood, C. Hoyos, E. Ibar, M. Jarvis, S. Maddox, M.J. Michałowski, E. Pascale, D. Scott, S. Serjeant, M.W.L. Smith, E. Valiante, P. van der Werf, H-ATLAS: The cosmic abundance of dust from the far-infrared background power spectrum, The Astrophysical Journal 768 (2013) 58.
[14] V.M. Zolotarev, R.K. Mamedov, A.N. Bekhterev, B.Z. Volchek, Spectral emissivity of a globar lamp in the 2-50-μm region, Journal of Optical Technology 74 (2007) 378.
[15] R.A. Friedel, A.G. Sharkey Jr., Comparison of glower and globar sources for infra-red spectrometry, Review of Scientific Instruments 18 (1947) 928.
[16] J.H. Booske, R.J. Dobbs, C.D. Joye, C.L. Kory, G.R. Neil, G.S. Park, J. Park, R.J. Temkin, Vacuum electronic high power terahertz sources, IEEE Transactions on Terahertz Science and Technology 1 (2011) 54.
[17] S. Perez, T. Gonzalez, D. Pardo, J. Mateos, Terahertz Gunn-like oscillations in InGaAs/InAlAs planar diodes, Journal of Applied Physics 103 (2008) 094–516.
[18] G. Dodel, On the history of far-infrared (FIR) gas lasers: thirty-five years of research and application, Infrared Physics and Technology 40 (1999) 127.
[19] X. Yin, et al., Terahertz Imaging for Biomedical Applications: Pattern Recognition and Tomographic Reconstruction, vol. 2, Springer Science Business Media, LLC, 2012, pp. 9–26.
[20] K.A. McIntosh, E.R. Brown, K.B. Nichols, O.B. McMahon, W.F. DiNatale, T.M. Lyszczarz, Terahertz photomixing with diode lasers in low temperature-grown GaAs, Applied Physics Letters 67 (1995) 3844.
[21] J. Horvat, R.A. Lewis, Peeling adhesive tape emits electromagnetic radiation at terahertz frequencies, Optics Letters 34 (2009) 2195.
[22] D.L. Cortie, R.A. Lewis, Terahertz surfoluminescence, Surface Science 606 (2012) 1573.
[23] K. Charrada, G. Zissis, M. Aubes, Two-temperature, two-dimensional fluid modelling of mercury plasma in high-pressure lamps, Journal of Physics D Applied Physics 29 (1996) 2432.
[24] Y.M. Shin, G.S. Park, G.P. Scheitrum, G. Caryotakis, Circuit analysis of an extended interaction klystron, Journal of the Korean Physical Society 44 (2004) 1239.
[25] S. Bhattacharjee, J.H. Booske, C.L. Kory, D.W. van der Weide, S. Limbach, S. Gallagher, J.D. Welter, M.R. Lopez, R.M. Gilgenbach, R.L. Ives, M.E. Read, R. Divan, D.C. Mancini, Folded waveguide traveling-wave tube sources for terahertz radiation, IEEE Transactions on Plasma Science 32 (2004) 1002.
[26] V.L. Bratman, Y.K. Kalynov, V.N. Manuilov, Large orbit gyrotron operation in the terahertz frequency range, Physical Review Letters 102 (2009) 245101.
[27] T. Idehara, T. Saito, I. Ogawa, S. Mitsudo, Y. Tatematsu, L. Agasu, H. Mori, S. Kobayashi, Development of terahertz FU CW Gyrotron series for DNP, Applied Magnetic Resonance 34 (2008) 265.
[28] A. Knyazev, G.N. Kulipanov, N.A. Vinokurov, Novosibirsk terahertz free electron laser: instrumentation development and experimental achievements, Measurement Science and Technology 21 (2010), 054-017.
[29] J. Lusakowski, W. Knap, N. Dyakonova, L. Varani, J. Mateos, T. Gonzalez, Y. Roelens, S. Bollaert, A. Cappy, K. Karpierz, Voltage tuneable terahertz emission from a ballistic nanometer In-GaAs/InAlAs transistor, Journal of Applied Physics 97 (2005) 064–307.
[30] Maestrini, J.S. Ward, J.J. Gill, C. Lee, B. Thomas, R.H. Lin, G. Chattopadhyay, I. Mehdi, A frequency-multiplied source with more than 1 mW of power across the 840–900-GHz band, IEEE Transactions on Microwave Theory and Techniques 58 (2010) 19–25.
[31] L. Ozyuzer, A.E. Koshelev, C. Kurter, N. Gopalsami, Q. Li, M. Tachiki, K. Kadowaki, T. Yamamoto, H. Minami, H. Yamaguchi, T. Tachiki, K.E. Gray, W.-K. Kwok, U. Welp, Emission of coherent THz radiation from superconductors, Science 318 (2007) 1291.
[32] H.W. Hubers, S.G. Pavlov, V.N. Shastin, Terahertz lasers based on germanium and silicon, Semiconductor Science and Technology 20 (2005) S211.
[33] Y. Chassagneux, R. Colombelli, W. Maineult, S. Barbieri, H.E. Beere, D.A. Ritchie, S.P. Khanna, E.H. Linfield, A.G. Davies, Electrically pumped photonic-crystal terahertz lasers controlled by boundary conditions, Nature 457 (2009) 174.
[34] R. Kohler, A. Tredicucci, F. Beltram, H.E. Beere, E.H. Linfield, A.G. Davies, D.A. Ritchie, R.C. Iotti, F. Rossi, Terahertz semiconductor-heterostructure laser, Nature 417 (2002) 156.
[35] S. Williams, Terahertz quantum-cascade lasers, Nature Photonics 1 (2007) 517.
[36] R.A. Friedel, A.G. Sharkey Jr., Erratum: comparison of glower and globar sources for infra-red spectrometry, Review of Scientific Instruments 19 (1948) 180.
[37] M. Mineo, C. Paoloni, Corrugated rectangular waveguide tunable backward wave oscillator for terahertz applications, IEEE Transactions on Electron Devices 57 (2010) 1481.
[38] X. Xu, Y. Wei, F. Shen, H. Yin, J. Xu, Y. Gong, W. Wang, A watt-class 1-THz backward-wave oscillator based on sine waveguide, Physics of Plasmas 19 (2012) 013113.
[39] W. He, C.R. Donaldson, L. Zhang, K. Ronald, P. McElhinney, A.W. Cross, High power wideband

gyrotron backward wave oscillator operating towards the terahertz region, Physical Review Letters 110 (2013) 165101.

[40] M.A. Dem'yanenko, D.G. Esaev, B.A. Knyazev, G.N. Kulipanov, N.A. Vinokurov, Imaging with a 90 frames/s microbolometer focal plane array and high-power terahertz free electron laser, Applied Physics Letters 92 (2008), 131116.

[41] J.M. Byrd, W.P. Leemans, A. Loftsdottir, B. Marcelis, M.C. Martin, W.R. McKinney, F. Sannibale, T. Scarvie, C. Steier, Observation of broadband self-amplified spontaneous coherent terahertz synchrotron radiation in a storage ring, Physical Review Letters 89 (2002) 224–801.

[42] X.L. Wu, S.J. Xiong, Z. Liu, J. Chen, J.C. Shen, T.H. Li, P.H. Wu, P.K. Chu, Green light stimulates terahertz emission from mesocrystal microspheres, Nature Nanotechnology 6 (2011) 103.

[43] H. Auston, Picosecond optoelectronic switching and gating in silicon, Applied Physics Letters 26 (1975) 101.

[44] Y.C. Shen, P.C. Upadhya, E.H. Linfield, H.E. Beere, A.G. Davies, Ultrabroadband terahertz radiation from low-temperature-grown GaAs photoconductive emitters, Applied Physics Letters 83 (2003) 3117.

[45] K.Y. Kim, J.H. Glownia, A.J. Taylor, G. Rodriguez, Coherent control of terahertz supercontinuum generation in ultrafast laser-gas interactions, Nature Photonics 2 (2008) 605.

[46] M. Kress, T. Loffler, S. Eden, M. Thomson, H.G. Roskos, Terahertz-pulse generation by photoionization of air with laser pulses composed of both fundamental and second-harmonic waves, Optics Letters 29 (2004) 1120.

[47] Beaurepaire, G.M. Turner, S.M. Harrel, M.C. Beard, J.Y. Bigot, C.A. Schmuttenmaer, Coherent terahertz emission from ferromagnetic films excited by femtosecond laser pulses, Applied Physics Letters 84 (2004) 3465.

[48] K. Kawase, M. Sato, T. Taniuchi, H. Ito, Coherent tunable THz-wave generation from $LiNbO_3$ with monolithic grating coupler, Applied Physics Letters 68 (1996) 2483.

[49] K. Radhanpura, S. Hargreaves, R.A. Lewis, L. Sirbu, I.M. Tiginyanu, Heavy noble gas (Kr, Xe) irradiated (111) InP nanoporous honeycomb membranes with enhanced ultrafast all-optical terahertz emission, Applied Physics Letters 97 (2010) 181921.

[50] S. Hargreaves, K. Radhanpura, R.A. Lewis, Generation of terahertz radiation by bulk and surface optical rectification from crystal planes of arbitrary orientation, Physical Review B: Condensed Matter 80 (2009) 195323.

[51] J.D. Rowley, J.K. Wahlstrand, K.T. Zawilski, P.G. Schunemann, N.C. Giles, A.D. Bristow, Terahertz generation by optical rectification in uniaxial birefringent crystals, Optics Express 20 (2012) 16968.

[52] M. Reid, I.V. Cravetchi, R. Fedosejevs, Terahertz radiation and second-harmonic generation from InAs: bulk versus surface electric-field-induced contributions, Physical Review B: Condensed Matter 72 (2005) 035201.

[53] Urbanowicz, A. Krotkus, R. Adomavičius, V.L. Malevich, Terahertz emission from femtosecond laser excited Ge surfaces due to the electrical field-induced optical rectification, Physica B: Condensed Matter 398 (2007) 98.

[54] J.N. Heyman, N. Coates, A. Reinhardt, G. Strasser, Diffusion and drift in terahertz emission at GaAs surfaces, Applied Physics Letters 83 (2003) 5476.

[55] S. Hargreaves, R.A. Lewis, Single-cycle azimuthal angle dependence of terahertz radiation from (100) n-type InP, Applied Physics Letters 93 (2008) 242101.

[56] H. Dember, A photoelectrical-motive energy in copper-oxide crystals, Physikalische Zeitschrift 32 (1931) 554.

[57] H. Dember, A crystal photocell, Physikalische Zeitschrift 32 (1931) 856.

[58] H. Dember, Forward motion of electrons induced by light, Physikalische Zeitschrift 32 (1931) 207.

[59] G. Klatt, F. Hilser, W. Qiao, M. Beck, R. Gebs, A. Bartels, K. Huska, U. Lemmer, G. Bastian, M.B. Johnston, M. Fischer, J. Faist, T. Dekorsy, Terahertz emission from lateral photo-Dember currents, Optics Express 18 (2010) 4939.

[60] G. Klatt, B. Surrer, D. Stephan, O. Schubert, M. Fischer, J. Faist, A. Leitenstorfer, R. Huber, T. Dekorsy, Photo-Dember terahertz emitter excited with an Er:fiber laser, Applied Physics Letters 98 (2011) 021114.

[61] J. Lloyd-Hughes, S.K.E. Merchant, L. Fu, H.H. Tan, C. Jagadish, E. Castro-Camus, M.B. Johnston, Influence of surface passivation on ultrafast carrier dynamics and terahertz radiation generation in GaAs, Applied Physics Letters 89 (2006) 232102.

[62] Y.-S. Lee, Principles of Terahertz Science and Technology, ch. 1, Springer US, 2009, pp. 1–7.

[63] H.B. Ye, Y.H. Zhang, W.Z. Shen, Carrier transport and optical properties in GaAs far-infrared/terahertz mirror structures, Thin Solid Films 514 (2006) 310.

[64] N. Krumbholz, K. Gerlach, F. Rutz, M. Koch, R. Piesiewicz, T. Kurner, D. Mittleman, Omnidirectional terahertz mirrors: a key element for future terahertz communication systems, Applied Physics Letters 88 (2006) 202905.

[65] M. Tecimer, K. Holldack, L.R. Elias, Dynamically tunable mirrors for THz free electron laser applications, Physical Review Accelerators and Beams 13 (2010) 030703.

[66] B. Scherger, M. Scheller, C. Jansen, M. Koch, K. Wiesauer, Terahertz lenses made by compression molding of micropowders, Applied Optics 50 (2011) 2256.

[67] B. Scherger, C. Jordens, M. Koch, Variable-focus terahertz lens, Optics Express 19 (2011) 4528.

[68] H.D. Hristov, J.M. Rodriguez, W. Grote, The grooved-dielectric Fresnel zone plate: an effective terahertz lens and antenna, Microwave and Optical Technology Letters 54 (2012) 1343.

[69] Siemion, A. Siemion, M. Makowski, J. Suszek, J. Bomba, A. Czerwiński, F. Garet, J.-L. Coutaz, M. Sypek, Diffractive paper lens for terahertz optics, Optics Letters 37 (2012) 4320.

[70] X.-Y. Jiang, J.-S. Ye, J.-W. He, X.-K. Wang, D. Hu, S.-F. Feng, Q. Kan, Y. Zhang, An ultrathin terahertz lens with axial long focal depth based on metasurfaces, Optics Express 21 (2013) 30030.

[71] L.J. Cheng, L. Liu, Optical modulation of continuous terahertz waves towards cost-effective reconfigurable quasi-optical terahertz components, Optics Express 21 (2013) 28657.

[72] H. Tao, N.I. Landy, C.M. Bingham, X. Zhang, R.D. Averitt, W.J. Padilla, A metamaterial absorber for the terahertz regime: design, fabrication and characterization, Optics Express 16 (2008) 7181.

[73] H.-T. Chen, W.J. Padilla, M.J. Cich, A.K. Azad, R.D. Averitt, A.J. Taylor, A metamaterial solid state terahertz phase modulator, Nature Photonics 3 (2009) 148.

[74] F. Alves, D. Grbovic, B. Kearney, N.V. Lavrik, G. Karunasiri, Bi-material terahertz sensors using metamaterial structures, Optics Express 21 (2013) 13256.

[75] F. Alves, D. Grbovic, B. Kearney, G. Karunasiri, Microelectromechanical systems bimaterial terahertz sensor with integrated metamaterial absorber, Optics Letters 37 (2012) 1886.

[76] B. Kearney, F. Alves, D. Grbovic, G. Karunasiri, Al/SiOx/Al single and multiband metamaterial absorbers for terahertz sensor applications, Optical Engineering 52 (2013) 013801.

[77] X. Yin, B.W.-H. Ng, D. Abott, Terahertz Imaging for Biomedical Applications Pattern Recognition and Tomographic Reconstruction, Springer Science Business Media, LLC, 2012, pp. 9–26 (Chapter 2).

[78] L.C. Roess, E.N. Dacus, The design and construction of rapid-response thermocouples for use as radiation detectors in infra-red spectrographs, Review of Scientific Instruments 16 (1945) 164.

[79] W.J.H. Moll, A thermopile for measuring radiation, Proceedings of the Physical Society 35 (1922) 257.

[80] R.W. Whatmore, Pyroelectric devices and materials, Reports on Progress in Physics 49 (1986) 1335.

[81] P.L. Richards, Bolometers for infrared and millimeter waves, Journal of Applied Physics 76 (1994) 1.

[82] J.R. Gao, J.N. Hovenier, Z.Q. Yang, J.J.A. Baselmans, A. Baryshev, M. Hajenius, T.M. Klapwijk, A.J.L. Adam, T.O. Klaassen, B.S. Williams, S. Kumar, Q. Hu, J.L. Reno, Terahertz heterodyne receiver based on a quantum cascade laser and a superconducting bolometer, Applied Physics Letters 86 (2005) 1.

[83] J. Yang, S. Ruan, M. Zhang, Real-time, continuous- wave terahertz imaging by a pyroelectric camera, Chinese Optics Letters 6 (2008) 29.

[84] Q. Wu, X.-C. Zhang, Design and characterization of traveling-wave electrooptic terahertz sensors, IEEE Journal of Selected Topics in Quantum Electronics 2 (1996) 693.

[85] J. Song, G. Aizin, Y. Kawano, K. Ishibashi, N. Aoki, Y. Ochiai, J.L. Reno, J.P. Bird, Evaluating the performance of quantum point contacts as nanoscale terahertz sensors, Optics Express 18 (2010) 4609.

[86] S. Pelling, R. Davis, L. Kulik, A. Tzalenchuk, S. Kubatkin, T. Ueda, S. Komiyama, V.N. Antonov, Point contact readout for a quantum dot terahertz sensor, Applied Physics Letters 93 (2008) 073501.

[87] D. Seliuta, I. Kašalynas, V. Tamošiunas, S. Balakauskas, Z. Martunas, S. Ašmontas, G. Valušis, A. Lisauskas, H.G. Roskos, K. Kohler, Silicon lens coupled bow-tie InGaAs-based broadband terahertz sensor operating at room temperature, Electronics Letters 42 (2006) 825.

[88] F. Liu, Y.J. Song, Q.R. Xing, M.L. Hu, Y.F. Li, C.L. Wang, L. Chai, W.L. Zhang, A.M. Zheltikov, C.Y. Wang, Broadband terahertz pulses generated by a compact femtosecond photonic crystal fiber amplifier, Photonics Technology Letters, IEEE 22 (2010) 814–816.

[89] J. Dai, B. Clough, I. Ho, X. Lu, J. Liu, X. Zhang, Recent progresses in terahertz wave air photonics, IEEE Transactions on Terahertz Science and Technology 1 (1) (Sept. 2011) 274–281.

[90] T. Zhou, et al., Terahertz imaging with quantum-well photodetectors, IEEE Photonics Technology Letters 24 (13) (July 1, 2012) 1109–1111.

[91] M.L.P. Bailey, et al., Narrow-band water-based absorber with high return loss for Terahertz spectroscopy, IEEE Transactions on Terahertz Science and Technology 5 (6) (Nov. 2015) 961–966.

[92] J. Dai, J. Liu, X. Zhang, Terahertz wave air photonics: terahertz wave generation and detection with laser-induced gas plasma, IEEE Journal of Selected Topics in Quantum Electronics 17 (1) (Jan–Feb. 2011) 183–190.

[93] Passive millimeter-wave imaging technology VI and radar sensor technology VII, in: R. Appleby, D.A. Wikner, R. Trebits, J.L. Kurtz (Eds.), Proceedings of SPIE 5077 (2003).

[94] [94a] D.A. Zimdars, J.S. White, Terahertz reflection imaging for package and personnel inspection, Proceedings of SPIE 5411 (2004), 78;
[94b] D.A. Zimdars, Fiber-pigtailed terahertz time-domain spectroscopy instrumentation for package inspection and security imaging, Proceedings of SPIE 5070 (2003), 5108.

[95] T. Yuan, H. Liu, J. Xu, F. Al-Douseri, Y. Hu, X. Zhang, Proceedings of SPIE 5070 (2003), 28.

[96] T.A. Heimer, E.J. Heilweil, Bulletin of the Chemical Society of Japan 75 (2002) 899–908.

[97] D.L. Woolard, et al., Journal of Applied Toxicology 17 (1997) 243.

[98] F.C. De Lucia, in: D. Mittleman (Ed.), Spectroscopy in the Terahertz Spectral Region Sensing with Terahertz Radiation, Springer, Berlin, 2003.

[99] W.R. Tribe, D.A. Newnham, P.F. Taday, M.C. Kemp, Hidden object detection: security applications of terahertz technology, Proceedings of SPIE 5354 (2004), 168.

[100] M.C. Kemp, P.F. Taday, B.E. Cole, J.A. Cluff, A.J. Fitzgerald, W.R. Tribe, Proceedings of SPIE 5070 (2003), 44.

[101] F. Huang, B. Schulkin, H. Altan, J. Federici, D. Gary, R. Barat, D. Zimdars, M. Chen, D.B. Tanner, Terahertz study of 1,3,5-trinitro-s-triazine (RDX) by time domain

spectroscopy and FTIR, Applied Physics Letters 83 (2003) 2477.

[102] D. Woolard, T. Globus, E. Brown, L. Werbos, B. Gelmont, A. Samuels, in: Proc. 5th Joint Conf., Stand-off Detection for Chemical and Biological Defense, 2001 (Williamsburg, vol. A).

[103] D.J. Cook, B.K. Decker, G. Maislin, M.G. Allen, Through container THz sensing: applications for explosive screening, Proceedings of SPIE 5354 (2004), 55.

[104] R.W. Cohen, G.D. Cody, M.D. Coutts, B. Abeles, Physical Review B: Condensed Matter 8 (1973) 3689.

[105] [105a] J.F. Federici, H. Grebel, Characteristics of nano-scale composites at THz and IR spectral regions sensing science and technology at THz frequencies, in: D. Woodard, M. Shur, W. Loerop (Eds.), Volume II. Emerging Scientific Applications & Novel Device Concepts, World Scientific, Hackensack, NJ, 2003;
[105b] H. Altan, F. Huang, J.F. Federici, A. Lan, H. Grebel, Optical and electronic characteristics of single walled carbon nanotubes and silicon nanoclusters by THz spectroscopy, Journal of Applied Physics 96 (2004) 6685.

[106] J.F. Federici, B. Schulkin, F. Huang, D. Gary, R. Barat, F. Oliveira, D. Zimdars, THz imaging and sensing for security applications-explosives, weapons and drugs, Semiconductor Science and Technology 20 (2005) S266–S280.

[107] [107a] R. Osiander, J.A. Miragliotta, Z. Jiang, J. Xu, X.C. Zhang, Mine field detection and identification using THz spectroscopic imaging, Proceedings of SPIE 5070 (2003), 1;
[107b] J.B. Spicer, P. Dagdigian, R. Osiander, J.A. Miragliotta, X.C. Zhang, R. Kersting, D.R. Crosley, R.K. Hanson, J. Jeffries, Proceedings of SPIE 5089 (2003), 1088;
[107c] Y. Chen, H. Liu, Y. Deng, D. Veksler, M. Shur, X.-C. Zhang, D. Schauki, M.J. Fitch, R. Osiander, Spectroscopic characterization of explosives in the far infrared region, Proceedings of SPIE 5411 (2004), 1.

[108] M.J. Fitch, D. Schauki, C.A. Kelly, R. Osiander, Terahertz imaging and spectroscopy for landmine detection, Proceedings of SPIE 5354 (2004), 45.

[109] A. Bandyopadhyay, A. Sengupta, F. Huang, J.F. Federici, R.B. Barat, D.E. Gary, M. Chen, D.B. Tanner, Impact of grain size dependent scattering on terahertz absorption spectra, Applied Optics (2005) (Submitted).

[110] K. Kawase, Y. Ogawa, Y. Watanabe, Non-destructive terahertz imaging of illicit drugs using spectral fingerprints, Optics Express 11 (2003) 2549.

[111] M.B. Campbell, E.J. Heilweil, Noninvasive detection of weapons of mass destruction using THz radiation, Proceedings of SPIE 5070 (2003), 38.

[112] B.M. Rice, G.F. Chabalowski, The Journal of Physical Chemistry A 101 (1997) 8720–8726.

[113] P.F. Taday, I.V. Bradley, D.D. Arnone, M. Pepper, Journal of Pharmaceutical Sciences 92 (2003) 831–838.

[114] Y. Watanabe, K. Kawase, T. Ikari, Component spatial pattern analysis of chemicals using terahertz spectral imaging, Applied Physics Letters 83 (2003) 800.

[115] J.E. Bjarnason, T.L.J. Chan, A.W.M. Lee, M.A. Celis, E.R. Brown, Millimeter-wave, terahertz, and mid-infrared transmission through common clothing, Applied Physics Letters 85 (2004) 519.

[116] E.R. Brown, Fundamentals of terrestrial millimeter-wave and THz remote sensing terahertz sensing technology, in: D.L. Woolard, W.R. Loerop, M.S. Shur (Eds.), Vol 2: Emerging Scientific Applications & Novel Device Concepts, World Scientific, Singapore, 2003.

CHAPTER 4

2D Materials as THz Generators, Detectors, and Modulators: Potential Candidates for Biomedical Applications

TANMOY BASU, PHD • AMIT BANERJEE, PHD • SAUMITRA VAJANDAR, PHD

INTRODUCTION

This chapter summarizes methods and setups for terahertz (THz) sources, modulators, and detectors with a specific focus on graphene and other 2D materials (2DMs) for biomedical applications. This chapter mainly provides a comprehensive review on some basic concepts on THz instrumentations and applications which will be helpful for both materials scientists and biologists. In addition, this chapter also gives an outlook on 2DMs for imaging, modulating, and sensing applications to overcome some of the present bottlenecks with THz conventional materials. THz radiation is nonionizing and many materials are transparent to it which implies its applicability biological tissue imaging (reaching submillimeter resolution). In addition, the spectra obtained from different materials can be used for composition identification. For instance, explosives, active pharmaceutical ingredients in medicines, and different narcotic materials have been properly detected using THz imaging method. Moreover, ultrashort THz radiation pulses can be used to measure the thickness, and density of materials can even be used to image embedded defect location.

Due to the advancement of nanofabrication technologies, various seemingly difficult applications are being accomplished by 2DMs recently. Similarly, 2DMs are a potential candidate for THz generators, detectors, and modulators and may be viable for future biomedical applications also. This chapter will briefly introduce some basics of graphene-based THz research, including devices for generating THz radiation, further works on THz detectors using graphene. A brief description of the advancement of THz modulation using graphene-based technology is also outlined followed by a short introduction on other 2DM-based THz research. Since its first successful separation from graphite in 2004, graphene has drawn much attention as it shows a new avenue to isolate atomically thin materials viz. graphene and other 2DMs [1]. Graphene is highly susceptive to chemical functionalization [2] due to the sp^2 hybridized of carbon atoms, having the highest edge atoms fraction for any allotrope. It demonstrates broadband light absorption including THz range [3]. Due to its unique band structure with the presence of Dirac point, graphene shows high degree of nonlinearities as compared with contemporary materials [4]. The ability of having a strong light interaction and plasmons in graphene makes it a special candidate for photonic applications [5,6]. For instance, graphene ribbons show broadband absorption at shorter wavelength scale [7]. In fact, the broadband absorption and plasmon excitation behavior by electrostatic gating has driven researcher to design many electro-optic modulators in THz to visible wavelengths. In addition, graphene-based metamaterials are finding importance for engineering polarization rotator in THz range [8]. Here various THz devices, e.g., emitters, detectors, and modulators, based on graphene will be discussed. In the following sections, we will describe the advances in the THz field in terms of generation, detection, and modulation. Later, we will discuss the use of THz toward biomedical application followed by an outlook toward the potential applications of 2DM-based THz devices in biomedical research.

GRAPHENE-BASED THZ EMITTERS

The heart of the entire THz system is to develop THz emitters which may lead to achieve THz waves of higher intensity and broader bandwidth. THz emitters can be categorized in three generations viz. photoconductive antennas [9], nonlinear electro-optic crystal [10], and

Terahertz Biomedical and Healthcare Technologies. https://doi.org/10.1016/B978-0-12-818556-8.00004-5

air plasma [11]. However, these sources fail to meet the present demand of having higher efficiency. In order to solve this issue, the concept of graphene-based THz emitters has been introduced in 2007 [12] where optically or electrically pumped graphene was projected [13] to show positive gain in selective wavelength ranges. For example, graphene-based THz laser was designed with Fabry-Perot resonant cavity [14] (Fig. 4.1) structure where optical excitation leads to electron and hole pair generation and subsequent acquire population inversion to generate THz radiation.

In another approach, the graphene-based current-injection THz emitter has been demonstrated which shows higher power. For instance, the work carried out by Tong et al. is worth mentioning where graphene has been coupled to a double-patch antenna and an on-chip silicon lens to fabricate THz sources operating at room temperature yielding significantly high power than conventional ones [15].

The device is schematically shown in Fig. 4.1A where a graphene piece is placed in-between the two metal patches made by palladium/gold (yellow color).

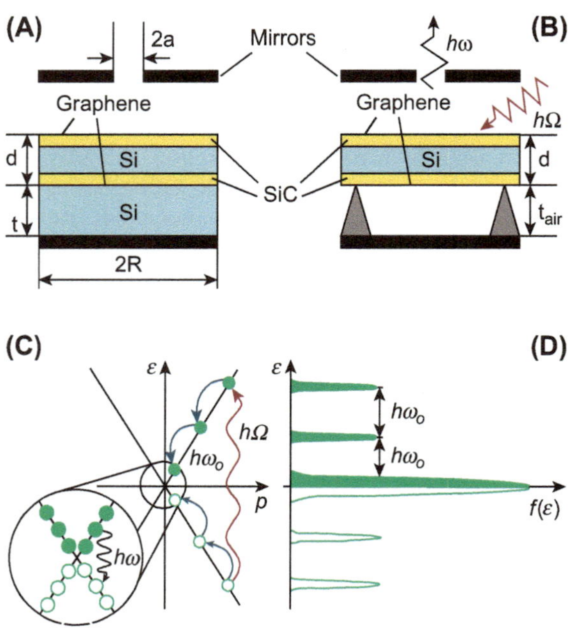

FIG. 4.1 Schematic view of the laser structures with Si separation layer **(A)** and with air separation layer **(B)**, as well as the laser pumping scheme **(C)** and electron and hole distribution functions **(D)**. (Figures reprinted with permission from ref. Adapted with permission J. Tong, M. Muthee, S.Y. Chen, S.K. Yngvesson, J. Yan, Antenna enhanced graphene THz emitter and detector, Nano Letters 15 (2015) 5295–5301. Copyright 2015, American Chemical Society.)

According to their simulation results, the impedance spectrum in Fig. 4.2B shows a peak frequency of 2.1 THz, while the electric field distribution at that frequency is shown in Fig. 4.2C. The details of the fabrication process can be found in Ref. [16]. In short, high resistivity silicon chip with a 300 nm-thick silicon oxide layer has been used as the platform where they are glued back-to-back on an elliptical silicon lens. The schematic of emission measurements is shown in Fig. 4.2D where I denotes the applied electric current to heat up the device. On the other hand, schematic of detection measurements is shown in Fig. 4.2E (which will be discussed later).

The top view of actual fabricated device is shown in Fig. 4.3A, while Fig. 4.3B shows the schematic of the whole structure. A Fourier-transform THz spectrometer has been employed to analyze the THz radiation (as shown in Fig. 4.3C). It may be noted that the experimentally measured radiation spectrum peaks around 1.9 THz (see Fig. 4.3D). The gate voltage dependence of the spectra can also be seen in Fig. 4.3D. Gate voltage introduces more holes into the device which can be revealed from the change in spectral weight around the peak. Fig. 4.3E shows total radiated power as a function of V_G using a silicon bolometer kept at cryogenic temperature, while DC electrical resistance depicts a monotonically increasing behavior. The results have been explained by invoking Drude model which predicts the existence of a THz radiative mechanism in the graphene field-effect transistors [17].

In addition, graphene-based p-i-n junction produced by chemical doping or gating was studied as well (in order to reduce excess heating) where self-excitation of THz lasing was demonstrated under proper experimental conditions [18]. Apart from these works, graphene-based plasmonic oscillator THz generators were also proposed. In addition, intrinsic plasmons of graphene can be tuned to generate radiation up to 1 THz (in case of optically pumped graphene). However, the absorption in graphene is 2.3% which limits the application of graphene as THz lasers.

DETECTORS

Due to its growing importance in the field of security, drug, biological imaging, and explosive detection, various THz detectors have been fabricated. For instance, THz detectors based on bolometers [19,20], Schottky barrier THz detectors [21], pair braking THz detectors [22], field-effect transistor (FET) THz detectors [23], etc., are noteworthy. It may be noted that the differences between detection at THz frequencies and

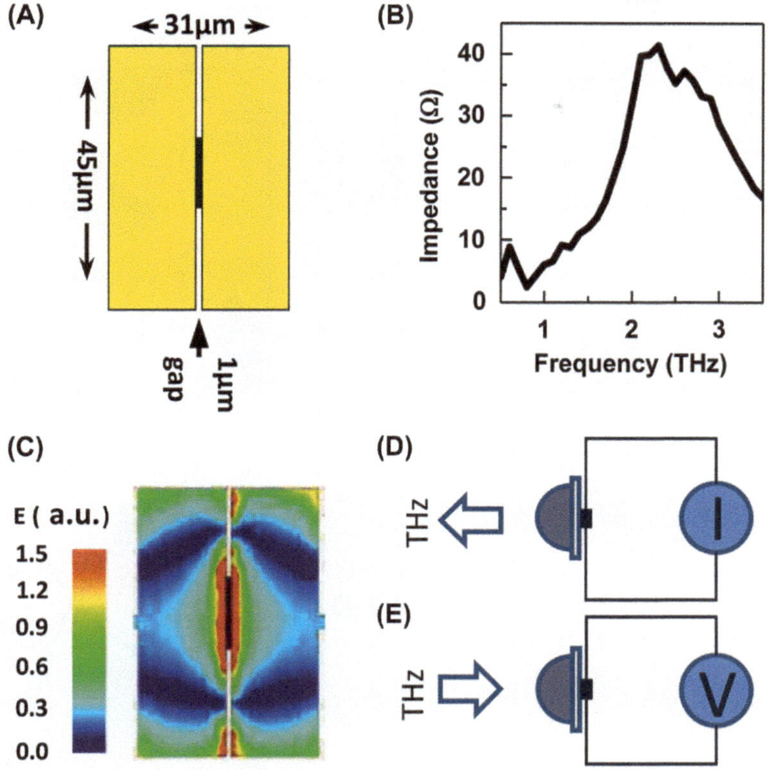

FIG. 4.2 **(A)** Design of the terahertz (THz) antenna-coupled graphene device. **(B)** HFSS-simulated frequency dependence of impedance. **(C)** Calculated distribution of THz electric field at 2.1 THz. **(D, E)** Schematic setup of the emission **(D)** and detection **(E)** experiments. (Adapted with permission J. Tong, M. Muthee, S.Y. Chen, S.K. Yngvesson, J. Yan, Antenna enhanced graphene THz emitter and detector, Nano Letters 15 (2015) 5295–5301. Copyright 2015, American Chemical Society.)

in the infrared (IR) range is more prominent at low photon energies (at around 4 meV) while the room temperature thermal energy lies around 26 meV. On the other hand, photon detectors can allow the detection of long wavelength limits which are comprised of solid solutions ($Hg_{1-x}Cd_xTe$) [24], doped semiconductors (Si and Ge here as dopants) [25], quantum well structures [26], etc.

The performance of a THz detector can be evaluated using two main parameters: the smallest detectable power or noise equivalent power (NEP) and detectivity [27]. Even after years of developments, THz detectors suffer from different shortcomings. For instance, bolometer-based detectors are susceptible to background radiation and temperature fluctuation. In addition, mechanical vibration and electrical interference plays critical role and deteriorates it performance [27]. To avoid these perturbations, cryogenic temperatures (restricting its usage in day-to-day basis) become unavoidable in most of the cases.

On the other hand, despite their poor sensitivity, uncooled Schottky barrier THz detectors are used due to their cost effectiveness, wide dynamic range, and ability to get integrated in arrays by integrated design. However, they are hard to design, fabricate, and operate. As an alternative, FET-based THz detector appears promising compared with other detectors because of their fast and high responsivity. Since the prediction of plasma oscillation-induced emission of THz radiation in FET channels [28,29], researcher demonstrated emission and detection of THz in both low and room temperatures where it was realized that the plasma frequency of the resonator can be tuned by varying the gate lengths [30].

However, graphene, with its gapless Dirac-cone structure and exceptional carrier mobility, offers great promise due to its potential applications in ultrafast and ultrasensitive broadband detection of electromagnetic radiation including THz frequency range [31–34]. In fact, the enhanced intraband absorption along with weak electron-phonon coupling graphene open a new

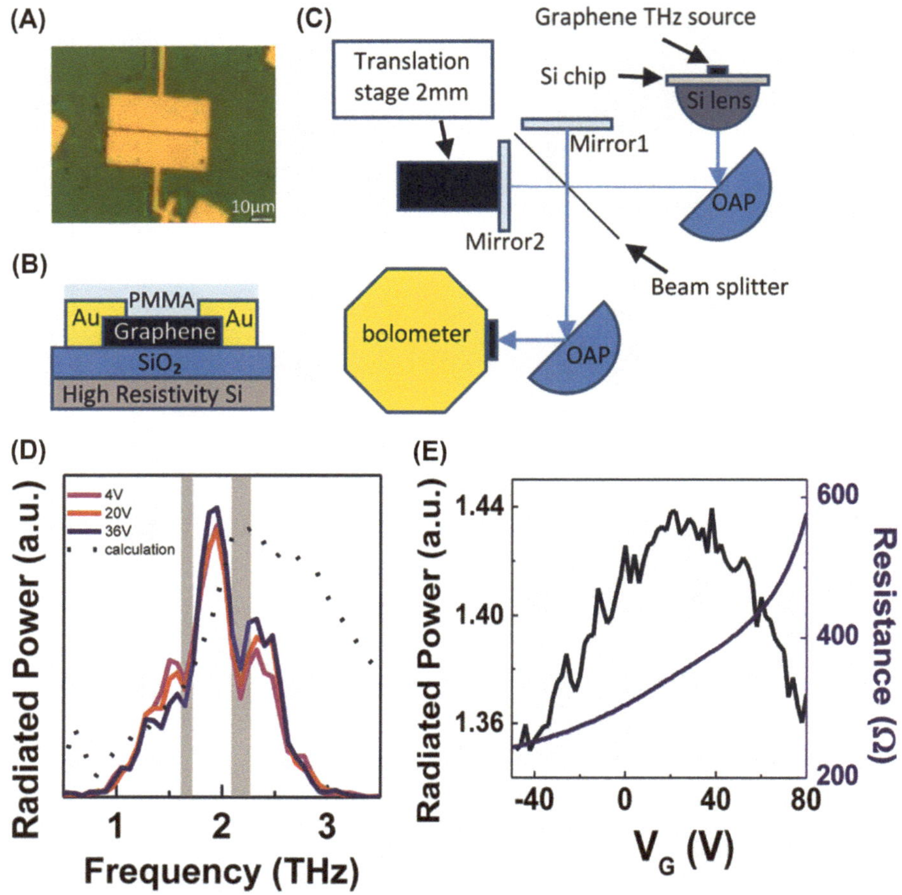

FIG. 4.3 **(A)** Optical image of the graphene field-effect transistor (GFET) emitter. **(B)** Schematic side view of GFET emitter. **(C)** Fourier-transform terahertz (THz) interferometer setup. **(D)** Measured (*solid lines*) THz radiation spectra from graphene at different gate voltages. The *dashed line* is the transmission spectrum calculated from HFSS simulation in Fig. 4.1B. The two gray bands indicate water absorption lines. **(E)** Comparison of VG-dependent GFET resistance (blue) and THz radiated power (black). (Adapted with permission J. Tong, M. Muthee, S.Y. Chen, S.K. Yngvesson, J. Yan, Antenna enhanced graphene THz emitter and detector, Nano Letters 15 (2015) 5295–5301. Copyright 2015, American Chemical Society.)

avenue for hot-electron photothermoelectric detection of THz [35] with high responsivity and large modulation frequency [15,36]. For instance, single-layer and bilayer graphene FET devices are employed for resonant THz detection where top-gate antenna-coupled setup has been used [17,37–43]. Guo et al. have proposed a new kind of graphene-based broadband THz detector with square-spiral antenna arrangement which can operate at room temperature [44] Fig. 4.4.

This configuration leads to a sensitivity over 28 $V W^{-1}$ at room temperature and NEP of less than 0.35 $nW/Hz^{0.5}$. The benefit is that the whole structure can be integrated in chip-based THz optoelectronics (optics letters). Some other works can also be found, where graphene-based transistors and photodetectors were demonstrated to detect THz range radiation [45–48].

In another work, 2D heterostructure approach has been adapted where h-BN layer has been incorporated in the FET structure. New tunnel transistors are formed by sandwiching h-BN layer in between two graphene layers to overcome the limitation of long carrier dwell time inside quantum well [40,49].

GRAPHENE-BASED THZ MODULATORS

Graphene-based THz modulators can be formed by tuning the Fermi level by various means [50], and later Gao et al. showed significant enhancement of the modulation depth and 50% amplitude modulation by using

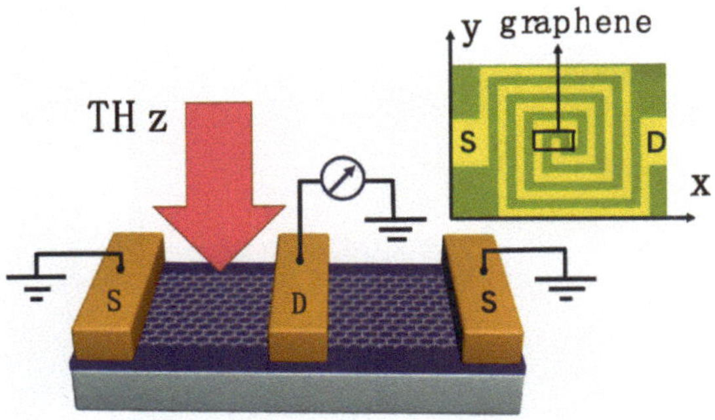

FIG. 4.4 Schematic of the graphene-based terahertz detector integrated with a square-spiral antenna. The source is the left electrode connected to the right one, and the middle electrode is the drain electrode. The inset shows a zoomed image of the terahertz detector in the center of the square-spiral antenna [44]. (Reprinted/adapted with permission from W. Guo, L. Wang, X. Chen, C. Liu, W. Tang, C. Guo, J. Wang and W. Lu, Graphene-based broadband terahertz detector integrated with a square-spiral antenna, Optics Letters 43 (2018) 1647. https://doi.org/10.1364/ol.43.001647. © The Optical Society.)

gated single-layer graphene with a metallic ring placed right above it [51]. This leads to 7 times near-field enhancement of THz absorption in graphene. Due to the presence of intrinsic plasmon in graphene, combining it with noble metal nanostructures can lead to modulation in THz regime [51]. In another note, Weis et al. have shown that simple graphene on Si can be used for attenuation and modulation of THz. In fact, wide band THz transmission with a maximum modulation depth of 99% was achieved [52]. Recently, Kakenov et al. have shown graphene-based THz phase modulator by electrically tuning graphene devices [53]. A schematic and a picture of the phase modulator are shown in Fig. 4.6 where graphene on porous polyethylene membrane with Au back reflector was used for the modulation study [53]. Graphene acts as a tunable-impedance surface modulating reflection phase with high attenuation capability in this configuration Fig. 4.5.

FEW OTHER 2D MATERIALS FOR THZ BIOMEDICAL APPLICATIONS

Here, we will discuss about the other 2DMs apart from graphene. Some of the candidates in this category are as follows: h-BN is a wide bandgap (5.9 eV) layered material [55], monolayer transition metal dichalcogenides (TMDs), black phosphorous, etc. [56–60]. Although they are 2DMs, they are different from graphene. For example, TMDs show higher optical absorption due to the presence of bandgap, while electron mobility in TMDs is low as compared with graphene. Molybdenum disulfide (MoS_2) is one of the important TMDs which is considered to be a potential candidate in THz application [61]. For instance, Guo et al. developed an ultrafast two-dimensional visible/far-IR spectroscopy based on IR/THz detection method and used this method to study relaxation dynamics of the photoexcited carriers in MoS_2 [62]. Sun et al. used ultrafast transient absorption measurements to identify exciton-exciton annihilation in MoS_2 [63]. Subsequently, optically tuned THz modulator with multilayer MoS_2 on silicon substrate was shown [16] where 87% of THz transmission has been modulated by varying the laser power. Chen et al. developed highly sensitive THz modulator using Si-grown MoS_2 nanosheets [54]. High modulation depth of 75% has been achieved with this configuration (chip integrable design), proving it to be more effective THz wave modulator.

In terms of THz detection using 2DMs, 2D heterostructure-based THz devices have been proposed which show a new avenue to THz technology-based research [64,65].

2DMs have been the focus of much research due to their highly diverse properties making them suitable for a wide spectrum of applications ranging not only from optical [66], electrical [67], energy storage [68], and semiconductors [69] but also biomedical applications such as drug delivery, bioimaging, diagnosis, and tissue engineering. Their low dimensional features (nanostructures) make them more suited to biomedical applications. For example, 2DMs have the highest specific surface areas suitable for drug delivery applications, considering high levels of small-scale surface interactions are critical. These materials are able to adsorb large numbers of drug molecules and hence give better control over release kinetics. 2DMs with extremely high surface-to-volume ratios, high modulus values, are good for enhancing mechanical characteristics of nanocomposites, at moderate concentrations, for biomedical applications. The very low thickness is extensively utilized in better understanding biosensing and gene sequencing. Graphene with its unparalleled properties has been at the forefront of 2DM research resulting in new classes of 2DMs that include TMDs, transition metal oxides, and layered double hydroxides. Here, we elaborate on some of the biomedical uses of graphene and TMDs.

Carbon-Based 2DMs

Graphene is the oldest and well-researched carbon 2DM material, having been first found in 2004 [1,70,71]. This research, more recently, has extended to the area of biomedical applications, where graphene has shown a strong future potential in the field of tissue

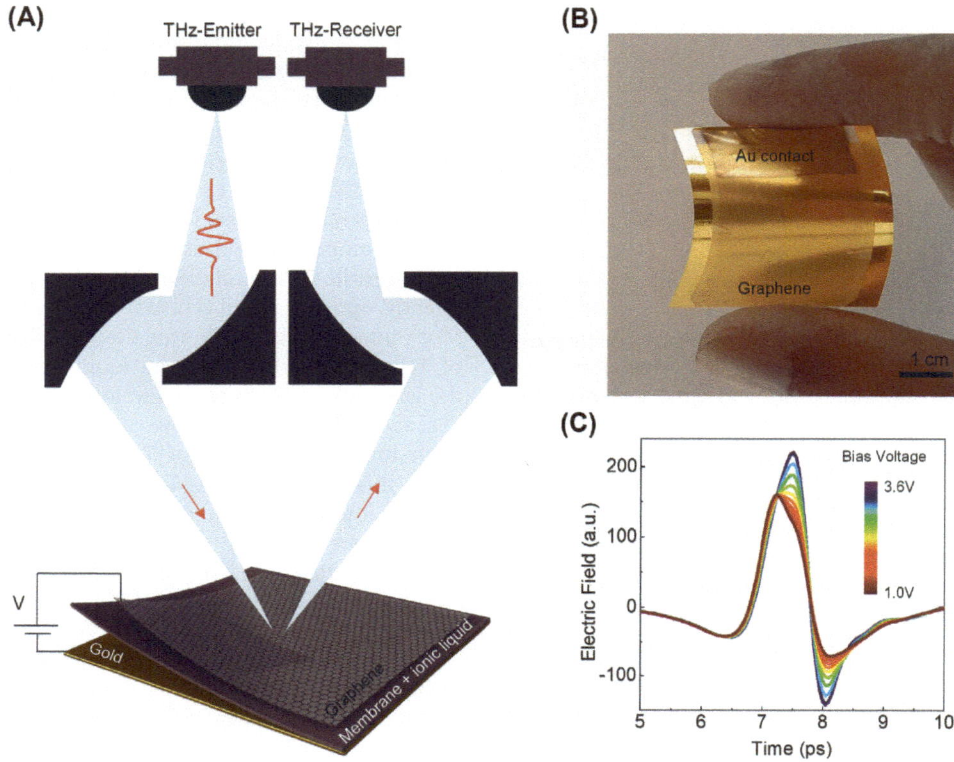

FIG. 4.5 Electrically tunable phase modulator. **(A)** Experimental setup used for the terahertz (THz) time-domain reflection measurements. THz pulses are generated by InGaAs photoconductive antenna and focused on the device by parabolic mirrors at 10 degrees incidence angle. The phase modulator consists of monolayer graphene on porous 20 μm-thin polyethylene membrane and gold reflector at the back. Ionic liquid electrolyte [deme][Tf2N] is injected into the membrane. **(B)** Photograph of the fabricated device. **(C)** Measured time-varying electric field of THz pulses at gate voltages between 1.0 and 3.6 V. The THz pulse is suppressed and shifted with varying applied voltage, indicating the phase modulation. Each color represents different gate voltage. (Reproduced from N. Kakenov, M.S. Ergoktas, O. Balci, C. Kocabas, Graphene based terahertz phase modulators, 2D Materials 5 (2018). https://doi.org/10.1088/2053-1583/aabfaa under Creative Commons Attribution-noncommercial 3.0 unported licence.)

engineering. In 2014, Qiu et al. [72] were able to synthesize a nanocomposite aerogel of poly (N-isopropylacrylamide) (PNIPAM) along with graphene. This aerogel had a highly interconnected architecture and exhibited a modulus that was an order of magnitude higher than graphene-free PNIPAM hydrogels [72]. Moreover, the researchers also found significant increase in electrical conductivity due to addition of graphene and the thermoresponsive properties of the nanocomposite aerogel compared with the graphene-free counterparts. They attributed this effect to the prefabrication of a graphene aerogel with superior conductivity in-between the graphene sheets. This method also eliminated the need to functionalize the graphene to the less conductive graphene oxide (GO) for solution dispersion.

Because of their high electrical conductivity, graphene-based nanocomposites have also been explored for tissue engineering applications that require an electrical stimulus for operation. Tang et al. reported graphene substrate as electrically conductive material and can direct cell fate by enhancing electrical interactions in neural stem cells [73]. The neuron density and excitability increased nearly two times on a graphene substrate in comparison to a tissue culture polystyrene control. This improvement makes graphene most favorable substrate for culturing neurons, creating biocompatible neural interfaces (Fig. 4.1, [73]), attributed to the enhanced electrical conductivity. For biomedical applications, suitable graphene surface can be made hydrophilic through an oxidative exfoliation method, resulting in the graphene oxidation to GO,

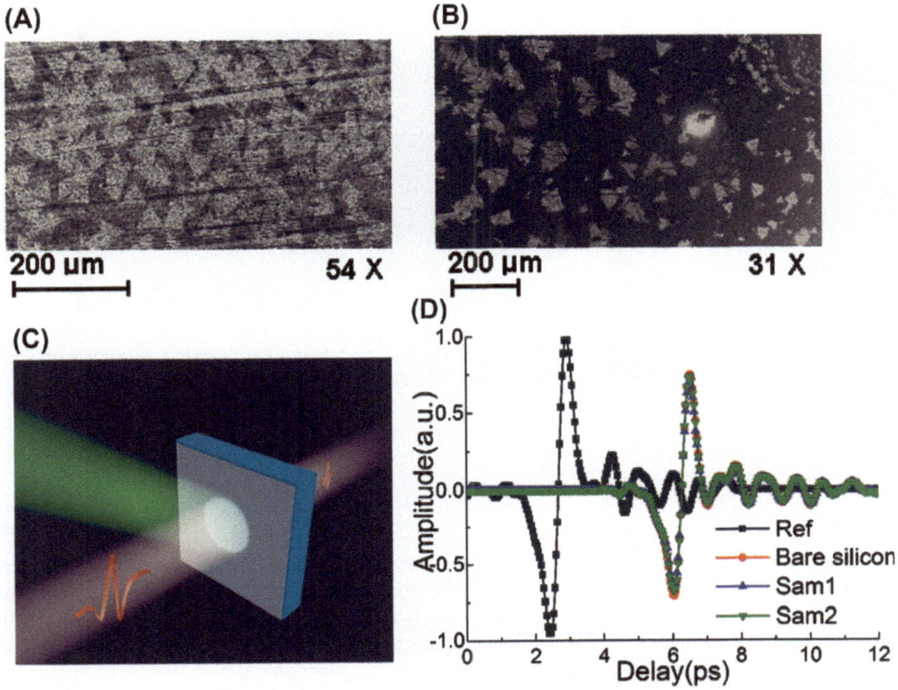

FIG. 4.6 SEM images of MoS_2 nanosheet samples: **(A)** Sam1 and **(B)** Sam2. Sam1 was grown for a longer time and has more MoS_2 molecules. **(C)** Illustration of the MoS_2 sample and experimental configuration. **(D)** Normalized THz time-domain signals of air (reference), bare Si substrate. (Reproduced with permission from S. Chen, F. Fan, Y. Miao, X. He, K. Zhang, S. Chang, Ultrasensitive terahertz modulation by silicon-grown MoS_2 nanosheets, Nanoscale 8 (2016) 4713–4719. https://ds.doi.org/10.1039/c5nr08101g.)

though this enables the surface of GO to interact with biomacromolecules such as proteins and certain drugs, but at the cost of electrical conductivity and mechanical strength. GO with its sheet like construction with hydroxyl groups on its surface can combine various synthetic and natural polymers that can provide physical strengthening [74,75], Fig. 4.7.

Additionally, GO with its superior electrical conductivity is ideal for making conductive patches for biomedical applications like tissue engineering (Fig. 4.1, [77,78]). A recent study showed the enhancement of electrical conductivity of nanocomposite hydrogels when GO was added to methacrylated gelatin [78]. The higher electrical conductivity of the nanocomposite hydrogel was yielded in a higher proliferation of cardiomyocytes seeded on the hydrogel surface, indicating GO can be useful for cardiac patch [77,78]. It is also reported that hydrogel stiffness was increased by modifying the GO surface with methacrylate groups. During polymerization, these groups covalently cross-link the surface of GO to methacrylated gelatin [79]. The addition of GO (small amount, $3\ mg\ mL^{-1}$) in gelatin hydrogels resulted in a two- to threefold increase in the mechanical stiffness of the hydrogel leading to enhanced cell viability, proliferation, and distribution in a 3D environment.

The reduction of GO results in the formation of reduced graphene oxide (rGO) sheets, another member of carbon-based 2DM family that is easy to fabricate and incorporates some inherent characteristics of pristine graphene. In rGo, most of the functional groups are removed from the sheets, leaving behind a bare carbon sheet with structural defects. Owing to convenient availability, superior electrical conductivity comparative to GO, rGO has found wide usage in biosensing applications. Moreover, with larger specific surface area, superior carrier mobility, rGO surface can trap higher densities of biomolecule receptors relative to single-dimensional materials, e.g., carbon nanotubes and silicon nanowires [80–83], making them a very viable choice for use in high-sensitivity, high-resolution biosensors. Various research groups [80–83] have used rGO in the fabrication of ultrasensitive FET biosensors to detect prostate specific antigens with very high specificity and without the need for labeling. The ease and low cost of fabrication with the added advantage

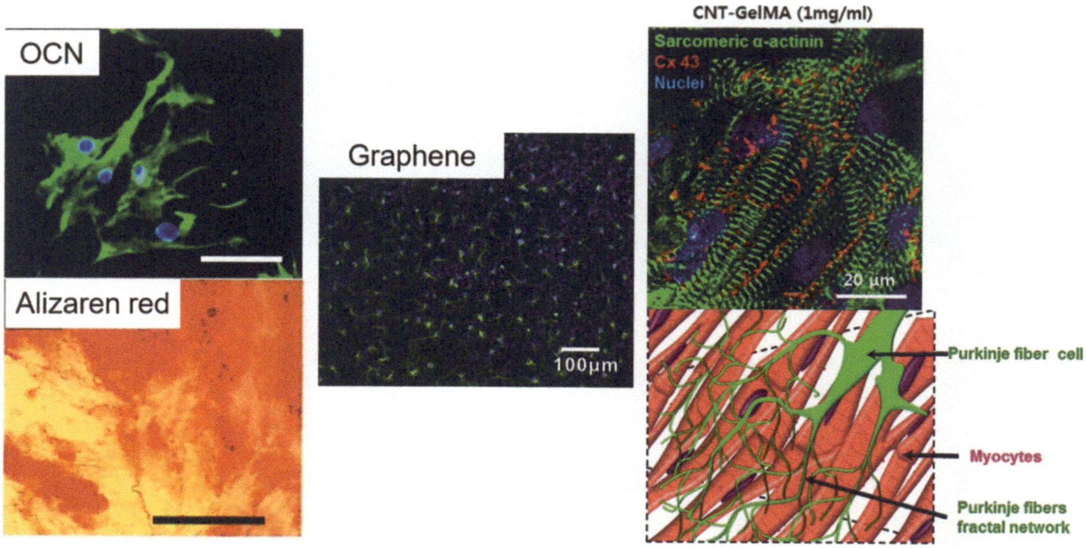

FIG. 4.7 Carbon 2D nanomaterial applications in tissue engineering, e.g., application of graphene/graphene oxide/reduced graphene oxide for control, direct cellular fate toward osteoblasts, scale bars are 100 μm [76], neural networks on graphene substrates [73] and cardiomyocytes [77]. (Osteoblasts images adapted with permission T.R. Nayak, H. Andersen, V.S. Makam, C. Khaw, S. Bae, X. Xu, P.-L.R. Ee, J.-H. Ahn, B.H. Hong, G. Pastorin, B. Özyilmaz, Graphene for controlled and accelerated osteogenic differentiation of human mesenchymal stem cells, ACS Nano 5 (2011) 4670–4678. https://ds.doi.org/10.1021/nn200500h. Copyright 2011, American Chemical Society. Neurons images adapted with permission M. Tang, Q. Song, N. Li, Z. Jiang, R. Huang, G. Cheng, Enhancement of electrical signaling in neural networks on graphene films, Biomaterials 34 (2013) 6402–6411. https://ds.doi.org/10.1016/j.biomaterials.2013.05.024. Copyright 2013, American Chemical Society. Cardiomyocytes images adapted with permission S.R. Shin, S.M. Jung, M. Zalabany, K. Kim, P. Zorlutuna, S. bok Kim, M. Nikkhah, M. Khabiry, M. Azize, J. Kong, K. Wan, T. Palacios, M.R. Dokmeci, H. Bae, X. Tang, A. Khademhosseini, Carbon-nanotube-embedded hydrogel sheets for engineering cardiac constructs and bioactuators, ACS Nano 7 (2013) 2369–2380. https://ds.doi.org/10.1021/nn305559j. Copyright 2013 American Chemical Society.)

of high sensitivity and specificity makes rGO a very attractive material for biosensing technologies that could result in better diagnostic techniques and eventually improved patient outcomes.

Transition Metal Dichalcogenides

TMDs, by definition, are two-dimensional nanoparticles made up of a single layer of transition metal atoms sandwiched between two layers of chalcogen atoms arranged in a hexagonal lattice [84]. Of the 60 known TMDs, there are only three that have shown significant potential: molybdenum disulphide (MoS_2), tungsten disulphide (WS_2), and titanium disulphide (TiS_2). TMDs are thin, flexible, and structurally much more rigid than their carbon counterpart. They also possess good catalytic properties, exhibit photoluminescence (PL), show optical absorption, and have a direct bandgap and very high wear resistance [85–87]. All of these properties combined make this class of 2DMs excellent biomaterial candidates for use in biosensors, nanocomposites, and bioimaging.

2D MoS_2 nanosheets possess tunable photoluminescent properties that make them ideal materials for biosensing applications. The PL effect of MoS_2 comes from the atomic orbitals (s, p, d) of molybdenum in MoS_2. Pumera et al. [87] have shown that the PL characteristics of MoS_2 can be modified through an electrical gating mechanism, via polarized light, a mechanical force, and cation intercalation. The resulting change in the PL potential has been used as a concentration detector of biologically important cations such as H^+, Li^+, Na^+, and K^+ in a wide range of bioprocesses. Fig. 4.2 highlights some of the PL characteristics of MoS_2 [88].

In a recent novel approach to FET biosensing, Sarkar et al. have fabricated low-cost, high-sensitivity 2D FETs using MoS_2 nanoparticles [89] in an effort to advance nanosensor-based diagnostics. These FETs were used as biotin sensors to detect a charged biomolecule on a biotin-functionalized surface. For instance, the transistor current output will drop due to the bound negative charge on the dielectric surface of the FET, if a

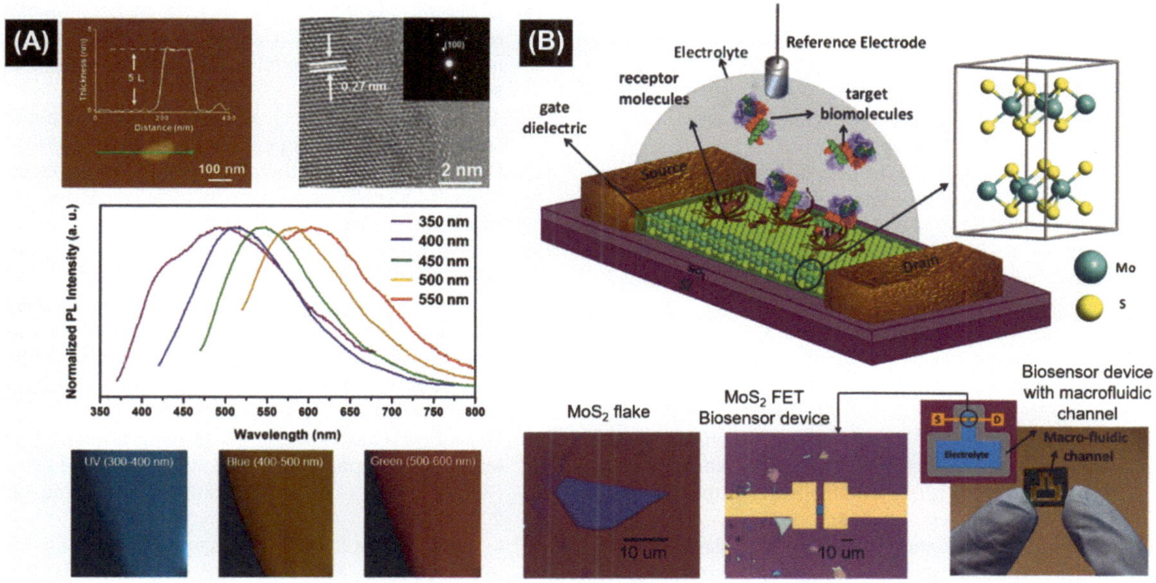

FIG. 4.8 Due to superior photoluminescence (PL) characteristics, transition metal dichalcogenide has application as biosensors. **(A)** AFM and HRTEM images of quasi-2D MoS_2 flake, with PL spectra at various excitation wavelengths, along with fluorescent images of MoS_2 thin films. **(B)** Schematics of a MoS_2 field-effect transistor biosensor device. (Reproduced with permission J.Z. Ou, A.F. Chrimes, Y. Wang, S. Tang, M.S. Strano, K. Kalantar-zadeh, Ion-driven photoluminescence modulation of quasi-two-dimensional MoS_2 nanoflakes for applications in biological systems, Nano Letters 14 (2014) 857–863. https://ds.doi.org/10.1021/nl4042356. Copyright 2014, American Chemical Society.)

negatively charged biomolecule entered the system Fig. 4.8

WS_2 is another 2D TMD material that has potential applications in biomedical imaging as contrast agents such as computed tomography (CT). In CT imaging, X-ray absorption contrast in the targeted areas is enhanced with the use of WS_2 due to their high opacity to X-ray absorption. This was demonstrated by Cheng et al. in their recent paper where they used biocompatible poly(ethylene glycol) (PEG)-functionalized WS_2 nanosheets as bimodal contrast enhancement agents for detection and imaging of tumors through CT.

TiS_2 is a relatively newer 2D TMD nanomaterial that is being explored in biomedical imaging. Qian et al. successfully used [90] PEG-modified TiS_2 nanosheets as contrast agents in photoacoustic tomography due to their high near-IR absorbance.

REFERENCES

[1] A.K. Geim, Graphene: status and prospects, Science 324 (2009) 1530–1535.

[2] D.W. Boukhvalov, M.I. Katsnelson, Chemical functionalization of graphene with defects, Nano Letters (2008).

[3] G. Lozano, J. Go, G. Pirruccio, L. Martı, Coherent and broadband enhanced optical absorption in graphene, ACS Nano (2013) 4810–4817, https://doi.org/10.1021/nn4012253.

[4] E. Hendry, P.J. Hale, J. Moger, A.K. Savchenko, Coherent nonlinear optical response of graphene, Physical Review Letters (2010) 097401, https://doi.org/10.1103/PhysRevLett.105.097401, 1–4.

[5] F. Xia, H. Yan, P. Avouris, The interaction of light and Graphene: basics, devices, and applications, Proceedings of the IEEE 101 (2013) 1717–1731, https://doi.org/10.1109/JPROC.2013.2250892.

[6] S.M. Rao, J.J.F. Heitz, T. Roger, N. Westerberg, D. Faccio, Coherent control of light interaction with graphene, Optics Letters 39 (2014) 5345–5347.

[7] X.I.S. Hi, L.G.E. Ixin, X.I.W. En, D.E.H. An, Y.A.Y. Ang, Broadband light absorption in graphene ribbons by canceling strong coupling at subwavelength scale, Optics Express 24 (2016) 151–156.

[8] X. Wen, J. Zheng, Broadband THz reflective polarization rotator by multiple plasmon resonances, Optics Express 22 (2014) 28292–28300, https://doi.org/10.1364/OE.22.028292.

[9] P.E. Smith, A.K. Isaac, Aspects oF chock shield support designs using a finite element technique, Mining Science and Technology 6 (1988) 255–266.

[10] Y. Jin, X.F. Ma, X. Zhang, Terahertz optical rectification from ⟨ 110 ⟩ zinc-blende crystals, Applied Physics Letters 1324 (2007) 1–4, https://doi.org/10.1063/1.111922.

[11] J. Dai, J. Liu, X. Zhang, Terahertz wave air photonics: terahertz wave generation and detection with laser-induced gas, Plasma 17 (2011) 183–190.

[12] T. Review, Graphene-based devices in terahertz, Journal of Physics D: Applied Physics (2012), https://doi.org/10.1088/0022-3727/45/30/303001.

[13] J.A. Phys, Negative dynamic conductivity of graphene, Journal of Applied Physics (2009) 083114, https://doi.org/10.1063/1.2717566.

[14] A.A. Dubinov, V. Aleshkin, M. Ryzhii, T. Otsuji, Terahertz laser with optically pumped graphene layers and fabri—perot resonator, Applied Physics Express (2009), https://doi.org/10.1143/APEX.2.092301.

[15] J. Tong, M. Muthee, S.Y. Chen, S.K. Yngvesson, J. Yan, Antenna enhanced graphene THz emitter and detector, Nano Letters 15 (2015) 5295–5301, https://doi.org/10.1021/acs.nanolett.5b01635.

[16] Y. Cao, S. Gan, Z. Geng, J. Liu, Y. Yang, Q. Bao, H. Chen, Optically tuned terahertz modulator based on annealed multilayer MoS_2, Nat. Publ. Gr. Scientific Report (2016) 1–10, https://doi.org/10.1038/srep22899.

[17] L. Vicarelli, M.S. Vitiello, D. Coquillat, A. Lombardo, A.C. Ferrari, W. Knap, M. Polini, Graphene field-effect transistors as room-temperature terahertz detectors, Nature Materials 11 (2012) 865–871, https://doi.org/10.1038/nmat3417.

[18] J.A. Phys, Double injection in graphene p-i-n structures, Journal of Applied Physics (2013) 244505, https://doi.org/10.1063/1.4812494.

[19] A. You, M.A.Y. Be, I. In, Terahertz heterodyne receiver based on a quantum cascade laser and a superconducting bolometer, Applied Physics Letters (2006) 244104, https://doi.org/10.1063/1.1949724, 2003–2006.

[20] L. Titanate, T. Film, C. Wang, Y. Chen, Micromachined infrared detectors based on pyroelectric thin films, Reports on Progress in Physics (2001).

[21] T. Yasui, A. Nishimura, Detection system operating at up to 7 THz using quasioptics and Schottky barrier diodes, Review of Scientific Instruments (2013) 066102, https://doi.org/10.1063/1.2206770, 1–4.

[22] A. You, M.A.Y. Be, I. In, Quantum-limited heterodyne detection of millimeter waves using superconducting tantalum tunnel junctions, Applied Physics Letters 2487 (2013) 1–4, https://doi.org/10.1063/1.104111.

[23] C.A. Saylor, L.C. Brunel, Nonresonant detection of terahertz radiation in field effect transistors, Journal of Applied Physics 9346 (2009), https://doi.org/10.1063/1.1468257.

[24] J.M. Doviak, A.F. Gibson, T. Grave, E. Scholl, H. Wurz, A.F. Gibson, P.N.D. Maggs, Two-photon absorption in InSb and Hg 1-x Cd x Te, Journal of Physics C: Solids State Physics (1979).

[25] G. Masini, L. Colace, G. Assanto, H. Luan, L.C. Kimerling, High-performance p-i-n Ge on Si photodetectors for the near Infrared: from, Model to Demonstration 48 (2001) 1092–1096.

[26] A. You, M.A.Y. Be, I. In, Quantum-Well Infrared Photodetectors, vol. 1, 2009, https://doi.org/10.1063/1.354252.

[27] O. Access, We are IntechOpen, the world's leading publisher of Open Access books Built by scientists, for scientists TOP 1 %, (n.d.).

[28] M. Dyakonov, M. Shur, Phys. Rev. Lett. 71 (1993) 2465–2469.

[29] M. Dyakonov, M. Shur, Phys. Rev. B 51 (1995) 341–345.

[30] M.I. Dyakonov, Boundary instability of a two-dimensional electron fluid, Low-Dimensional System 42 (2008) 984–988, https://doi.org/10.1134/S1063782608080186.

[31] H. Zhao, Q. Guo, F. Xia, H. Wang, Two-dimensional materials for nanophotonics application, Nature Photonics (2015) 128–142, https://doi.org/10.1515/nanoph-2014-0022.

[32] J. Kong, F. Xia, Coupling-enhanced broadband mid-infrared light absorption in graphene plasmonic nanostructures, ACS Nano (2016), https://doi.org/10.1021/acsnano.6b06203.

[33] M. Badioli, A. Woessner, K.J. Tielrooij, S. Nanot, G. Navickaite, T. Stauber, F.H.L. Koppens, Phonon-mediated mid-infrared photoresponse of graphene, Mesoscale and Nanoscale Physics (2014), https://doi.org/10.1021/nl502847v.

[34] A. Phys, D. Spirito, D. Coquillat, S.L. De Bonis, A. Lombardo, M. Bruna, C. Andrea, V. Pellegrini, A. Tredicucci, W. Knap, M.S. Vitiello, D. Spirito, D. Coquillat, S.L. De Bonis, A. Lombardo, M. Bruna, A.C. Ferrari, V. Pellegrini, A. Tredicucci, W. Knap, M.S. Vitiello, High performance bilayer-graphene terahertz detectors, Applied Physics Letters (2017) 061111, https://doi.org/10.1063/1.4864082.

[35] X. Deng, Y. Wang, Z. Zhao, Z. Chen, Terahertz-induced photothermoelectric response in graphene-metal contact structures, Journal of Physics D: Applied Physics (2016), https://doi.org/10.1088/0022-3727/49/42/425101.

[36] V. Ryzhii, M. Ryzhii, M.S. Shur, V. Mitin, A. Satou, T. Otsuji, Resonant plasmonic terahertz detection in graphene split-gate field-effect transistors with lateral p − n junctions, Journal of Physics D: Applied Physics (2016), https://doi.org/10.1088/0022-3727/49/31/315103.

[37] J.A. Phys, Single-particle tunneling in doped graphene-insulator-graphene junctions, Journal of Applied Physics (2016) 043711, https://doi.org/10.1063/1.3686639.

[38] V. Ryzhii, T. Otsuji, M. Ryzhii, M.S. Shur, Double graphene-layer plasma resonances terahertz detector, Journal of Physics D: Applied Physics (2012), https://doi.org/10.1088/0022-3727/45/30/302001.

[39] L. Britnell, R. V Gorbachev, A.K. Geim, L.A. Ponomarenko, A. Mishchenko, M.T. Greenaway, T.M. Fromhold, K.S. Novoselov, L. Eaves, Resonant tunnelling and negative differential conductance in graphene transistors, Nature Communications 4 (2013) 1794–1795, https://doi.org/10.1038/ncomms2817.

[40] A. Mishchenko, J.S. Tu, Y. Cao, R. V Gorbachev, J.R. Wallbank, M.T. Greenaway, V.E. Morozov, S. V Morozov, M.J. Zhu, S.L. Wong, F. Withers, C.R. Woods, Y. Kim, K. Watanabe, T. Taniguchi, E.E. Vdovin, O. Makarovsky, T.M. Fromhold, V.I. Fal, A.K. Geim, L. Eaves, K.S. Novoselov, Twist-controlled resonant tunnelling in graphene/boron nitride/graphene heterostructures, Nature Nanotechnology 9 (2014) 7–12, https://doi.org/10.1038/nnano.2014.187.

[41] B. Fallahazad, K. Lee, S. Kang, J. Xue, S. Larentis, C. Corbet, K. Kim, H.C.P. Movva, T. Taniguchi, K. Watanabe, L.F. Register, S.K. Banerjee, E. Tutuc, Gate-tunable resonant tunneling in double bilayer graphene heterostructures, Nano Letters (2015) 1–6, https://doi.org/10.1021/nl503756y.

[42] A. Phys, M. Polini, Photocurrent-based detection of terahertz radiation in graphene Photocurrent-based detection of terahertz radiation in graphene, Mesoscale and Nanoscale Physics (2014) 211120, https://doi.org/10.1063/1.4831682.

[43] A. Phys, Graphene-insulator-graphene active plasmonic terahertz devices, Applied Physics Letters (2014) 123109, https://doi.org/10.1063/1.4821221.

[44] W. Guo, L. Wang, X. Chen, C. Liu, W. Tang, C. Guo, J. Wang, W. Lu, Graphene-based broadband terahertz detector integrated with a square-spiral antenna, Optics Letters 43 (2018) 1647, https://doi.org/10.1364/ol.43.001647.

[45] F. Schwierz, Graphene transistors, Nat. Publ. Gr. Nature Nanotechnology 5 (2010) 487–496, https://doi.org/10.1038/nnano.2010.89.

[46] Y. Wu, Y. Lin, A.A. Bol, K.A. Jenkins, F. Xia, D.B. Farmer, Y. Zhu, P. Avouris, Diamond-like carbon, Nature 472 (2011) 74–78, https://doi.org/10.1038/nature09979.

[47] Y. Wu, K.A. Jenkins, A. Valdes-garcia, D.B. Farmer, Y. Zhu, A.A. Bol, C. Dimitrakopoulos, W. Zhu, F. Xia, P. Avouris, Y. Lin, State-of-the-Art graphene high-frequency electronics, Nano Letters (2012), https://doi.org/10.1021/nl300904k.

[48] M. Ryzhii, N. V Baryshnikov, V.E. Karasik, V. Mitin, T. Otsuji, I. Engineering, Terahertz and infrared photodetectors based on multiple graphene layer and nanoribbon structures, Opto-Electronics Review 20 (2012) 15–25, https://doi.org/10.2478/s11772.

[49] Y. Kawano, Wide-band frequency-tunable terahertz and infrared detection with graphene, Nanotechnology (2013) 1–7, https://doi.org/10.1088/0957-4484/24/21/214004.

[50] L. Ren, Q. Zhang, S. Nanot, I. Kawayama, M. Tonouchi, Terahertz dynamics of quantum-confined electrons in carbon nanomaterials, Journal of Infrared, Millimeter and Teraherts Wave (2012) 846–860, https://doi.org/10.1007/s10762-012-9916-8.

[51] W. Gao, J. Shu, K. Reichel, D.V. Nickel, X. He, G. Shi, R. Vajtai, P.M. Ajayan, J. Kono, D.M. Mittleman, Q. Xu, High-contrast terahertz wave modulation by gated graphene enhanced by extraordinary transmission through ring apertures, Nano Letters (2014), https://doi.org/10.1021/nl4041274.

[52] P. Weis, J.L. Garcia-pomar, M. Ho, B. Reinhard, A. Brodyanski, M. Rahm, Spectrally wide-band terahertz wave modulator based on optically tuned graphene, ACS Nano (2012) 9118–9124, https://doi.org/10.1021/nn303392s.

[53] N. Kakenov, M.S. Ergoktas, O. Balci, C. Kocabas, Graphene based terahertz phase modulators, 2D Materials 5 (2018), https://doi.org/10.1088/2053-1583/aabfaa.

[54] S. Chen, F. Fan, Y. Miao, X. He, K. Zhang, S. Chang, Ultrasensitive terahertz modulation by silicon grown MoS_2 nanosheet, Nanoscale 8 (2016) 4713–4719, https://doi.org/10.1039/c5nr08101g.

[55] A. You, M.A.Y. Be, I. In, Hydrogen in mechanically prepared nanostructured h-BN: a critical comparison with that in nanostructured graphite, Applied Physics Letters 318 (2008) 12–15, https://doi.org/10.1063/1.1432447.

[56] V.K. Kumar, S. Dhar, T.H. Choudhury, S.A. Shivashankar, S. Raghavan, A predictive approach to CVD of TMDs: the case of MoS_2, Nanoscale (2015) 7802–7810, https://doi.org/10.1039/c4nr07080a.

[57] A. Phys, Optical study of local strain related disordering in CVD-grown $MoSe_2$ monolayers, Applied Physics Letters (2017) 253106, https://doi.org/10.1063/1.4972782.

[58] S. Tongay, W. Fan, J. Kang, J. Park, U. Koldemir, J. Suh, D.S. Narang, K. Liu, J. Ji, J. Li, R. Sinclair, J. Wu, Tuning interlayer coupling in large-area heterostructures with CVD- grown MoS_2 and WS_2 monolayers, Nano Letters 2 (2014), https://doi.org/10.1021/nl500515q.

[59] W. Yang, J. Shang, J. Wang, X. Shen, B. Cao, N. Peimyoo, Electrically tunable valley-light emitting diode (vLED) based on CVD-grown Monolayer WS_2, Nano Letters (2016), https://doi.org/10.1021/acs.nanolett.5b04066.

[60] J. Qiao, X. Kong, Z. Hu, F. Yang, W. Ji, High-mobility transport anisotropy and linear dichroism in few-layer black phosphorus, Nature Communications 5 (2014) 1–7, https://doi.org/10.1038/ncomms5475.

[61] C. Zhang, H. Wang, W. Chan, C. Manolatou, F. Rana, Absorption of light by excitons and trions in monolayers of metal dichalcogenide MoS_2: experiments and theory, Physical Review B (2014) 205436, https://doi.org/10.1103/PhysRevB.89.205436, 12–16.

[62] J.C. Phys, Electron-phonon interactions in MoS_2 probed with ultrafast two-dimensional visible/far-infrared spectroscopy, The Journal of Chemical Physics (2015) 212447, https://doi.org/10.1063/1.4921573.
[63] A.R. Harutyunyan, T.F. Heinz, Observation of rapid exciton – exciton annihilation in monolayer molybdenum disulfide, Nano Letters (2014), https://doi.org/10.1021/nl5021975.
[64] L. Viti, J. Hu, D. Coquillat, A. Politano, C. Consejo, W. Knap, M.S. Vitiello, Heterostructured hBN-BP-hBN nanodetectors at terahertz frequencies, Advanced Materials (2016) 7390–7396, https://doi.org/10.1002/adma.201601736.
[65] A. Autere, H. Jussila, Y. Dai, Y. Wang, H. Lipsanen, Z. Sun, Nonlinear optics with 2D layered materials, Advanced Materials (2018) 1705963, https://doi.org/10.1002/adma.201705963, 1–24.
[66] F. Xia, H. Wang, D. Xiao, M. Dubey, A. Ramasubramaniam, Two-dimensional material nanophotonics, Nature Photonics 8 (2014) 899, https://doi.org/10.1038/nphoton.2014.271.
[67] A.H. Castro Neto, F. Guinea, N.M.R. Peres, K.S. Novoselov, A.K. Geim, The electronic properties of graphene, Reviews of Modern Physics 81 (2009) 109–162, https://doi.org/10.1103/RevModPhys.81.109.
[68] P. Bollella, G. Fusco, C. Tortolini, G. Sanzò, G. Favero, L. Gorton, R. Antiochia, Beyond graphene: electrochemical sensors and biosensors for biomarkers detection, Biosensors and Bioelectronics 89 (2017) 152–166, https://doi.org/10.1016/j.bios.2016.03.068.
[69] Chalcogenides fill the gap, Nature Materials 13 (2014) 1073, https://doi.org/10.1038/nmat4163.
[70] A.K. Geim, K.S. Novoselov, The rise of graphene, Nature Materials 6 (2007) 183–191.
[71] K.S.G. Novoselov, A.K. Geim, S.V. Morozov, D. Jiang, et al., Two-dimensional gas of massless dirac fermions in graphene, Nature 438 (2005) 197–200.
[72] L. Qiu, D. Liu, Y. Wang, C. Cheng, K. Zhou, J. Ding, V.-T. Truong, D. Li, Mechanically robust, electrically conductive and stimuli-responsive binary network hydrogels enabled by superelastic graphene aerogels, Advanced Materials 26 (2014) 3333–3337, https://doi.org/10.1002/adma.201305359.
[73] M. Tang, Q. Song, N. Li, Z. Jiang, R. Huang, G. Cheng, Enhancement of electrical signaling in neural networks on graphene films, Biomaterials 34 (2013) 6402–6411, https://doi.org/10.1016/j.biomaterials.2013.05.024.
[74] S. Goenka, V. Sant, S. Sant, Graphene-based nanomaterials for drug delivery and tissue engineering, Journal of Controlled Release 173 (2014) 75–88, https://doi.org/10.1016/j.jconrel.2013.10.017.
[75] C. Shuai, W. Guo, P. Wu, W. Yang, S. Hu, Y. Xia, P. Feng, A graphene oxide-Ag co-dispersing nanosystem: dual synergistic effects on antibacterial activities and mechanical properties of polymer scaffolds, Chemical Engineering Journal 347 (2018) 322–333, https://doi.org/10.1016/j.cej.2018.04.092.
[76] T.R. Nayak, H. Andersen, V.S. Makam, C. Khaw, S. Bae, X. Xu, P.-L.R. Ee, J.-H. Ahn, B.H. Hong, G. Pastorin, B. Özyilmaz, Graphene for controlled and accelerated osteogenic differentiation of human mesenchymal stem cells, ACS Nano 5 (2011) 4670–4678, https://doi.org/10.1021/nn200500h.
[77] S.R. Shin, S.M. Jung, M. Zalabany, K. Kim, P. Zorlutuna, S. bok Kim, M. Nikkhah, M. Khabiry, M. Azize, J. Kong, K. Wan, T. Palacios, M.R. Dokmeci, H. Bae, X. Tang, A. Khademhosseini, Carbon-nanotube-embedded hydrogel sheets for engineering cardiac constructs and bioactuators, ACS Nano 7 (2013) 2369–2380, https://doi.org/10.1021/nn305559j.
[78] S.R. Shin, B. Aghaei-Ghareh-Bolagh, T.T. Dang, S.N. Topkaya, X. Gao, S.Y. Yang, S.M. Jung, J.H. Oh, M.R. Dokmeci, X. Tang, A. Khademhosseini, Cell-laden microengineered and mechanically tunable hybrid hydrogels of gelatin and graphene oxide, Advanced Materials 25 (2013) 6385–6391, https://doi.org/10.1002/adma.201301082.
[79] C. Cha, S.R. Shin, X. Gao, N. Annabi, M.R. Dokmeci, X. Tang, A. Khademhosseini, Controlling mechanical properties of cell-laden hydrogels by covalent incorporation of graphene oxide, Small 10 (2014) 514–523, https://doi.org/10.1002/smll.201302182.
[80] B. Cai, S. Wang, L. Huang, Y. Ning, Z. Zhang, G.-J. Zhang, Ultrasensitive label-free detection of PNA–DNA hybridization by reduced graphene oxide field-effect transistor biosensor, ACS Nano 8 (2014) 2632–2638, https://doi.org/10.1021/nn4063424.
[81] D.-J. Kim, I.Y. Sohn, J.-H. Jung, O.J. Yoon, N.-E. Lee, J.-S. Park, Reduced graphene oxide field-effect transistor for label-free femtomolar protein detection, Biosensor and Bioelectronics 41 (2013) 621–626.
[82] J. Chang, S. Mao, Y. Zhang, S. Cui, G. Zhou, X. Wu, C.-H. Yang, J. Chen, Ultrasonic-assisted self-assembly of monolayer graphene oxide for rapid detection of *Escherichia coli* bacteria, Nanoscale 5 (2013) 3620–3626.
[83] B. Zhan, C. Li, J. Yang, G. Jenkins, W. Huang, X. Dong, Graphene field-effect transistor and its application for electronic sensing, Small 10 (2014) 4042–4065.
[84] M. Xu, T. Liang, M. Shi, H. Chen, Graphene-like two-dimensional materials, Chemical Reviews 113 (2013) 3766–3798.
[85] V. Nicolosi, M. Chhowalla, M.G. Kanatzidis, M.S. Strano, J.N. Coleman, Liquid exfoliation of layered materials, Science 340 (2013), 1226419.
[86] V. Sorkin, H. Pan, H. Shi, S.Y. Quek, Y.W. Zhang, Nanoscale transition metal dichalcogenides: structures, properties, and applications, Journal Critical Reviews in Solid State and Materials Sciences 39 (2014) 319–367.

[87] M. Pumera, A.H. Loo, Layered transition-metal dichalcogenides (MoS_2 and WS_2) for sensing and biosensing, TrAC Trends in Analytical Chemistry 61 (2014) 49–53.

[88] J.Z. Ou, A.F. Chrimes, Y. Wang, S. Tang, M.S. Strano, K. Kalantar-Zadeh, Ion-driven photoluminescence modulation of quasi-two-dimensional MoS_2 nanoflakes for applications in biological systems, Nano Letters 14 (2014) 857–863, https://doi.org/10.1021/nl4042356.

[89] D. Sarkar, W. Liu, X. Xie, A.C. Anselmo, S. Mitragotri, K. Banerjee, MoS_2 field-effect transistor for next-generation label-free biosensors, ACS Nano 8 (2014) 3992–4003, https://doi.org/10.1021/nn5009148.

[90] X. Qian, S. Shen, T. Liu, L. Cheng, Z. Liu, Two-dimensional TiS_2 nanosheets for in vivo photoacoustic imaging and photothermal cancer therapy, Nanoscale 7 (2015) 6380–6387, https://doi.org/10.1039/C5NR00893J.

CHAPTER 5

Terahertz Technology—Emerging Trends and Application Viewpoints

SUBAL KAR, MTECH, PHD (TECH)

INTRODUCTION

Terahertz (THz) covers the electromagnetic (EM) frequency spectrum from the upper edge of microwaves (>300 GHz) and going up to the lower edge of infrared (<or = 10 THz): typically from 0.5 THz to 10 THz (1 THz = 10^{12} Hz) with wavelengths from 160 to 30 μm and photon energy from 2 to 40 meV—that overlaps both the electronics and photonics (vide Fig. 5.1). Some industries, however, consider >100 GHz as the beginning of the THz regime with wavelength in the range from 3 mm to 30 μm.

Though THz radiation received attention from scientists since 100 years ago, the so-called "THz gap" of the EM spectrum remained unutilized till 1980s. This is because of the nonavailability of active and passive components for THz system development—as the THz region needs two different approaches for its development, the "electronics" and "photonics" of the EM radiation. On one side of the THz spectrum are the "radio waves" and "microwaves," that use antenna/aerial to radiate out and receive the EM signal, and electronics technology is used for signal generation and manipulation. On the other side is our well-known "visible light" that depends upon the electron transition between orbits of an atom giving rise to absorption or emission of photon; the light wave can be steered with mirrors and transmitted via well-known optical fiber. Since the THz frequencies are extremely high for electronics technology and also too low for optical technology, none of these technologies can be used as it is. In other

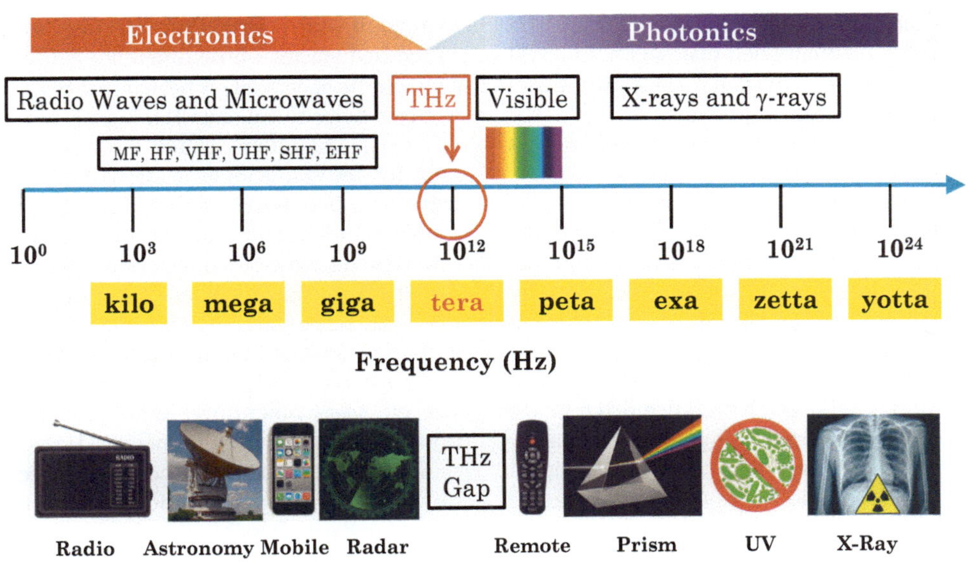

FIG. 5.1 Electromagnetic spectrum showing the location of terahertz (THz) frequency range and some applications in various other frequency ranges.

Terahertz Biomedical and Healthcare Technologies. https://doi.org/10.1016/B978-0-12-818556-8.00005-7

words, the THz region cannot use either microwave/millimeter-wave (MMW) devices and circuits, or optical devices and circuits directly. THz technology rather requires a combination of electronics and optics (i.e., photonics)—thus it a quasioptic domain. Till the end of 20th century, the technology required for THz band was much less mature than the technology for the region near 100 GHz (i.e., MMW). However, from the beginning of this century, especially during the last decade, the "THz gap" has no more remained as a gap and has become a frontier area for research in physics, chemistry, biology, medicine, and so forth with a lot of possible and emerging applications.

Anyway, it is worth mentioning that from the last 2 decades of 20th century, cataloging and mapping of thermal emission lines for a wide variety of lightweight molecules using THz spectroscopy were carried out by the Earth and planetary scientists including chemists. Many of the thermal emission lines were found to peak in the sub-MMW range, especially between 300 GHz and 2.5 THz, for gases that appear in the Earth's stratosphere and upper troposphere. It may be noted that, we receive a lot of information about these chemical species only in THz region and not anywhere else in the EM spectrum. The cold dust in the interstellar medium in the Milky Way galaxy and also in distant starburst galaxies is at 10 −20 K and it is known that the THz radiation is emitted as black body radiation from anything with temperatures greater than 10 K. Thus, astronomers are engaged in THz spectroscopy from the very beginning of the development of THz technology. It may be mentioned that, a ground-based interferometric telescope, Atacama Large Millimeter Array, located in the Atacama desert of Chile has recently planned to make stellar spectrometric studies at frequencies around 1.5 THz.

THz radiation are invisible to naked eye but can pass through cloths including paper, wood, cardboard, masonry, plastic, and ceramics, the penetration depth being much less than that of microwave/MMW radiation. They are reflected by metals and scattered by sharp edges even of plastic knives (similar to microwaves and MMW), hence they can be used for concealed weapon detection (CWD); but with much better image resolution as they are much higher in frequency compared with microwaves and MMW. THz signal has the advantages of radio waves (penetrating power in zero visibility) and also of optical waves (spectroscopic, i.e., chemical-discriminating capability). Thus, such rays can be used for standoff detection (meaning: "to see with its radio eye" a few meters/tens of meters away) of contraband, i.e., explosives (say RDX) which may otherwise seem identical to talcum powder visually or touching by hand. Water soaks up THz radiation, thus human tissue which has large water content absorbs it strongly. The healthy tissue and malignant tissues differ by large water content, and hence THz signal with its strong absorptivity and spectroscopic capability can help in early detection of cancer, especially the skin and breast cancer. But unlike X-rays (that has photon energy of hundreds of electron volt, eV), the THz radiation is nonionizing (photon energy: 2−40 meV), noninvasive, and known to be safe and harmless; if the exposure is not for too long a time and the power of THz radiation is not too high. Further, T-rays have very small skin depth, i.e., cannot penetrate much beyond our skin, and its photon energy lacks the capability to ionize molecules in human tissue (unlike X-rays, which are ionizing radiation); so it cannot cause cancer by smashing up our DNA. Moreover, the power levels of most T-ray imagers used for medical diagnosis are lower than that of the infrared LED used in our TV remote control and hence are practically harmless at any count.

THz signal generation is a real challenge as the commonly used junction and bulk semiconductor devices or tube devices used at RF and microwave/MMW frequencies cannot be simply scaled down in size to operate at THz frequency. Thus, various novel techniques have been developed during last 2 decades to generate THz signal most of which are based on optical techniques in some form or the other. Optical heterodyning, in which signal from two laser sources (tuned to the frequencies whose difference is the desired THz signal to be generated) is beated in a photodiode/photomixer, helps to generate THz signal in microwatt power level. Quantum cascade laser (QCL) is also an attractive technique for generation of milliwatt level power at THz frequency with broad bandwidth. However, for few hundred milliwatt to watt level THz signal generation accelerator-based technique (free-electron laser [FEL]) may be used to generate THz signal over a broad frequency range. Each technique has its own advantages and disadvantages in terms of the level of power being generated, cost, complexity, need for cryogenic cooling, size, etc. Many other novel techniques are also coming up every new morning to generate THz signal.

THz detection/sensing and also image reconstruction with THz imaging technique is again a challenging field of research. Possibly THz detector/sensor development has progressed faster than any other sub-MMW technology. Detection of THz signal can be done either by latest generation Schottky diode or by quantum-limited detectors similar to photodetectors used at optical frequencies. Both of these detection techniques have relative advantages and disadvantages. It may be mentioned that detection is only the first step of image making—the image reconstruction is a more involved process of signal processing which uses various algorithmic and digital signal processing techniques.

In this chapter, we would first discuss the limitations of the conventional RF, microwave, and MMW approach of designing THz signal generators on the basis of size scaling with frequency of operation. Then we would discuss in detail how optical heterodyning technique, QCL technique, FEL technique, and many other optical techniques can solve the problem of generating THz signal. In addition to signal generation, the techniques of THz signal detection/sensing will also be discussed including some THz components. In addition to a brief discussion on THz time-domain spectroscopy (THZ-TDS), the application potential of THz frequency for security, medical, and other emerging purposes will also be discussed. The development of THz metamaterial and their application possibilities will also be addressed as in the recent times metamaterials are opening up a vast new possibility of the design of THz sensors and other components with improved performance and size miniaturization.

LIMITATIONS OF CONVENTIONAL RF, MICROWAVE, AND MILLIMETER-WAVE TECHNIQUES FOR THZ SIGNAL GENERATION

RF, microwave, and MMW signal is conventionally generated by electronic technique by mounting the device in a suitably designed cavity. Signal generation at GHz frequency is not a big deal—IMPATT device can generate even up to 480 GHz signal; but it's quite challenging to build a circuit that oscillates at THz rate (i.e., trillions of times per second). In the following, we would discuss in brief the electronic techniques for generation of microwave and MMW signal using solid-state devices like Gunn (a bulk semiconductor device) and IMPATT (IMPact Avalanche Transit Time, a semiconductor junction device) and would comment on the limitations of such electronic techniques for THz signal generation. In a Gunn device, electrons are nucleated at the cathode and after traversing/transiting via the length of the bulk semiconductor (GaAs/InP) quenches at the anode, while in an IMPATT device electrons are generated by avalanche process under high-field effect and then transit via the transit-time region. In both the cases, negative resistance is realized as the generated RF current lags behind the applied voltage by 180degrees and thus operates as negative resistance oscillator/amplifier. In both Gunn and IMPATT devices, the length of the transit-time zone determines the frequency of oscillation which becomes smaller with increasing frequency of operation.

The Gunn/IMPATT device mounting in waveguide cavity may either be done through a bias-post in a reduced-height waveguide and connected to load via a taper/stepped impedance transformer for impedance matching (vide Fig. 5.2A) or through a resonant-cap in a full-height waveguide (vide Fig. 5.2B) for microwave/MMW signal generation [1]. Post mounted oscillators are not very efficient due to the lack of proper impedance matching between the device and the circuit in which the device is embedded. In resonant-cap oscillator, the radius of the cap structure determines the oscillation frequency. The cap structure acts as a quarter-wave impedance transformer between the resonant-cap cavity (formed between the bottom surface of the cap and the bottom wall of the waveguide acting as radial transmission line) and the full-height waveguide in which the device and the cap structures are mounted. Oscillator tuning is done by the back-short tuner as shown in Fig. 5.2.

Yet another way to design an IMPATT-based MMW oscillator is to mount the device in a coaxial-waveguide cavity. This provides broadband operation of the oscillator by generating the MMW signal in the coaxial structure realized with the coaxial spacers (vide Fig. 5.3). The coaxial spacers help to match the impedance of the device with the iris in the center of the bottom wall of the reduced-height waveguide. The holes in the spacers

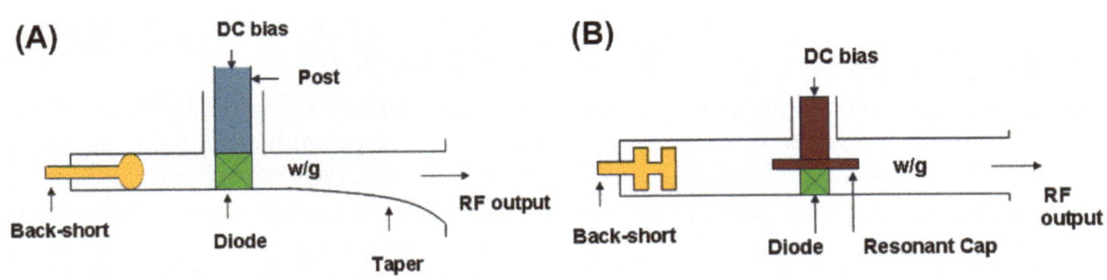

FIG. 5.2 Microwave/millimeter-wave oscillator configurations. **(A)** Post mounted oscillator, **(B)** resonant-cap mounted oscillator [1].

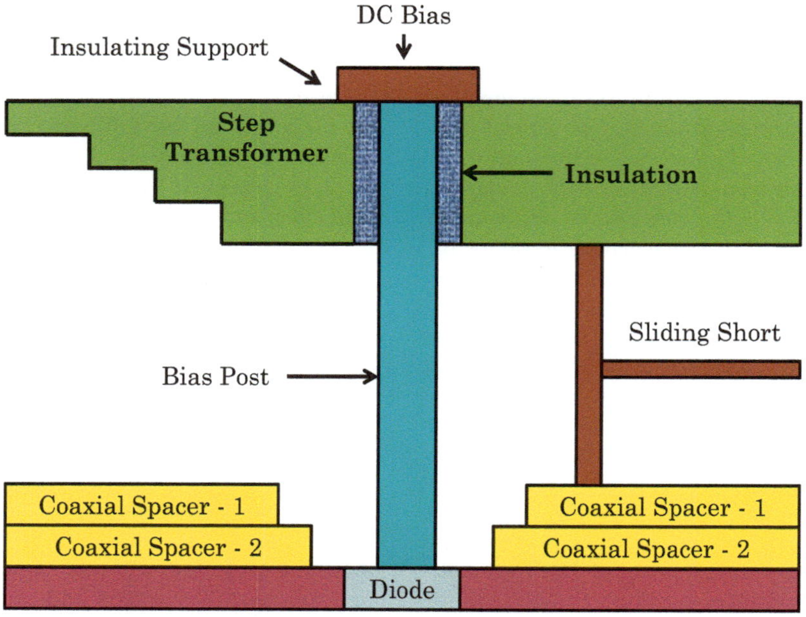

FIG. 5.3 Coaxial-waveguide cavity mount for millimeter-wave signal generation [2].

help to optimize the coupling of the signal from the device to the circuit. The coaxial-waveguide mount shown in Fig. 5.3 can provide a tuning bandwidth of 20% at 34.25 GHz having a power output of nearly 1.0 Watt using GaAs DDR IMPATT diode [2].

However, sub-MMW and especially the THz signal generation with reasonable phase noise required for communication applications has not yet been possible due to inherent technical limitations of electronic techniques. Though solid-state source like Gunn, especially IMPATT may be used in conjunction with Schottky multiplier for THz signal generation but that is only of the order of microwatt with narrow bandwidth at 1.5 THz. Commercially available IMPATT-Schottky multiplier-based THz sources are available at 300 GHz having milliwatt power levels [3]. Reactive mixing is used for such Schottky multipliers with frequency doubler/tripler configuration. Comb generators or higher-order multipliers are not used due their higher conversion loss. In space applications, InP MMIC (Monolithic Microwave Integrated Circuit) amplifiers and spatial power combined IMPATT sources with Schottky multiplier chain is used rather than bulky power-hungry lasers (optical technique) or short-lived very-heavy kilovolt-driven tube sources. Tube devices like carcinotron (a form of backward-wave oscillator), klystron, and gyrotron tubes can generate few hundred GHz signal but again THz signal generation has not yet been possible in the true sense with any of these devices that operate with electronic technique. The reason for this may be understood as follows. For Gunn device, the length of the bulk device determines the frequency of operation thus to generate THz signal it would demand an impractically small length of the semiconductor sample which cannot be fabricated with due accuracy. For IMPATT device, similarly the length of the transit-time zone will become impractically small at THz frequency. Thus, traditional electronic solid-state sources (oscillators/amplifiers) at microwave and MMW frequencies based on semiconductors are limited by transit times and also reactive parasitic at THz frequencies becomes excessively high causing high-frequency roll-off a problem. Tube sources are limited by simple physical scaling problems including metallic losses, and the need for extremely high fields (both magnetic and electric), as well as high current densities at THz frequency. However, research is going on to develop innovative techniques to generate THz signal with semiconductor devices either with single device (especially with IMPATT device) or using power combining technique.

OPTICAL MEANS OF THZ SIGNAL GENERATION

It is difficult to generate THz signal with solid-state laser which is very common at optical frequency. This is because the irradiative recombination of conduction band electrons with valence band holes across the bandgap of the active material is easily realizable with photon energy available at optical frequency. But at THz frequency range, the photon energy is only in meV range and suitable narrow bandgap semiconductors are not available at THz frequency range. Thus, successful techniques for generating THz power with optical means may be either with heterodyning of laser sources or with QCL or with irradiation of photoconductive material or electro-optic or other nonlinear crystal with femtosecond laser and so forth. In this section, we would discuss the principle of THz signal generation with various such optical techniques.

Optical Heterodyning for THz Signal Generation

There are various optical heterodyning techniques for THz signal generation of which we would discuss two of the techniques in Figs. 5.4 and 5.5.

Injection locking or optical phase locking of two laser sources

Here two laser sources (the slave laser I and slave laser II) can be injection locked (IL) to the two selected sidebands of a frequency modulated (FM) master laser or the two selected FM sidebands of the master laser after being processed through optical phase-lock loops (OPLLs) are beated in a photodetector to produce the MMW/THz signal [4,5]. Since the two beating optical signals are either injection or phase locked to a reference source (master laser), the generated beat signal (MMW/THz signal) will have low phase noise. The low phase noise (or equivalently the low time jitter) is of advantage for high data-rate communication which the THz communication system is capable of. It may be noted that in the IL system the locking range is restricted by stability considerations, while OPLL system is limited by the requirement of very short loop propagation delay.

A novel modified OPLL system

Here judicious use of cascaded Mach-Zehnder modulators has been made whose output consists of optical carrier having amplitude J_0 (X) and sideband amplitudes are J_2 (X), J_4 (X) …, which is at twice the modulation frequency. This reduces the sideband pulling and pushing effect normally found in conventional IL system thereby increasing the locking capability of the signal. Further, the requirement of subnanosecond loop delay of conventional OPLL is overcome by using additional phase modulator incorporated in the loop. This reduces the effective phase error resulting in better noise rejection capability and also the frequency of cycle slips is considerably reduced making the system highly stable [6].

The methods discussed above can generate tens of microwatts of THz signal. The key factor in the development of such THz generator is the photomixer/photodetector, made of InGaAs (indium gallium arsenide), which can mix lasers of two different frequencies efficiently and that can be easily carried on optical fibers. Channeling the lasers on optical fibers (instead of going for carefully alignment of laser beams with expensive optics) has greatly simplified THz imagers [7] and also has the added benefit of driving down their cost.

Quantum Cascade Laser for THz Signal Generation

Bell Labs team headed by Jérôme Faist and Federico Capasso first demonstrated the QCLs in 1994 [7,8]. The difference between an ordinary light emitter and a laser is that in the latter case there are always more electrons in the excited state in the upper energy level than in the lower energy level (known as population inversion) realized by pump signal. The pumping may be either optical pumping or electronic pumping, the former being used in solid-state laser like ruby laser, while the latter is used in gas laser like helium-neon laser and so forth. However, conventional laser sources be it semiconductor diode laser or gas laser are inherently narrowband as their operational frequencies are determined by specific molecular transitions.

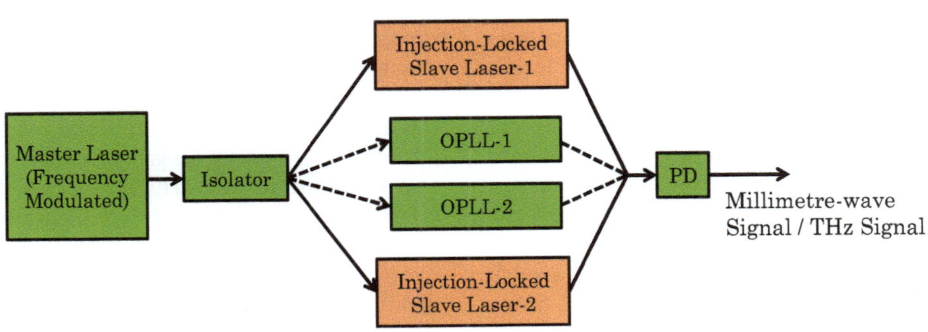

FIG. 5.4 Injection locking or optical phase locking of two slave lasers for millimeter-wave/THz signal generation [4,5].

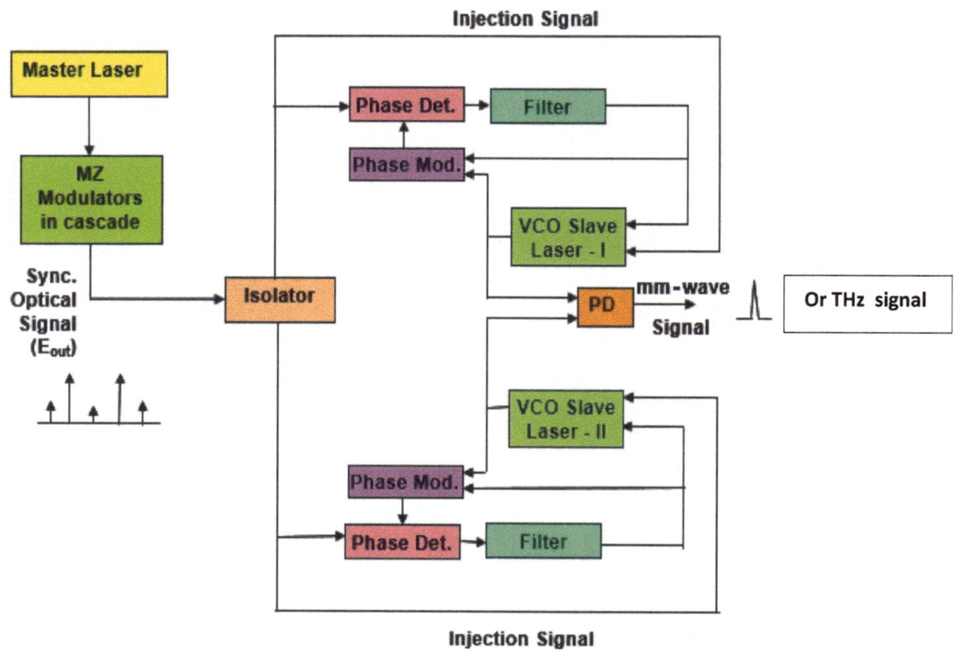

FIG. 5.5 A novel modified optical phase-lock loop system for millimeter-wave/THz signal generation [6].

A totally different principle of coherent signal generation is followed in QCL. Here the photon is not being generated due to interband transition of electron, from conduction band to valance band, and the electron does not get annihilated by combining with hole in the valance band by emitting a photon. Lasing action in QCL is achieved through the use of intersubband transitions of only one type of carrier, the electrons, which takes place in a multiple quantum-well heterostructures and hence QCLs are unipolar, unlike conventional laser which is bipolar (where both electrons and holes are involved in the process of laser signal generation). As quantum wells are very thin structures, from an electrons perspective, they are considered to be two dimensional.

In QCL, there are three energy levels (or quantum wells), each nanometer thick. When an electron is injected into the highest energy level, it falls to the lower one, emitting radiation (photon) of frequency that is determined by the thickness of the quantum well. The electron then immediately falls into the still lower energy level, the third state, when a quantum of heat called phonon is emitted. It is possible to engineer a population inversion between two subbands in the system (which is required in order to achieve laser emission) by suitably designing the layer thickness (which determines the thickness of the quantum well). Since, it is not the material property but the thickness of the layer that determines the position of the energy levels in the system, it is possible to tune the emission frequency of QCLs over a wide frequency range (i.e., broadband operation) in the same material.

Unlike conventional laser, a QCL does not use bulk semiconductor materials in its optically active region. It consists of a periodic series of thin layers of varying material composition forming a superlattice. The first QCL was fabricated in the GaInAs/AlInAs material system lattice matched to an InP substrate. In QCL, once an electron has undergone an intersubband transition and emitted a photon in one period of the superlattice, it can tunnel into the next period of the structure (through the quantum well) where another photon can be emitted (vide Fig. 5.6). It is important to note that the above-mentioned three-layered structure can be repeated a number of times and at each structure the electron goes through the same dance, emitting the same color (i.e., frequency) photon. This process of a single electron causing the emission of multiple photons as it traverses through the QCL structure gives rise to the name *cascade* and makes the quantum efficiency of the device greater than unity possible which leads to higher output powers than semiconductor laser diodes.

QCL has become more attractive than optical heterodyning technique as they are broadband and capable to give higher power (of the order of milliwatts) THz signal. However, initial systems desired cryogenic cooling for higher THz signal generation but now-a-days room-temperature QCLs are under development at THz frequency.

Other Laser-based Techniques for THz Signal Generation

These are mostly dependent on nonlinear interaction of optical laser pulses with crystals. These methods suffer from the drawback of low levels of power generated (no more than 100 mW per pulse/microwatt CW power) and low tunability of optical lasers. Since the THz pulses are produced in these methods in an optically nonlinear crystal, the spectral range is also limited by the material properties.

One of these optical techniques for producing THz energy is based on using a short pulse (femtosecond) optical laser (argon laser-pumped Ti:sapphire laser), in which the photon energy is greater than the bandgap of the material. Here the laser pulse illuminates a gap between two closely spaced electrodes on a photoconductor: silicon on sapphire or low-temperature-grown (LTG)-GaAs, InP, generating carriers, which are then accelerated with the help of an applied DC electric field [9–12], vide Fig. 5.7A. The photoexcited carriers constitute a transient current pulse, whereby THz radiation is produced in accordance with Maxwell's equations. THz radiation thus generated is being coupled out via a lens antenna as shown in Fig. 5.7B.

This photoconduction approach is capable to produce relatively large average THz power of 40 μW at 3 THz. This operates with low input power but the beam is stable with good temporal characteristics. Thus, it is useful for spectroscopy and THz imaging technologies.

Another technique of THz signal generation is based on short laser pulses being applied to an electro-optic crystal (ZnTe) having large second-order susceptibility (field-induced polarization) [10,13]. Since the higher-order susceptibility terms have nonlinear response, mixing occurs, producing a time-varying polarization with a frequency-response representative of the pulse length, i.e., THz oscillation. This technique can produce nW to μW power output of THz signal.

Yet another pulsed laser technique capable of producing relatively high levels of THz output power uses

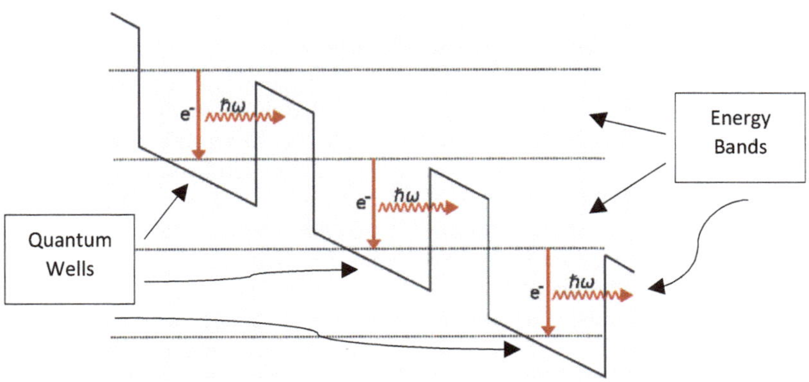

FIG. 5.6 Transition of electron via different quantum wells in quantum cascade laser emitting a photon in each case (https://commons.wikimedia.org/w/index.php?curid=2647294).

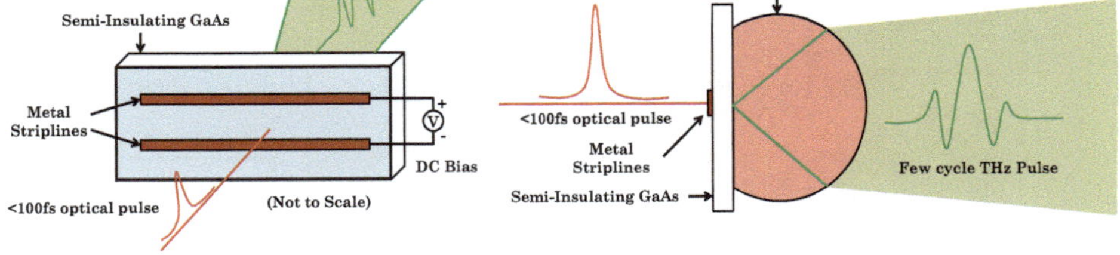

FIG. 5.7 Laser-based photoconduction approach of THz signal generation. **(A)** Side view of scheme. **(B)** Top view of scheme (Picture from the presentation entitled Outline on THz Applications of Junji Urakawa, KEK, Japan, 06–09 March, 2018; who referred Paul A. George of Cornell University, US.)

a switched Nd:YAG laser to illuminate a LiNbO sample causing optical parametric oscillation via the crystal. The parametric process creates a near-IR frequency close in wavelength to that of the Nd:YAG pump and a THz difference signal. A prism coupler helps to extract the THz power and tuning can be realized by changing the incident angle of the Nd:YAG laser. The system is capable to produce pulsed power output as high as 3 mW at 1.8 THz [10,14].

THz signal may also be generated with IR-pumped gas lasers. This technique uses grating tuned CO_2 pump lasers (20−100 W) injected into low-pressure flowing-gas cavity that lase to produce the THz signals. Power levels of 1−20 mW are common depending on the line being used, with one of the strongest being that of methanol at 2522.78 GHz [10].

Every new morning it is seen that new techniques of THz signal generation is coming up—a resonant tunneling diode is capable of generating THz signal that may be used in next-generation THz communication systems [15].

ACCELERATOR TECHNOLOGY-BASED THZ SIGNAL GENERATION

Most of the THz-wave sources in current use are based on semiconductor technology using either optical heterodyning or QCL or other novel techniques like the nonlinear interaction of optical laser pulses with crystals and so on. The primary drawbacks of these methods include the low level of power that can be generated (microwatt to milliwatt level power) and the lack of tunability in some cases. However, FEL based on accelerator technology can produce high-power (hundreds of milliwatt to watt level) coherent radiation in the THz region [16]. In such sources, frequency can be tuned continuously, the pulse length can be very short, and very high intensities can be realized. These characteristics make FEL an extremely attractive source of coherent THz radiation. However, these appealing features of FELs (i.e., their tunability and high power) are usually counterbalanced by some drawbacks, such as large size, high cost, and system complexity. But, FEL-based THz signal is powerful enough to penetrate some distance into the ground and can detect landmines and improvised explosive device at a distance. Thus, US defense use such FEL-based T-ray imagers with typically hundreds of milliwatts to watt range power or so for security purposes in today's society plagued with security hazards.

Unlike conventional laser, where electrons are bound into the atoms and molecules, in FEL, coherent radiation is produced from a beam of free electrons that are accelerated very close to the velocity of light before being passed through a periodic arrangement of magnets with alternating poles (known as undulators) placed across the path of the electron beam. The lasing medium in FEL is the very high-speed electrons, and since they move freely through the magnetic structure, the term "free electron." The FEL is broadly tunable, covering the frequency range from microwaves, through THz radiation, and going up to soft X-ray frequency. The frequency of the emitted radiation can be readily tuned by adjusting the energy of the electron beam or the magnetic field strength of the undulators. John Madey of Stanford University invented FEL in 1971.

The direction of the electron beam shot through the so-called undulator or wiggler system is longitudinal, while the direction of the magnetic field of the undulator is perpendicular to the path of electron beam, as shown in Fig. 5.8. A structure consisting of a series of dipole magnets of alternating magnetic fields B is known as undulator. The electrons shot through the undulator is guided along a sinusoidal path transverse to the magnetic field (follows from Lorentz force, causing electron beam to wiggle, i.e., "twist" transversely to the magnetic field) (vide Fig. 5.8). When electrons get accelerated in each magnet, a series of radiation pulses are emitted. In an undulator, these

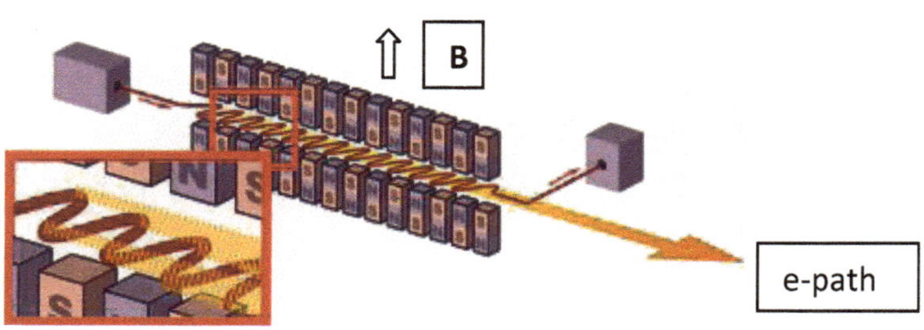

FIG. 5.8 Schematic representation of an undulator at the core of a free-electron laser (https://en.wikipedia.org/wiki/Free-electron_laser#/media/File:FEL_principle.png).

pulses interfere constructively at the radiation wavelength. A properly designed undulator can emit intense THz radiation when the electrons get "bunched" in the undulator thereby emitting radiation coherently [17].

When lightweight charged particles (electrons/positrons) are speeded up to the relativistic velocities, they experience transverse acceleration in the magnetic field of the undulator, thereby emitting photons, i.e., synchrotron radiation (SR). These radiations are monochromatic (i.e., with single frequency) but still incoherent, because in this situation EM wave is generated by constructive/destructive interference of electrons those are distributed with random phase. But if by some means one can realize lock-synchronism of electrons, then coherent emission of radiation is possible and the electric field grows linearly with the number of electrons unlike scaling of radiated power with number of electrons (N) in nonsynchronized situation. The power then varies with the square of the field, and if N is very large, one can realize an enormous gain in emitted power and thus very high-power output is possible with such laser system.

To realize lock-synchronization of electrons, either an external excitation may be provided in the system or mirrors may be placed at each end of the undulator to create an optical cavity causing radiation to form standing waves. In either case, the SR becomes sufficiently strong and the electric field of the radiation beam interacts with the transverse electron current created by the sinusoidal wiggling motion. Due to this interaction of radiation beam and electron current, some electrons will gain and others will lose energy to the optical field. This energy modulation of electrons will result in electron density (current) modulation once per cycle at the optical frequency. The electrons thus form "microbunches" on being longitudinally clumped separated by one optical wavelength along the axis. In the undulator alone, the electrons were radiating randomly (i.e., incoherently), but now the radiation emitted by the "bunched electrons" is in phase, and the fields add together coherently. The radiation intensity continuously grows in this way, causing additional microbunching of the electrons, which radiates in phase with each other. Until the electrons are completely microbunched (that may contain of the order of several hundred million electrons), this process of microbunching continues and the radiation reaches a saturated power several orders of magnitude higher than that of the radiation that was possible with the undulator alone with unbunched (i.e., randomly moving) electrons.

With near-infrared FELs, beam energies of the order of 40 MeV are realizable. For a longer wavelength machine, the beam energy may be in the range of 10–15 MeV. Lowering the beam energy requirement significantly below 15 MeV needs reduced shielding complexity, and thus lowers the cost and space requirements. THz FELs are therefore cheaper and thus have lower technical risk compared with FELs operating at shorter wavelengths of optical frequency.

Significantly low-cost, portable FELs are also available in the THz region. A compact, monochromatic, tunable, and high-power THz source is expected to be one of the key technologies in THz applications of the future. Several works have been reported that can realize compact THz FEL. A relatively high-power table-top THz FEL has been designed [18] useful for security inspection at airports, in public facilities, and also in principal buildings. The size of the system is typically $1 \times 2\ m^2$ and uses a 600 mm long helical undulator and a compact 4 MeV microtron accelerator based on magnetron oscillator. The average THz power is 1 W, with a tunable wavelength range from 200 to 600 μm (i.e., from 0.5 THz to 1.5 THz). Although the power of these compact devices is not very high, some users prefer such table-top sources because of their compactness, low cost, and convenience of use.

THZ SIGNAL DETECTION/SENSING AND IMAGE RECONSTRUCTION TECHNIQUES

The signal detection at THz frequency can be done either by semiconductor sensors like Schottky diode detector or quantum-limited detectors (similar to photodetectors at optical frequency). It is expected that individual photon counters would soon be available as THz detectors just as photomultipliers do for optical frequencies. Single photon detection has been realized for signals in the range of 1.4–1.7 THz [10].

For applications where low to medium sensitivity of detection suffices, the semiconductor-based honeycomb Schottky diode mixer is used as downconverter for THz frequency range. Such a diode mixer with fully integrated planer geometry [10] has been designed and space qualified up to 2.5 THz. Receivers based on room-temperature Schottky diode mixers typically have radiometric sensitivities near 0.05 K at 500 GHz and 0.5 K at 2.5 THz for a one-second integration time and a 1-GHz predetection bandwidth. This is sufficient for detecting many naturally occurring thermal emission lines for astronomical and atmospheric studies [10]. For high sensitivity detection in the THz range cryogenic cooling is used. Several superconducting heterodyne detectors including those based on the Josephson effect, superconductor-semiconductor barriers (super-Schottky), and bolometric devices have also been developed. However, the superconducting equivalent of the Schottky diode downconverter (in terms of widespread use below 1 THz) is the superconductor-insulator-superconductor (SIS) tunnel junction mixer [10]. An alternative to THz SIS mixers that has also become important during last few years is the transition-edge or hot-electron bolometer (HEB) mixer. Modern HEB mixers are based on extremely small microbridges of niobium, niobium-nitride, or niobium-titanium–nitride that respond thermally to THz radiation [10].

The problem with the detection of THz signal compared with optical frequencies using quantum-limited device similar to photodiode lies in the low photon energies (2–40 meV) of the former. Due to this, as the naturally emitted narrowband signals are always dominated by ambient background thermal noise, the requirement of either cryogenic cooling of the detector elements or long integration-time radiometric techniques or both becomes essential. Also some form of matched director (antenna) is required to be placed between the signal and the sensor element. The antenna for detection purpose performs just the opposite function than that is done for radiating the signal from an antenna. Here the photosensitive antenna irradiated by the THz pulse creates short-lived electrons and holes. Under the influence of the electric field of the incident THz waves, these electrons then flow through the antenna. So the current in the antenna, which is eventually amplified, acts as a measure of THz radiation. Because the detector is sensing T-rays only during the picosecond pulse duration, several pulses are required to get the full waveform of the incoming T-rays which is done by signal processing in a computer. The same scheme works when pairs of tuned laser are used instead of pulses in which the lasers are tuned so that the difference in their frequency is equal to the desired THz frequency. In this situation, when T-rays hit the antenna, they mix with the THz frequency generated by the combined lasers to produce a DC signal which is the eventual indicator of the input THz signal.

Anyway, detection is only the first step for image formation. The actual image formation is more involved, one of the techniques for actual image formation is raster scanning that records the phase and amplitude of the T-rays reflected from each scanning point of the object. Such scanning may be at the rate of 100 pixels per second; this is, however, not sufficient for video and only marginal for scanning a bag on a conveyor belt. In an effort to get speed and spectrometry, interferometric imaging technique may be used [7]. This method relies on the spatial Fourier transform, which is a common mathematical concept used in image processing technology. According to Fourier theory, any signal can be broken into the sum of many sinusoidal waves of different frequencies, phases, and amplitudes—an image is also known to be defined by these parameters. Instead of obtaining the image itself, an interferometric imager derives a pictures spatial Fourier transform from a measure of the electric field sensed by the detectors when a THz wave reaches a pair of detectors. Then the transformation is reversed in a computer to get the real image. In an interferometric imager, spatial frequencies are represented by the distance between two detectors on an array and the number of spatial frequencies can be increased by increasing the number of detectors which improves the image resolution. An imager made of 12 detectors arranged in a spiral pattern on a 1-meter disc can measure 66 spatial frequencies which can resolve a 2.5-centimeter square of RDX plastic explosive at a standoff distance of 50 m [7]. The Fourier image is acquired almost instantly, and the main limit on the image formation is the time it takes the computer to digitize the data from the detected signal and perform the necessary calculation. The resolution of a reversed transformed image comes from the number and arrangement of spatial frequencies represented in the transform—higher the spatial frequency, i.e., larger the detecting cameras, better is the image resolution.

THZ SYSTEM COMPONENTS

Both quasioptical and waveguide system (commonly used in microwave and MMW technology) are used at THz frequency to realize THz system components like couplers, resonators, polarizers, filters, antennae, etc. However, quasioptical components are expensive but readily available (as optical technology is more mature than THz technology as of today). To make a THz system smaller, lighter, and cheaper, waveguide structures offer distinct advantages like better isolation, wider choice of implementation solution, and integration with active devices over their quasioptical counterparts; the later also demands critical alignment accuracy. However, the THz systems operating all over the world are still using quasioptical-based systems in a number of applications.

High-performance guided-wave technologies used at THz frequencies may be all metal, metal-dielectric combination, or even all dielectric [19]. In general, since dielectrics can provide much lower losses compared with that is possible with room-temperature conductors, lower loss (i.e., high quality factor) passive components can be realized by minimizing conduction current densities and avoiding the use of metals altogether. However, in practice, hollow monolithic metal-pipe waveguides and horn antennas are still very much in use. A recent report [20] shows a 3 THz meandered metal-pipe rectangular waveguide with H-plane horn antenna coupling, which is manufactured using conventional surface micromachining and with electroplated gold walls. Silver-coated PTFE circular waveguides are also in use for 1.0–1.6 THz frequency range.

Conventional optical components can be used in the THz frequency region; however, they have inferior performance and have higher cost compared with that possible at much shorter optical wavelengths. As a result, a significant improvement in design and further development for ultra-broadband THz applications is needed. For example, in many quasioptical benches, a polarizer with high extinction ratio and broadband performance is an essential requirement. The wire-grid polarizer that is popularly used at present in THz frequencies has inferior extinction ratio and they are also more expensive than those in the optical region [19]. In recent times, new THz polarizer that has been developed using exotic materials such as liquid crystals and carbon nanotubes offers extinction ratios as high as 50 dB, which is comparable with those at shorter wavelengths. Filters are known to be indispensable components in spectroscopy. Metal-mesh filters are in use for a long time at MMW frequencies, which has recently been extended to the sub-MMW (i.e., THz) region; these are now understood to be a class of metamaterials or metasurfaces [21].

"Tunable metamaterials" have the potential to be an effective solution to develop practical THz quasioptics. Metamaterials are artificial metal-dielectric structures that can be engineered for the user-based control of microwave/MMW and THz waves. Good conductors have lower losses at THz frequencies compared with those at optical frequencies. Thus, the basic concept of the metal-mesh filter can be extended to other forms of metamaterials that can be used to realize high-performance THz quasioptics. Moreover, both MEMS and photoexcitation technologies may have a future role to play in realizing tuneable metamaterial properties at THz frequency [22] for passive component development.

THZ TIME-DOMAIN SPECTROSCOPY

In the THz frequency range (particularly >1 THz), many materials exhibit characteristic spectral features thereby enabling THz spectroscopy to be used as a tool to uniquely identify chemical species. In addition to addressing the intramolecular vibrational modes, THz spectroscopy can also excite intermolecular vibrations. Due to these reasons, the THz spectroscopy is found to have potential to provide both chemical and structural information of the object being studied.

During the last 2 decades, the most intriguing application for commercializing THz technology has been in the area of THz-TDS or T-ray imaging. T-ray imaging is a very attractive tool for the medical community, as well as for nondestructive probing of biological materials for pharmacists. The investigation of illegal materials and drugs and explosives for security purposes has also become the most important applications of THz imaging in recent times. Many companies around the world, Picometrix and Teraview in the United States, have commercialized it.

In the Picometrix system, in situ measurements of the reflected and transmitted THz energy incident upon the sample are processed to get the spectral content, refractive index, amplitude, and phase of the imaged signal. Fig. 5.9 shows the scheme of such a TDS system.

Here the generation and detection of THz EM transients produced in a photoconductor irradiated with femtosecond optical laser pulses are carried out [10,23]. The laser pulses are then beam-split and are synchronized through a scanning optical delay line

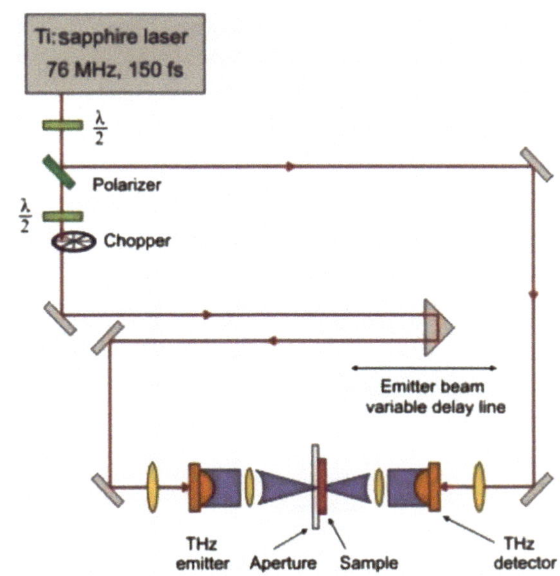

FIG. 5.9 Terahertz (THz) time-domain spectroscopy using photoconductive technique of signal generation and detection. (Picture from the presentation entitled "Outline on THz Applications" of Junji Urakawa, KEK, Japan, 06–09 March, 2018.)

which is finally made to strike the THz generator and detector in known phase coherence. A time-dependent waveform proportional to the THz field amplitude and containing the frequency response of the sample is thus obtained by scanning the delay line and simultaneously gating or sampling the THz signals incident on the detector. Here the photoconductive effect in LTG GaAs or radiation-damaged silicon on sapphire is used for both the generator and detector (vide Fig. 5.9). Though the experimental details might vary between different systems, however, in this example two vacuum-evaporated NiCr/Au electrodes, separated by a submillimetre-wide gap, fabricated on a 1-mm-thick LTG GaAs layer (which is grown on an undoped GaAs substrate itself) comprises the emitter. Suitably annealed LT-GaAs is an ideal material for this application which provides short photocarrier recombination lifetimes (a few hundred femtoseconds), together with both high resistivity (which allows high electric fields to be used) and high carrier mobility. A bias voltage of around 100 V, modulated at a few kilohertz, is applied between the emitter electrodes. The femtosecond optical pulses are currently derived from expensive Ti:Sapphire lasers (but much effort is being placed to get it done with solid-state devices). The Ti:sapphire laser beam, typically of a few hundred milliwatts average power (100 fs pulse width, 800 nm center wavelength), is focused onto the edge of one of the two electrodes of the photoconductor, and THz pulses are generated as described previously (vide Fig. 5.7). The RF signals produced by the optical pulses in present systems typically peak in the 0.5–2 THz range and have average power levels in the microwatt range and peak energies around a femtojoule.

The teraview system is based on the ultrafast Pockels effect in which an electro-optical sampling detection crystal (e.g., <110> ZnTe) is irradiated with THz signal [11,12]. The THz field induces an instantaneous birefringence in the electro-optic medium, which can be probed with a second visible/near-IR beam, initially split from the pump beam. The ellipticity of the probe beam is modulated with birefringence, which is measured using a quarter-wave ($\lambda/4$) plate, a Wollaston polarization splitting prism, and two balanced photodiodes. Using the modulated bias field of the photoconductive emitter as a reference, one can measure the photodiode signal using lock-in technique. Further, the electric field in the THz pulse in the time domain can be obtained by measurement of the signal as a function of time delay between the arrival of the THz signal and the probe pulse at the electro-optic crystal using a variable delay line. Finally, the Fourier transform gives the frequency spectrum of the THz radiation; the scheme of the TDS system together with time-domain to frequency-domain conversion of the output signal is shown in Fig. 5.10.

APPLICATION VIEWPOINTS OF T-RAYS

Security Applications

Concealed weapon detection

In controlled access settings like airports, entrances to sensitive buildings, and public events manual screening procedures for detecting concealed weapons such as handguns, knives, and explosives are still a common practice. However, it has long been an important obstacle to the improvement of the security of the general public as well as the safety of public assets like

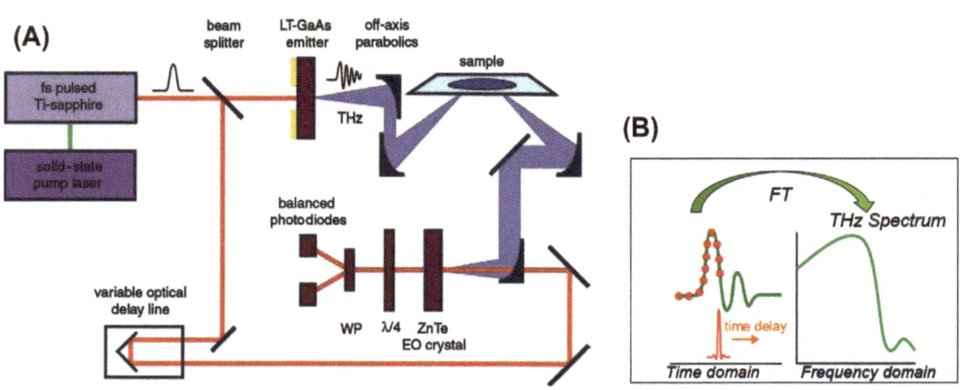

FIG. 5.10 **(A)** Schematic of terahertz (THz) time-domain spectroscopy system based on electro-optic crystal. **(B)** Time-domain to frequency-domain conversion of output signal. (**(A)**. Reprinted/Adapted with permission from A.G. Davies, A.D. Burnett, W. Fan, E.H. Linfield, J.E. Cunningham, Terahertz spectroscopy of explosives and drugs, Materials Today 11(3) (2008) 18–26 ©. Elsevier Ltd.)

airports and heritage buildings in detecting weapons concealed underneath a person's clothing, especially for heavy clothing. It is necessary in many situations to detect concealed weapons from a standoff distance, especially when it is impossible to arrange the flow of people through a controlled procedure. Thus, deployment of automatic detection and recognition of concealed weapons is an absolute necessity for security purposes. Innovative solutions in sensor technologies and image processing are essential to address such technological challenge. A number of sensor-based technologies as well as image processing techniques have been developed during last two to three decades using MMWs and THz radiation to make standoff detection of weapons underneath people's clothing or detection of concealed explosives/drugs, etc.

MMW active imaging systems are available for short range 3−10 m standoff detection of concealed weapons using FM-CW active radar imaging system [24]. The system is portable enough to be located in an entry point of school, airport, and sensitive building. The image processing can be done and evaluated at a colocated workstation or the system could be plugged into a building network and concealed weapon data may be viewed and analyzed at a central monitoring center.

The heart of the scanning system as shown in Fig. 5.11A is a 91 GHz Gunn oscillator. The output of the oscillator is mixed with a 2−4 GHz ramp generated from a voltage controlled oscillator (VCO). The upconverted mixer output signal thus obtained is transmitted through a circulator and radiated out through an antenna as (93−95) GHz signal. Lower band (87−89) GHz energy is filtered in the upconverter and band limited by the circulator preventing it from getting radiated by the antenna. The returned energy from the target propagates through the circulator and is then mixed with another portion of the 91 GHz Gunn oscillator output to obtain downconverted signal via the designated mixer and after filtering again mixed in another mixer with the 2−4 GHz ramp signal from the VCO. The output from this final mixer stage is then filtered and amplified for data acquisition. With such MMW

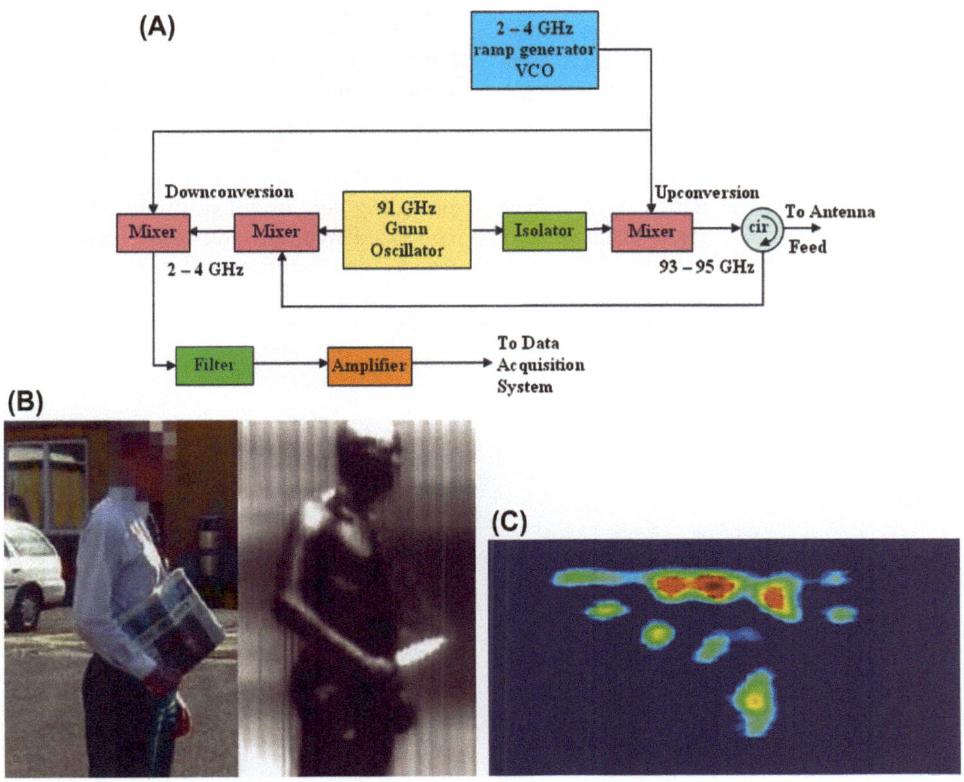

FIG. 5.11 Millimeter-wave (94 GHz) imaging system. **(A)** Gunn diode-based system block diagram (https://www.ncjrs.gov/pdffiles1/nij/grants/189918.pdf). **(B)** and **(C)** Image of a concealed weapon. (**(B** and **C)** Photographs taken from the presentation entitled Outline on THz Applications by Junji Urakawa, KEK, Japan.)

imaging system CWD can be done, as shown in Fig. 5.11B (where a person is trying to hide the knife covered by the newspaper) and Fig. 5.11C for a pistol/ handgun. However, as the MMW does not have any spectroscopic capability detection and identification capability, this scheme cannot be used for identification/detection of explosives or drug, etc.

Though MMW has the capability to penetrate better through some barrier materials compared with THz signal; however, there are two important considerations that favor THz scanning over MMW scanning for security applications: (a) spatial resolution and (b) spectroscopic signatures. THz detection system provides approximately 10 times better spatial resolution compared with MMW systems simply because the frequency of THz radiation is roughly 10 times higher than MMW radiation. Consequently, images of suspicious objects such as concealed metallic/plastic pistols or knives are imaged with much sharper contour and more readily identified with THz scanners [25], vide Fig. 5.12.

Standoff detection of explosives

The penetrating power of radio waves with spectroscopic capability of optical waves makes THz radiation unique for standoff detection of contraband (i.e., explosives, drugs, etc.). The analysis of THz spectrum of an image would help to identify concealed contents and potential threats through known characteristic of THz spectra of biological and chemical agents and illegal drugs including explosives [25]. As the trafficking of illegal drugs increasingly develops as a systemic threat and also the plastic explosives, fertilizer bombs and chemical and biological agents are becoming strategic weapons of war and terrorism, an effective means for detection and identification of these threats are very much required in the present society plagued by such security challenges. Use of THz EM waves to spectroscopically detect and identify concealed materials through their characteristic transmission or reflectivity spectra in the range of 0.5−10 THz appears to be an effective means for locating, detecting, and characterizing concealed threats. Many explosives like PETN, RDX, Semtex, Metabel, etc., and illegal drugs like Cocaine, MDMA, Heroin, etc., have characteristic absorption in the THz range [11,25] (vide Fig. 5.13) that could be distinguishable from other materials such as clothing, coins, and human skin, and even from talcum powder.

When compared with nonhazardous items, these materials are exhibited with different "colors" to the THz detector. Thus, using THz spectroscopy it becomes possible to detect explosives or drugs even if they are concealed, as the THz radiation is readily transmitted through plastics, clothing, luggage, paper products, and other nonconductive (nonmetallic) materials. One may identify the presence of these agents and distinguish them from benign objects by comparing measured reflectivity of THz spectra with known calibration spectra.

THz imaging for CWD or standoff detection of contraband can be done with THz-TDS; the commonly used systems for that have been discussed earlier (vide Figs. 5.9 and Fig. 5.10). Such imager can offer a standoff scanning distance of 10 −50 m and an image refresh rate of 10 Hz (10 images per second) or more, thereby providing very useful real-time imaging capability of concealed weapons and contrabands. The THz radiation is also significantly less susceptible to scattering than infrared, allowing improved reconstruction fidelity.

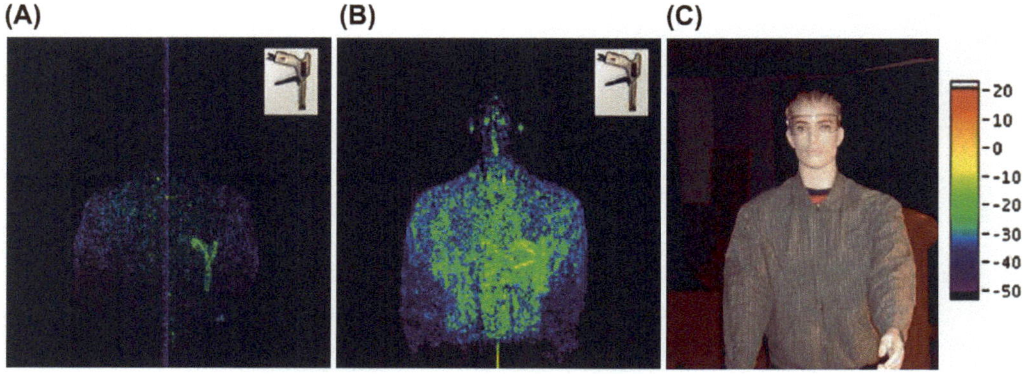

FIG.5.12 Concealed weapon detection imaging under heavy clothing with **(A)** THz signal, **(B)** millimeter-wave signal, and **(C)** optical image of the person having concealed weapon under heavy clothing. (Photographs taken from the presentation entitled Outline on THz Applications by Junji Urakawa, KEK, Japan.)

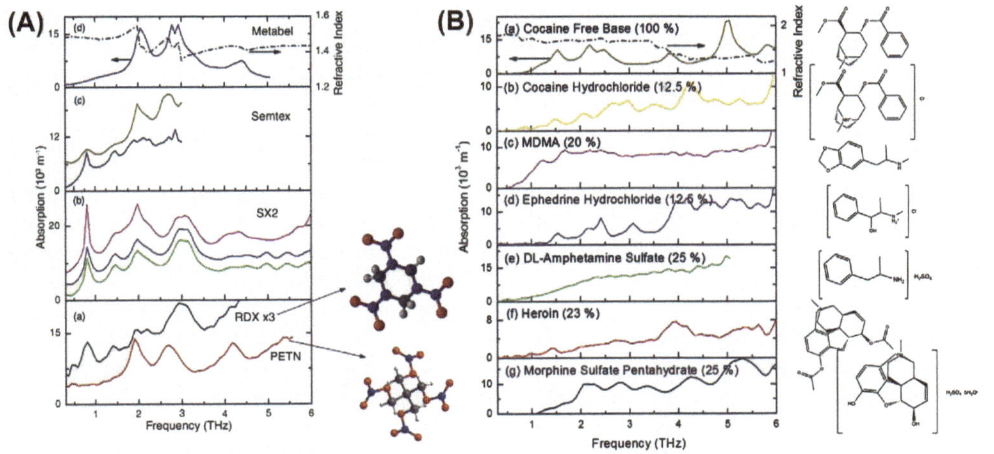

FIG. 5.13 Terahertz (THz) absorption spectra of **(A)** common explosives and **(B)** common abusive drugs [11,25]. (Reprinted/Adapted with permission from A.G. Davies, A.D. Burnett, W. Fan, E. H. Linfield, J.E. Cunningham, Terahertz spectroscopy of explosives and drugs, Materials Today 11(3) (2008) 18–26.© Elsevier Ltd.)

It may be mentioned herewith that no detection or imaging technology can reliably find every threat to security. Each technology has its own strength and weaknesses. But when several techniques are used together as a security sensing suit, their collective strengths are integrated and makes a wide ranged security scrutiny. For example, consider the security screening of trucks at a port or other check points. For monitoring nuclear radiation, we have standard detection systems, and X-ray system could penetrate through the trucks metal walls to probe the contents inside the truck. But how the driver is to be screened for possible concealed weapon, bomb, a trigger mechanism for a weapon hidden in the truck, or other threats? It is with invisible THz signal having its penetrating power of radio waves and spectroscopic capability of optical waves.

Pharmaceuticals and Medical Applications

There are, however, lots of uses of T-rays outside the security arena too; of which the application by pharmaceutical industry and for medical diagnosis are most important. The mundane job of checking the contents of a box without opening can be done effectively by pharmaceutical manufacturers using T-ray imaging (as THz has spectroscopic capability and can provide high resolution of the image of the object being imaged). Drug companies use T-ray imagers to distinguish good pills from bad ones by studying their spectral signature. To give a simple example let us talk about T-rays to characterize the uniformity of tablet coating, both within a single tablet and across an entire batch to develop an understanding of the functional analysis of the final product [26]. It is important to note that tablet coating is done to regulate the controlled release of active ingredients from the tablet to the body. In addition to bioavailability of a particular drug or combination of drugs during certain times and locations, the tablet coating can also protect the stomach from high concentrations of active ingredients. Also the improvement of tablet's visual appeal and the extension of the shelf life, by protecting the ingredients from degradation by moisture and oxygen, are guaranteed by good quality of tablet coating. Some of the conventional techniques that provide useful information in this regard are atomic force microscopy, confocal laser microscopy, X-ray photoelectron spectroscopy, and so on. However, all these methods are either destructive to the tablet or cannot be readily implemented for rapid online measurement. 3D analysis on tablets can be done effectively by THz imaging which helps to determine coating integrity and thickness, detect and identify localized chemical or physical defects of the structure. THz measurements may well become the primary method for the nondestructive determination of coating thickness, requiring little or no calibration for most coatings and substrates.

In this connection, it may also be mentioned that, invisible defects in the wings of the protective coatings of an aircraft's wing may also be detected with T-rays. NASA now-a-days use T-ray scanner to investigate for the presence of any tiny holes and other structural failing inside the foam that lines the external fuel tanks in the space shuttle fleet. It may be mentioned that a chunk of that foam fell away in 2003 and led to the death of seven astronauts and the fiery destruction of the *Columbia* space mission.

THz radiation has low photon energies so that it has no or very little chance of causing harmful photo ionization in biological tissues making THz tomography a better choice than infrared and X-ray tomography for medical imaging. THz images of cancer cells have revealed contrast between diseased and healthy cells both for breast and skin cancer. Using the strong absorption property of THz signal in the water content of tissues and the THz pulse imaging apparatus such studies have been successfully carried out.

Basal cell carcinoma is the most common form of skin cancer worldwide in white populations and has a reported annual incidence of over 1 million in the United States [26]. Several different imaging techniques are being evaluated as diagnostic tools for skin lesions and tumor margin assessment. The THz frequency is of particular interest as it excites the intermolecular interactions, such as vibrational modes of molecules providing spectroscopic information. Terahertz pulse imaging (TPI) is a noninvasive, coherent imaging modality with which both phase and amplitude information can be obtained, thereby providing absorption and refractive index. Through examination of the THz images, TPI may prove advantageous in distinguishing type, lateral spread, and depth of tumors. It may be seen from Fig. 5.14 that imaging with THz pulse imaging system (using one shown in Fig. 5.10) the absorbance/refractive index clearly shows the difference between the healthy and deceased cells that help in early diagnosis of skin cancer [26].

The difference of absorbance/refractive index between cancer and normal tissue is the potential of the THz imaging for early and better diagnosis of skin cancer that depends on small penetrative property and fingerprint spectrum provided by THz images. As may be seen from Fig. 5.14, the photo images of the sample appears in first column in which the red marked area gives the possible locations of cancer tissues which were previously identified with the pathological diagnostics. The second and the third columns show the THz images of the absorbance and the refractive index, respectively, taken at 1.7 THz; in which cancer tissues are more accurately located (note the red portions in the diagram of absorbance).

In dentistry, the dental carries or tooth decay is one of the most common disorders that are bothering dentists for a long time [27]. Carries proceed due the creation of a subsurface lesion in the enamel of the tooth. The lesion has the possibility to extend to the next tissue in the layer of the teeth, the dentine; and this breakdown or microcavity formation at the tooth surface may not be visible even with microscope. Thus, the early detection of tooth decay becomes difficult due to such nonavailability of visual features of the decayed tooth surface. One of the commonly used methods is to take an X-ray photograph of the decayed tooth surface, however, that only reveals the problem at a relatively later stage, when drilling and filling is the only method available to take care of the decay. If an early detection of the decay becomes possible, then it might be under the control of the dentist to reverse the process without the need for drilling by the use of either fissure sealing or remineralization. THz imaging has the capability to distinguish between the different types of tissue in a human tooth; detect carries at an early stage in the enamel layers of human teeth and monitor early erosion of the enamel at the surface of the tooth. Fig. 5.15 shows the dental image with TPI system that clearly indicates the formation of the cavity [27].

Epithelium is the place where more than 85% of all cancers originate. The gold standard for cancer diagnosis is excision biopsy in which tissue from the body is removed and examined under a microscope. THz technology has the advantage that it can greatly improve the conventional biopsy technique and associated surgery as it can more precisely identify the areas to be excised thereby reducing the number of procedures and facilitating earlier and more accurate diagnosis. As the technology develops, it may be possible to perform biopsies using live THz imaging of affected area which might be a great boon for oncology [26].

THz in Communication Applications

We may now discuss some emerging communication applications with THz signal. It is believed by many that THz technology will be very important for next-generation wireless communication. THz waves have higher frequencies or shorter wavelength compared with MMWs. Thus, THz signal is capable of providing more transmission bandwidth and hence can carry more data (of the order of terabit). However, THz signal will not be able to propagate a long distance like radio waves and microwaves because the Earth's atmosphere strongly absorbs THz radiation in some specific water vapor absorption bands, as may be seen from Fig. 5.16. Thus, THz radiation will not be useful for long-distance communications. However, at distances up to 50 m or so, the band may still allow many useful applications in imaging and construction of high bandwidth wireless networking systems, especially for indoor communication.

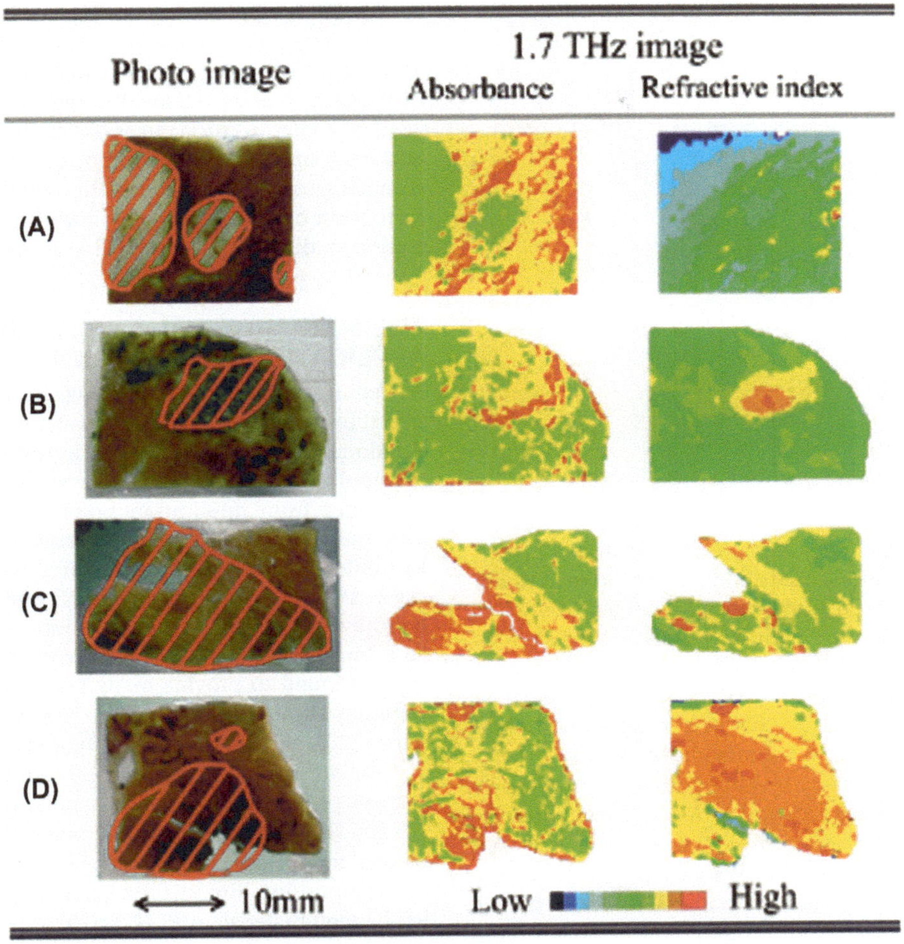

FIG. 5.14 The photo images and the terahertz (THz) images of samples **(A–D)** [26]. The first column shows photographs of the samples, with the cancer areas marked by redline. The second and the third columns show maps of the absorbance and the refractive index at 1.7 THz, respectively, in the same scale as the photographs. The absorbance is shown in color, from 0 to 2.0 for samples A, B and D and from 0 to 0.7 for sample C. The value of the refractive index is shown in color from 1.0 to 1.7 for all samples. (Reprinted/Adapted with permission from S. Nakajima, H. Hoshina, M Yamashita, C. Otani, N. Miyoshi, Terahertz imaging diagnostics of the cancer tissues with Chemometrics technique, Applied Physics Letters 90 (2007) 041102. © American Institute of Physics.)

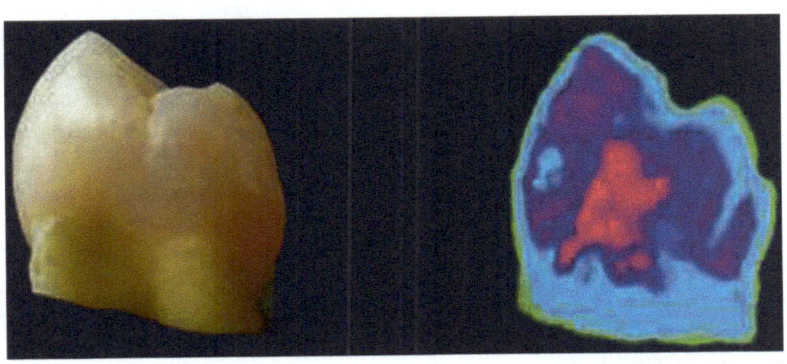

FIG. 5.15 Dental image (a tooth cavity shows up clearly in red). (Photograph taken from the presentation entitled Outline on THz Applications by Junji Urakawa, KEK, Japan, who referred Teraview Ltd.)

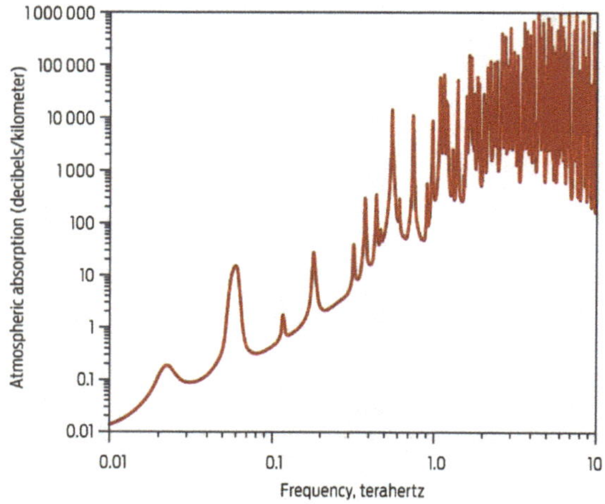

FIG. 5.16 Atmospheric absorption of terahertz signal.

In general, this means that use of THz waves in mobile communication could address many areas in which even the recently implemented 5G is not able to deliver high enough data throughput. We know that 1G provided us with mobile telephony, while 2G expanded on that and addressed some of the shortcomings of its predecessor. 3G and 4G did the same with mobile data and now that we are moving on to 5G, it is expected to support many new applications. It is believed that using THz frequency and with additional improvements in cellular technology, we will someday see thousand-dollar smart phones that have the computational power of the human brain. Of course, it's all highly speculative at this point, but if past trends continue, we can expect to see service providers harnessing THz waves for communications purposes we have not yet dreamt of.

At present, we might not hear much talk about THz communications (though fundamental developments are going on as undercurrent) because the electronics and communication industry is currently preoccupied with MMW frequency bands (30–300 GHz) to offer multi-gigabit-per-second (Gbps) data rates with 5G mobile devices. It has already been seen that, similar to MMWs, THz communication has the problem of propagation loss, but of severe magnitude, caused by a tremendous amount of signal attenuation due to atmospheric absorption of EM waves by oxygen and water molecules; thereby limiting the communication covering range. However, THz bands can be used as mobile backhaul for transferring much larger bandwidth signals, compared with MMWs, between base stations. Also, THz bands can be employed in close-in communications, known as whisper radio applications. There are also possible applications of THz in high-resolution spectroscopy and imaging and communication studies that require short-range communications in the form of massive channel bandwidth and having practically zero error rates in crucial areas like coding, redundancy, and frequency diversity. Additionally, THz bands can complement MMW communications in the commercial realization of indoor wireless networks, position localization studies, and gigabyte Wi-Fi support of Internet.

THZ METAMATERIAL AND THEIR APPLICATION POSSIBILITIES

In recent times, artificially designed subwavelength structures known as metamaterials have revolutionized the domain of microwave/THz/optical frequencies to manipulate EM waves and to provide different functionalities from application point of view. Material properties such as permittivity, permeability, and refractive index can be engineered/tailored with such artificially structured periodic array of unit cells that is typically called "meta-atoms"—both of "electrical" and "magnetic type." A periodic collection of metaatoms is found to provide many fascinating and exotic effects/applications like negative refraction [28], perfect lenses [29], perfect absorbers [30], and cloaking [31].

Properties of EM waves can be controlled by natural materials (also known as right-handed materials: as **E**, **H**, and **k** of propagating EM wave forms a right-handed triad in such materials) by changing their chemical composition. But in metamaterials (also known as left-handed material: as **E**, **H**, and **k** of propagating EM wave forms a left-handed triad in such materials), the researchers can manipulate the EM properties of an incident EM wave just by altering the geometry (spacing and shape) of the artificially designed constituent electric and magnetic atoms of such metamaterial. This unique advantage of metamaterials to independently manipulate their effective constitutive parameters, i.e., permittivity and permeability, makes them suitable for many emerging applications not possible with natural materials. In particular, the control of magnetic activity by tailoring the permeability of metamaterials results in the implementation of various circuit components with improved performance and size miniaturization in the higher parts of the EM spectrum, since the magnetism tends to vanish in the THz and higher frequencies.

During the first experimental realization of negative refractive index with metamaterial in 2001 at UCSD, US [28] (vide Fig. 5.17A), the constituent electric and magnetic atoms were realized with thin-wire (TW) and split-ring resonator (SRR). The first plasmonic

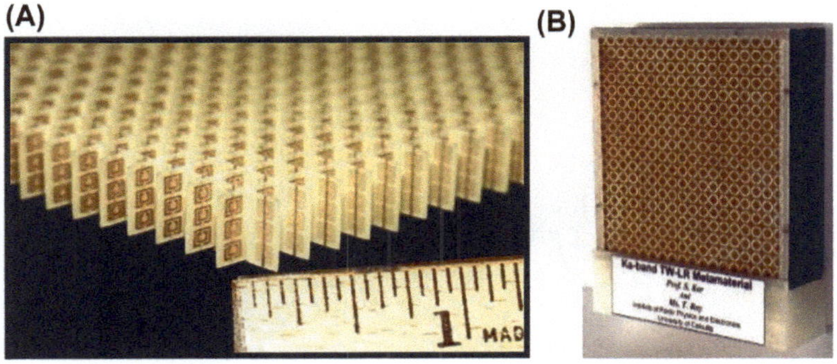

FIG. 5.17 **(A)** First metamaterial fabricated in United States (2001) [28]. **(B)** First metamaterial fabricated in India (2009) [1].

metamaterial in India was fabricated by our group at Calcutta University in collaboration with SAMEER, Kolkata Centre, and BARC, Mumbai, in 2009 (vide Fig. 5.17B) [32] using TW and labyrinth resonator (LR). Since metamaterial is fabricated with subwavelength structures (unit cells having dimension of the order of $\lambda/10$), the passive components (like antenna, couplers, filters, etc.) designed with metamaterial lead to size miniaturization [1].

Though initially metamaterials were developed to suggest the possibility of negative-index "superlens," the research agenda then shifted toward achieving tunable, switchable, nonlinear, and sensing functionalities. Thus, we now talk of "metadevices" where we define the devices as having unique and useful functionalities that are realized by structuring of functional entities on the subwavelength scale [22]. Such metadevice has also revolutionized the THz domain especially in the design of high-quality sensors and other passive components.

Since THz frequency spectrum is situated above the microwave and below the infrared radiation, the absorption of THz rays in molecular and biomolecular systems is dominated by the excitation of intramolecular and intermolecular vibrations. Thus, THz technology is expected to be an effective tool for the design of high-quality sensors. The poor sensitivity of free-space THz detectors limits their sensing applications—which can be significantly improved with metamaterial-inspired structures. Metamaterials can result in localized electric/magnetic field enhancement and result in large values of quality factor (Q factor) and are thus capable of showing high sensitivity to minor changes that occurs in the sample to be sensed.

The ubiquitous metallic SRR that acts as a highly resonant magnetic inclusion structure in metamaterial design at microwave frequency, along with TW structure (vide Fig. 5.18), can easily be scaled to THz frequency (though above 200 THz metal does not behave as metal any more). At microwave/MMW frequency, strong magnetic response is obtained with the incident signal polarization being parallel to the plane of SRR (vide Fig. 5.18(A) (ii)) [1].

However, the configuration of THz SRR is such that to realize effective magnetization at these frequencies, it needs to have vertical orientation of the SRR units with the polarization of the incident THz signal as indicated in Fig. 5.19 [33]. Here the SRR is of square shape and has two cuts forming the so-called LR (or double-split resonator) that does not suffer from bi-anisotropy problem (caused by asymmetric placement of slits in the two rings resulting in imbalance of the current in the two rings) prevalent with single-split conventional SRR structures [1]. Absence of bi-anisotropy in double SRR or more aesthetically called LR helps to achieve LC resonance of high quality factor.

Using THz signal, the sensing action is determined in terms of the resonances of various molecular vibrations in the sample to be sensed. As metamaterial magnetic inclusion structure (SRR/LR) is a highly resonant structure, it aids in enhancing the resonances and hence leads to better sensing with metamaterial assistance. More the Q (quality factor) of the metamaterial resonators, better is the sensing capability. Effective sensing is evaluated by measuring the resonant response differences of the metamaterial unit cells—thereby identifying and detecting minute amounts of differences in chemical and biochemical substances. In the structure shown in Fig. 5.19, the Q-value of 30 has been realized with maximum refractive index sensitivity of 788 GHz/RIU or 1.04×105 nm/RIU.

Use of metal structure for metamaterial design has inherent losses and hence the Q factor gets compromised. But if we use perfect absorbers designed with

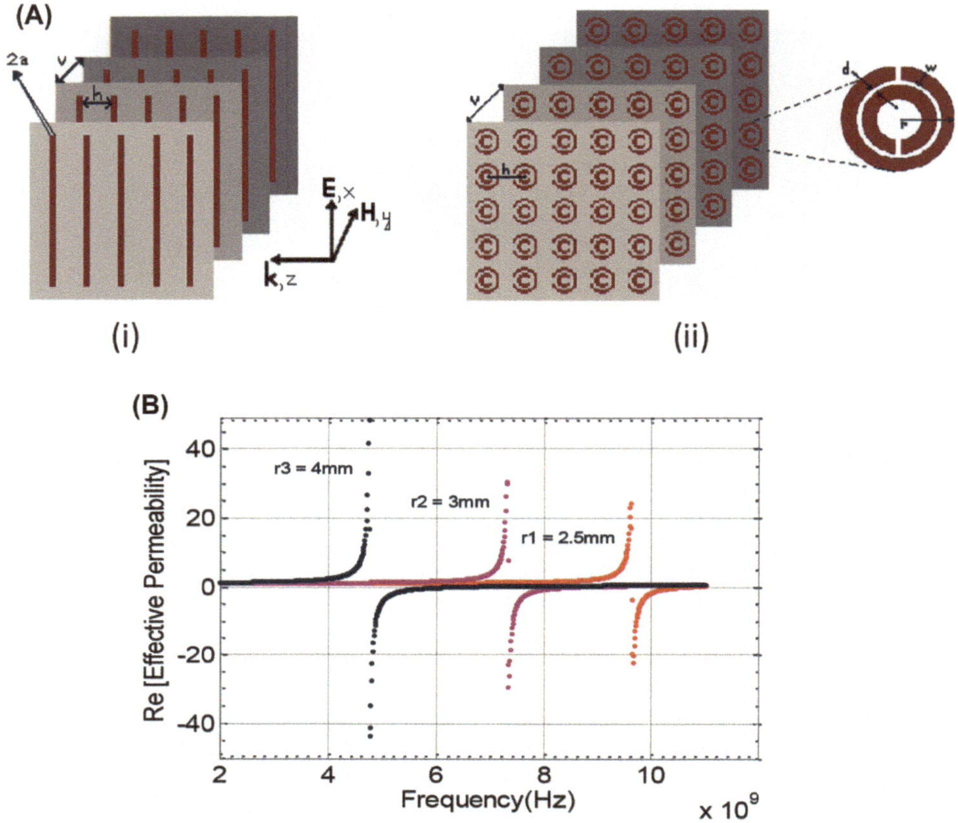

FIG. 5.18 **(A)** (i) 1D array of thin-wire that exhibit effective negative permittivity below electrical plasma frequency. **(A)** (ii)1D matrix of split-ring resonator that exhibit effective negative permeability below magnetic plasma frequency. **(B)** Magnetic resonance characteristics exhibited by split-ring resonator [1].

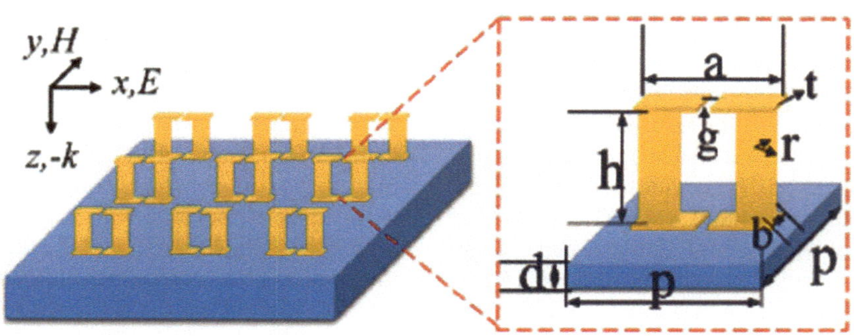

FIG. 5.19 3D schematic drawing of the proposed metamaterial sensor and a single enlarged unit cell with its geometrical dimensions. (Reprinted/Adapted with permission from W. Wang, F. Yan, S. Tan, H. Zhou, Y. Hou, Ultrasensitive terahertz metamaterial sensor based on vertical split-ring resonators, Photonics Research 5 (6) (2017) 571–577.© Chinese Laser Press.)

metamaterial, then we can have higher Q factor. The realization of high quality factor resonance in these structures leads to the enhancement of the sensing sensitivities to detect minute frequency shifts.

Bimaterial sensors with metamaterial absorbers have been used for sensor design, vide Fig. 5.20 [34]. This consists of a sensing element (absorber) that converts incoming THz radiation to heat which is eventually

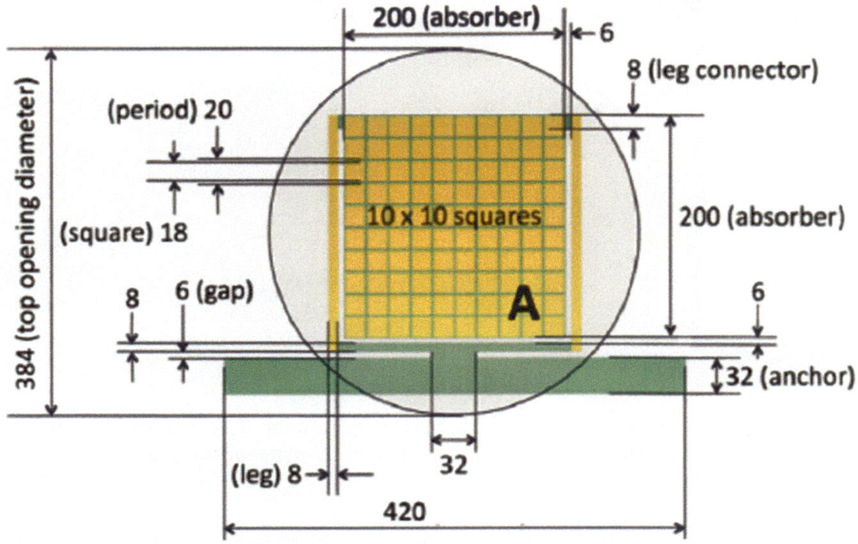

FIG. 5.20 Structure of bimaterial terahertz sensor using metamaterial absorber. (Reprinted/Adapted with permission from F. Alves, F. Grbovic, B. Kearney, N. V. Lavrik, G. Karunasiri, Bi-material terahertz sensors using metamaterial structures", Optics Express 21 (11) (2013) 13256–13271, https://doi.org/10.1364/OE.21.013256. © The Optical Society.)

transmitted by conduction to two symmetrically located bimaterial legs connected to the host substrate (heat sink) with supporting structures of lower thermal conductance (anchors). Temperature rise caused by absorption of incident THz radiation results in deformation of bimaterial legs. The deformation can be probed by different approaches of which optical readout is a simple technique that requires a reflective surface which is embedded into the absorber. Such sensors have responsivity values as high as 1.2deg/μW and time constants as low as 200 m. Minimum detectable power on the order of 10 nW and the sensors can operate with low-power THz sources.

A "perfect" absorber can be constructed with the proper design of structural parameters [34]. The challenge remains in the design of a metamaterial film that is thin enough to provide low thermal capacitance, while providing structural strength, low stress, and a flat reflective surface for an optical readout. It may be seen from Fig. 5.21 that a typical metamaterial absorber consists of a periodic array of Al square elements separated from an Al ground plane by a SiOx layer, a single unit cell being shown in Fig. 5.21A. Such a combination allows matching to the free-space impedance at specific frequencies, eliminating the reflection. Fig. 5.21B shows a periodic array of such metamaterial absorber [34].

Dynamic tuning of THz metamaterial can be done by manufacturing the metamaterial array on a MEMS-driven silicon platform [35]. This is basically a reconfigurable metamaterial which is realized by reconfiguring the unit cell, that consists of a pair of asymmetric split-ring resonators (ASRR) [35]. Bidirectional micromachined actuators help to tune the coupling distance between the pair of ASRRs.

Because the ASRRs are asymmetric in nature, a normally incident THz wave can excite the inductive-capacitive resonance in the metamaterial structure. In addition to its broadband tuning capability (up to 31% and 22% for the TE and the TM polarization, respectively), the reconfigurable metamaterial can also produce a high quality factor resonance and an in-phase magnetic-dipole oscillation for the TE polarization. In the process of dynamic tuning, the reconfigurable metamaterial can be switched from the polarization-dependent state to the polarization-independent state. Such metamaterial has many potential applications such as in transformation optics devices, sensors, intelligent detectors, tunable frequency-selective surfaces, and spectral filters at THz frequency.

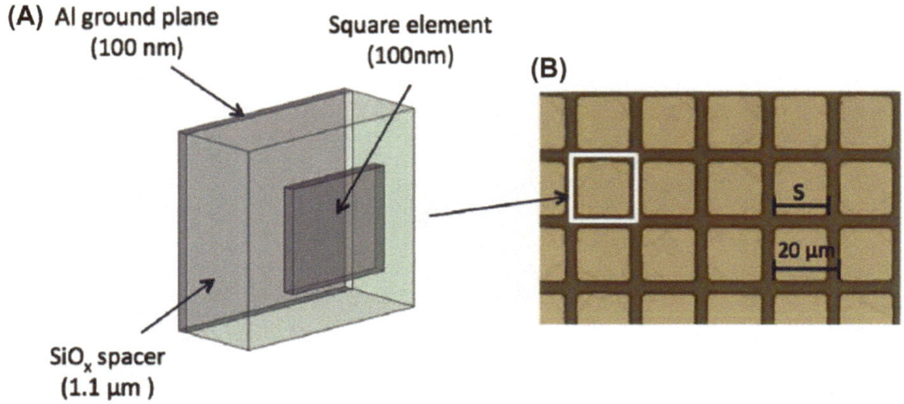

FIG. 5.21 Metamaterial absorber. **(A)** Unit cell and **(B)** 1D periodic array. (Reprinted/Adapted with permission from F. Alves, F. Grbovic, B Kearney, N. V.Lavrik, G. Karunasiri, Bi-material terahertz sensors using metamaterial structures, Optics Express 21 (11) (2013) 13256–13271, https://doi.org/10.1364/OE.21.013256. © The Optical Society.)

CONCLUSION

Though THz technology was used for some limited applications by radio astronomers in the end of the last century, the "THz gap" remained a least used chunk of the EM spectrum due to the lack of the availability of sources, detectors, passive components, etc., till the beginning of this century. However, with the advancement of MMW technology beyond 100 GHz and optical technology during last 2 decades, there has been a new vigor of development of THz technology as THz frequency spectrum demands the expertise of both electronic and optical technology. THz signal generation can now be done from nanowatt to milliwatt level by optical heterodyning of laser sources, using QCL, irradiation of photoconductive, and electro-optic material including other nonlinear crystals with femtosecond laser. FEL-based accelerator techniques can generate even watt level THz signal with relatively expensive system; however, low-cost portable systems are also possible with lower output power. THz signal detection can be done either by semiconductor Schottky diode or super-Schottky diode including HEB mixer. Optical techniques are also used where photosensitive antenna is coupled with the detector system. Image formation can be done either with raster scanning or interferometric imager. THz system components can be either quasioptical type or waveguide based; however, the former one is more common even these days, while the latter ones offer distinct advantages like better isolation, wider choice of implementation solution, and integration with active devices over their quasioptical counterparts. THz being a nonionizing radiation with the advantage of radio waves for penetration into materials of different types and spectroscopic capability of optical waves has opened up a number of applications for security purposes and also in medical and communication domain with its inherently high image resolution and broadband capability compared with MMWs. For security purposes, THz imaging is capable of better CWD than with MMWs, while standoff detection of explosives and illegal drugs is its unique capability. T-ray imager helps significantly in pharmaceutical industry and also in early detection of skin and breast cancer including applications in dentistry. New and emerging applications are coming up for advanced communication systems. Recent trend of metamaterial-inspired passive component development especially in the design of sensor, filter, etc., is expected to benefit THz technology immensely in near future.

REFERENCES

[1] S. Kar, Microwave Engineering—Fundamentals, Design, and Applications (Chapter 15), Universities Press, 2016.
[2] S. Kar, Design and characterization of a 34 GHz IMPATT oscillator using novel coaxial-waveguide cavity, Engineering Transactions (MUT) (2007) 1–5.
[3] Terasense Group Inc., San Jose, CA 95110, USA.
[4] J.J. O'Reilly, P.M. Lane, M.H. Capstick, Optical generation and delivery of modulated mm-wave for mobile communication, Analog Optical Fiber Communications, IEEE (1995) 229–256.
[5] S. Kar, M. Ghosh, S. Das, A. Saha, Optical heterodyning of injection-locked laser sources — a novel technique for millimetre-wave signal generation, International Journal of Electronics and Communication Engineering 8 (7) (2014) 1048–1051 (ISNI:0000000091950263).

[6] B.N. Biswas, A. Banerjee, A. Mukherjee, S. Kar, Lightwave technique of mm-wave generation for broadband mobile communication, PIERS Online 3 (7) (2007) 1071–1075.

[7] J.F. Federici, D. Gary, R. Barat, Z.H. Michalopoulou, T-rays versus terrorists, IEEE Spectrum (July 2007) 39–44.

[8] J. Faist, F. Capasso, D.L. Sivco, C. Sirtori, A.L. Hutchinson, A.Y. Cho, Quantum cascade laser, Science 264 (1994) 553–556.

[9] E.R. Brown, K.A. McIntosh, K.B. Nichols, C.L. Dennis, Photomixing up to 3.8 THz in low-temperature-grown GaAs, Applied Physics Letters 66 (3) (1995) 285–287.

[10] P.H. Siegel, Terahertz technology, IEEE Transactions on Microwave Theory and Techniques 50 (3) (2002) 910–928.

[11] A.G. Davies, A.D. Burnett, W. Fan, E.H. Linfield, J.E. Cunningham, Terahertz spectroscopy of explosives and drugs, Materials Today 11 (3) (2008) 18–26.

[12] D. Arnone, C. Ciesla, M. Pepper, Terahertz imaging comes into view, Physics World (April 2000) 35–40.

[13] H.A. Hafez, X. Chai, A. Ibrahim, S. Mondal, D. Férachou, X. Ropagnol, T. Ozaki, Intense terahertz radiation and their applications, Journal of Optics 18 (2016) 1–48, https://doi.org/10.1088/2040-8978/18/9/093004.

[14] K. Kawase, M. Sato, T. Taniuchi, H. Ito, Coherent tunable terahertz-wave generation from LiNbO with monolithic grating coupler, Applied Physics Letters 68 (18) (1996) 2483–2485.

[15] S. Diebold, K. Tsuruda, M. Fujita, T. Nagatsuma, J. Kim, T. Mukai, Terahertz resonant tunnelling diode systems for next generation wireless communication, in: 2015 IEEE International Meeting for Future of Electron Devices, 4–5 June 2015, Kyoto, Japan, 2015, https://doi.org/10.1109/IMFEDK.2015.7158534.

[16] T. Ping, H. Jiang, L.K. Feng, X.Y. Qian, F.M. Wu, Terahertz radiation sources based on free electron lasers and their applications, Science China, Information Sciences 55 (1) (2012) 1–15, https://doi.org/10.1007/s11432-011-4515-1.

[17] A.S. Müller, M. Schwarz, Synchrotron Light Sources and Free-Electron Lasers, Springer International Publishing, Switzerland, 2015, pp. 1–31, https://doi.org/10.1007/978-3-319-04507-8_6-1.

[18] Y.U. Jeong, G.M. Kazakevich, S.H. Park, et al., High power table-top THz free electron laser and its application, Nuclear Instruments and Methods 575 (2007) 58–59.

[19] S.S. Dhillon, et al., The 2017 terahertz science and technology roadmap, Journal of Physics Applied Physics (2017) 1–50, 043001.

[20] C.D. Nordquist, M.C. Wanke, A.M. Rowen, C.L. Arrington, A.D. Grine, C.T. Fuller, Properties of surface metal micromachined rectangular waveguide operating near 3 THz, IEEE Journal of Selected Topics in Quantum Electronics 17 (1) (2011) 130–137.

[21] S.A. Kuznetsov, et al., Development and characterization of quasi-optical mesh filters and metastructures for subterahertz and terahertz applications, Key Engineering Materials 437 (2010) 276–280, https://doi.org/10.4028/www.scientific.net/KEM.437.276.

[22] N.I. Zheludev, Y.S. Kivshar, From metamaterials to metadevices, Nature Materials 11 (2012) 917–924.

[23] D.M. Mittleman, R.H. Jacobsen, M.C. Nuss, T-ray imaging, IEEE Journal of Selected Topics in Quantum Electronics 2 (1996) 679–692.

[24] Y.W. Chang, M. Michael Johnson, Portable Concealed Weapon Detection Using Millimetre Wave FMCW Radar Imaging, U.S. Department of Justice, (unpublished). https://www.ncjrs.gov/pdffiles1/nij/grants/189918.pdf.

[25] J.F. Federici, B. Schulkin, F. Huang, D. Gary, R. Barat, F. Oliveira, D. Zimdars, THz imaging and sensing for security applications—explosives, weapons and drugs, Semiconductor Science and Technology 20 (2005) 266–280, https://doi.org/10.1088/0268-1242/20/7/018.

[26] S. Nakajima, H. Hoshina, M. Yamashita, C. Otani, N. Miyoshi, Terahertz imaging diagnostics of the cancer tissues with chemometrics technique, Applied Physics Letters 90 (2007) 041102.

[27] A.Y. Pawar, D.D. Sonawane, K.B. Erande, D.V. Derle, Terahertz technology and its applications, Drug Invention Today 5 (2013) 157–163, https://doi.org/10.1016/j.dit.2013.03.009.

[28] R.A. Shelby, D.R. Smith, S. Schultz, Experimental verification of a negative index of refraction, Science 292 (2001) 77.

[29] J.B. Pendry, Negative refraction makes a perfect lens, Physical Review Letters 85 (2000) 3966.

[30] L.H.N.I. Tao, C.M. Bingham, X. Zhang, R.D. Averitt, W.J. Padilla, A metamaterial absorber for the terahertz regime: design, fabrication and characterization, Optics Express 16 (2008) 7181–7188.

[31] D. Schurig, J.J. Mock, B.J. Justice, S.A. Cummer, J.B. Pendry, A.F. Starr, D.R. Smith, Metamaterial electromagnetic cloak at microwave frequencies, Science 314 (2006) 977, https://doi.org/10.1126/science.1133628.

[32] B. Das, India Joins Metamaterial Club, Nature (India), August 20, 2009 http://www.nature.com/nindia/2009/090820/full/nindia.2009.273.html.

[33] W. Wang, F. Yan, S. Tan, H. Zhou, Y. Hou, Ultrasensitive terahertz metamaterial sensor based on vertical split-ring resonators, Photonics Research 5 (6) (2017) 571–577.

[34] F. Alves, F. Grbovic, B. Kearney, N.V. Lavrik, G. Karunasiri, Bi-material terahertz sensors using metamaterial structures, Optics Express 21 (11) (2013) 13256–13271, https://doi.org/10.1364/OE.21.013256.

[35] Y.H. Fu, A.Q. Liu, W.M. Zhu, X.M. Zhang, D.P. Tsai, J.B. Zhang, T. Mei, J.F. Tao, H.C. Guo, X.H. Zhang, J.H. Teng, N.I. Zheludev, G.Q. Lo, D.L. Kwong, A micromachined reconfigurable metamaterial via reconfiguration of asymmetric split-ring resonators, Advanced Functional Materials 21 (2011) 3589–3594.

CHAPTER 6

THz Medical Imaging: Current Status and Future Outlook

M. MUKHERJEE, MSC, MTECH, PHD (TECH), PDF •
SULAGNA CHATTERJEE, MSC, MTECH, PHD (TECH)

INTRODUCTION

Terahertz (THz) technology is rapidly progressing all over the world owing to its various application possibilities in the field of basic natural science, engineering, and medicine. The THz wavelength lies in between 1000 and 100 μm (100 GHz−10 THz). In spite of its huge scientific interest since 1920s, THz spectrum range is still list tapped region of the EM spectrum. THz band lies in between microwave and optical technologies and very limited atmospheric propagation is possible. Since last three decades, THz domain is in focus of active research throughout the world of scientific community. Till 1980s, the work advancement in this field remained relatively insignificant. A few noticeable research was done before 1980, namely the development of THz gas laser by Gebbie et al. [1−3] in the year 1960, generation of THz signal through nonlinear optics in 1970 [4,5], and advanced technologies for infrared spectroscopy [6,7]. Thereafter, several technological challenges in generation and suitable detection of THz radiation have entered in the research domain worldwide, and the term "Tera-gap" became a wide spread phrase within scientific community. The phrase explains the unavailability of suitable source and detectors in this domain. In the late 1980s, invention of advanced spectroscopic tool helped the researcher immense. Auston et al. at Bell laboratory and Grischkowsky at IBM lab first developed technique for femtosecond laser source to generate and detect THz pulses [8−11]. This point was a start of new era in the field of THz source and detector development activity. This research eventually decreased cost and complexity of femtosecond laser pulse sources available commercially in market. Research groups in this field of THz time-domain spectroscopy (THz TDS) started exploring since 1990 and became several dozens by 2010. This way THz technology started spreading more extensively into research areas and especially in biological science owing to its some unique features suitable for biological applications. In the last decade, potentially better THz sources, including THz quantum cascade lasers (QCLs) [12,13], Si-based ICs on III-V semiconductors, started to immerge [14]. In the year 1995, THz TDS was used first time for generation of images [15], and with this scientists started thinking about the application of THz technology outside scientific and engineering applications, i.e., in biomedical imaging and sensor. Before 2010 and after 1990, researchers continued to explore various physical aspects of THz field toward new application possibilities [16−20]. The development of integrated THz system is still continuing and in future this will enable various new applications of this promising domain of EM spectrum. Already considered and standardized possibilities include THz wireless communication, high data rate transfer, and THz spectroscopy [21,22]. In this chapter, the authors will present a brief review on (I) available THz sources, (II) THz detectors, and (III) application of THz systems in biomedical imaging. Section I will deal with various different ways of generating THz power using optical/electronic means. Relative advantages and disadvantages of the available sources will be discussed thoroughly, followed by various physical phenomena that could be implemented in future source development to make it more compact and cheaper. Section II will deal with the various types of detection mechanisms available for commercial use, as well as in research domain that could be implemented successfully. Section III will deal with the possibilities of THz imaging in medicine. Various observations, new researches,

Terahertz Biomedical and Healthcare Technologies. https://doi.org/10.1016/B978-0-12-818556-8.00006-9

and pros and cons of THz imaging will be described thoroughly in light of medical applications. This chapter will work as a compact review and ready reference for all scientists and engineers who are working with the development of THz source and system for the betterment of mankind.

THZ SOURCES AND DETECTORS—REVIEW

During last years [23], research has been carried out for the development of suitable sources in this frequency regime worldwide. There are two technology roadmaps for THz solid-state devices. In the lower frequency range of the THz regime, electronic devices such as resonant-tunneling diode (RTD), Gunn diode, and field-effect transistors (FETs) based on plasma wave, are widely investigated for T-ray generation. From upper range of the THz frequency spectrum, the photonic device, i.e., QCL extends its emission wavelength to THz spectral range [23]. Another approach for T-ray generation is by using femtosecond LASER incident either on materials with nonlinear optical properties or on photoconductors made up with InP.

Most of the research works are made for effective generation of THz signals. Market available THz sources are bulky and complex. On the other hand, QCL has the advantage of small size, although they need low temperature arrangement for direct generation of THz pulses. The market study indicates that there is a void of compact size efficient THz source to serve a useful purpose. Thus, the development of low-cost, compact, and high-power semiconductor sources in THz region has attracted the attention of scientists working in this domain. Extensive research has already been carried out on wide bandgap (WBG) **IMP**act Ionization **A**valanche **T**ransit **T**ime (IMPATT) in the MM-wave region and those are published in standard literature [24–29]. Most of the devices are focused on fundamental frequency of oscillation and in few cases harmonic power generations are also being incorporated [30]. On-chip development of IMPATT power sources are still challenging domain of research. Series resistance and parasitic issues in generation of high power creates serious challenges and that has also been taken into account for its fruitful realization.

Necessity and Significance of IMPATT Diodes as THz Sources

Operating frequency range of various potential applications including RADAR, broadband wireless access, security, indoor communication, and instrumentation applications is expected to be extended to MM-wave region (30–300 GHz). The potential advantages of this wave region could be exploited in the scientific, commercial, and defense areas with the advancement of semiconductor sources. Till date, various solid-state sources such as GUNN and ATT (IMPATT, TRAPATT, and BARITT) are developed for MM-wave generation. Among all the available room temperature semiconductor devices, IMPATT oscillators are the most efficient and powerful device oscillator for MM-wave power system [30]. Also with the incorporation of doping and structural changes, the devices could be used for suitable biomedical applications in terms of power and efficiencies.

In present electronic industries, ATT devices are gaining significance in MM-wave communications, advanced RADAR, and missile seekers. The conventional Si (silicon) and GaAs (gallium arsenide) ATT devices have power limitations, constraints related to operating temperature and operating frequency. Therefore, nowadays a global demand is there for high-frequency biocompatible applications of these ATT devices, and thus there is a requirement for new class of ATT oscillators which would be able to outperform conventional Si- and GaAs-based ATT oscillators.

In the recent past, IMPATT-based research has mainly focused on the improvement of device performance through suitable modification related to structure and doping. As a result, efficient and powerful structures that include double drift region diode, high-low, and low-high-low IMPATT structures have evolved. In epitaxial growth techniques, technological advancements are achieved through rapid thermal annealing and ion implantation in last decades. Research focus is therefore in searching of suitable base materials for developing ATT oscillators. High-power and high-frequency capabilities of ATT oscillators mostly depend upon the inherent electrical, electronic, and thermal properties of base materials from which the devices would be fabricated. Different base materials are characterized by its unique optical, electronic, and thermal properties that could be suitably exploited for fabricating high-power electronic devices. The optimum base semiconductor for THz operation of ATT devices should have high saturation drift velocity (v_s) of charge carriers, critical electric field (E_C), as well as high thermal conductivity (K). It is so due to the fact that RF power output from an IMPATT diode is directly proportional to $E_C^2 \times v_s^2$. A higher operating frequency is a subsequent outcome of such higher saturated drift velocity. The consequent higher thermal conductivity results in the generated heat to be removed and, therefore, allows high-power operations to persist for greater extents of time. Thus, the demand for such high-power IMPATT devices that are capable of efficiently generating MM-wave power in extreme harsh environments has started a quest for really compatible semiconductors.

WBG semiconductor materials in context to the development of devices for high-power and high-frequency devices capable of high-temperature operations are being investigated by the research community currently [31–34]. A number of research reports have appeared covering different directions of WBG materials and their applications. Among all such WBG semiconductors, gallium nitride (GaN) and silicon carbide (SiC) have received maximum attention of researchers in the last decade for wide spread applications starting from high-power, high-frequency oscillators to short wavelength lasers and solid-state lighting. While the inherent material properties impart excellent performance advantages over conventional semiconductors, for example, Si and GaAs, however, choice of such advanced materials includes disadvantages such as underdeveloped material quality and immature application markets, therefore, rendering them not cost-effective to justify significant complexities in manufacturing processes. Yet the market scenario is changing with the technological advancement of WBG materials into advanced electronic applications [35]. Comparison of material parameters of WBG GaN, SiC, and diamond with other conventional semiconductors like Si, GaAs, and InP is summarized in Table 6.1. Among all of these materials, diamond has highest breakdown electric field and widest bandgap energy, and thus it shows promises for high-power device operations. However, fabrication complexities have not yet been solved. Diamond needs high processing temperature because of its high melting point and thus limited research activities have been carried out as of now.

SiC exist in various polytypes including cubic (C), hexagonal (H), and rhombohedral (R), and the number will vary between 150 and 250 as far as the current published literature is concerned [35]. Two types of structures are available such as alpha (α) and beta (β). The "α" category is primarily hexagonal and rhombohedral, on the other hand "β" category is cubic or zinc blende type. Due to the technical difficulty in growth mechanism associated with β-SiC, researchers are mostly concentrating on α-SiC, particularly on 4H-SiC and 6H-SiC. The two widely available polytypes of GaN are wurtzite (WZ) and zinc blende (ZB). Table 6.1 shows that 4H and 6H types of SiC and WZ and ZB type GaN form the most suitable alternative to conventional Si for high-power and temperature applications resulting from the inherent advantages due to better material properties such as high saturation drift velocity, WBG, and high thermal conductivity. Besides, capacitive loading at high frequencies in WBG materials is reduced due to their low dielectric constants. Therefore, there lies a potential of WBG semiconductors to develop a new generation of MM-wave and sub-MM-wave oscillators capable of operating at elevated temperatures with considerable output power at high frequencies.

TABLE 6.1
Figures of Merits of Different Semiconductors in Comparison to Si.

Material	JFM $(E_C v_s/\pi)^2$	KFM $(\lambda.(v_s/\varepsilon_r)^{1/2})$	BFM (μE_C^2)
Si	1	1	1
GaAs	7.1	0.45	11
SiC	278	5.1	29
GaN	756	1.6	77.8
InP	30	0.80	11
Diamond	2540	32.1	470

Figure of Merit (FOM) is a parameter which indicates an assessment of expected performances of WBG devices; this has been shown in Table 6.1. In the table, the numbers are normalized with respect to conventional Si. Apart from FOM, *Johnson's Figure of Merit* (JFM) is a measure to evaluate the power gain of transistors as well as their frequency performance by employing the product of the breakdown voltage with the saturation velocity. Besides the mentioned ones, there are also *Keyes's Figure of Merit* (KFM) and *Baliga's Figure of Merit* (BFM) which provide, respectively, for measuring thermal limitation to the switching behavior and high-frequency and high-power capability of devices, with ε being the dielectric constant and c the velocity of light. These parameters are important for evaluating high-frequency applications. The *FOMs* present a quantitative comparison of the semiconductors. The *FOM* values for diamond are a remarkable 40–50 times better than any other semiconductors as can be seen in the table. BFM and JFM for Si are taken as unity, whereas for GaAs those are 11.0 and 7.1, respectively, again for SiC are 29.0 and 278 and for GaN are 77.8 and 756 [35]. This comparison clearly shows that SiC and GaN are the most viable options for developing high-power and high-frequency ATT devices.

However, detailed investigations on the high-frequency behavior of SiC ATTs are not available despite of the fact that the fabrication of SiC IMPATTs has been reported in 2000–05 [24–26]. Theoretical work by I. Mehedi et al. [27] in 1988 has predicted that SiC IMPATT devices can offer spectacular high-power performance compared with conventional options. But their analysis has not accounted for the critical material parameters which were not considered at that stage. Later, Zhao et al. [28] in 2000 reported some simulation results on the 4H-SiC-based *hi-lo* IMPATT diode at around 200 GHz. But detailed analysis of the IMPATT characteristics, such as the electric field profile, current density profiles, nature of distribution of device negative resistivity in the avalanche and drift region of the diodes, device-admittance characteristics, and device-impedance characteristics were not available from their study. Recently, S. R. Pattanaik [29] in 2005 reported the performance of 6H-SiC IMPATT diodes at a window frequency (140 GHz). However, a systematic and detailed study on the MM-wave characteristics of 4H-SiC-based IMPATT diodes is still lacking. This has prompted the author to make an extensive study on various aspects of IMPATTs based on SiC in order to support the ongoing and future experimental works. One of the major purposes of the present thesis is to thoroughly investigate the static and dynamic performances of the WBG 4H-SiC IMPATT diodes operating at MM-wave atmospheric window frequencies 35, 140, and 220 GHz.

On the other hand, no experimental reports on another WBG device, GaN IMPATT, have yet been published. Panda et al. [30] in 2001 reported the DC and high-frequency characteristics of GaN-based IMPATTs at 140 GHz. But the values of RF power output, device negative conductance, and efficiency, as obtained from their simulation, did not predict the expected high potential of these devices. Improved modeling of MM-wave GaN IMPATT diodes incorporating all the latest available experimental data of material parameters in GaN, as well as corresponding high-frequency characteristics of these devices, is thus addressed in the thesis.

THz waves, occupying a large portion of the electromagnetic spectrum (300–10,000 GHz) between the millimeter (MM)-wave and infrared bands (Fig. 6.1), are the next frontier in basic natural science, medicine, and especially in technology. The so-called "Terahertz-gap" implies that a big challenge still occurs for THz technology since it is in the margin of electronics and photonics technologies. The THz regime is unique as it has the potential for developing innovative sensing and imaging technology which is unavailable in other portions of the electromagnetic spectrum [36,37]. The recent advancement of THz technology will impact wide variety of the potential applications including improvised explosive device detections [38,39], chemical and biological sensing [40,41], and medical diagnostics [42]. Compared with microwaves, the far-infrared or THz frequency range has significant reductions in antenna sizes [43,44] and greater communication bandwidth [45]. THz imaging can be employed for "Homeland Defense" and for contraband

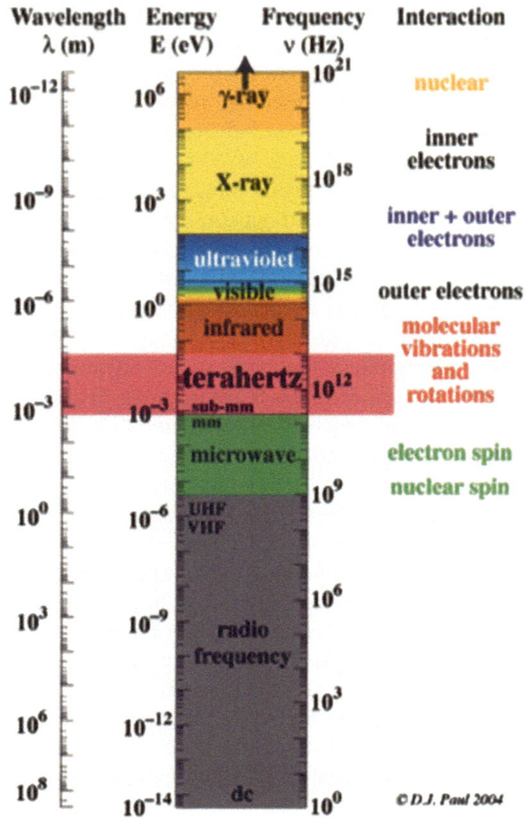

FIG. 6.1 Electromagnetic spectrum.

detection [46,47]. This is one of the critical technologies for defense against suicide bombers and other terrorist activities. Systems for rapidly emerging applications at THz frequencies thus require reliable high-power sources. In the last few years [23], the development of suitable sources for this frequency regime is being extensively explored worldwide. There are broadly two technology roadmaps for THz semiconductor devices. Approaching from the lower frequency range in the THz regime, electronic devices such as Gunn diode, RTD, and nanometer FETs based on plasma wave have been widely investigated for THz frequency generation. From higher portion of the THz frequency spectrum, the photonics-based device QCL extends the emission wavelength to THz spectral range [23]. The other approach to THz generation is through femtosecond lasers incident on materials with nonlinear optical properties or on photoconductors such as InP. Parametric amplifiers are also being used for the purpose.

All the above efforts are to pursue the effective generation of THz signals. Most of the available THz

TABLE 6.2
Material Properties of Si, GaAs, InP, and Important Wide Bandgap Semiconductors.

Semiconductor	Si	GaAs	6H-SiC	4H-SiC	3C-SiC	WZ-GaN	ZB-GaN	InP	Diamond
Bandgap (E_g) (eV)	S1	1.42	3.03	3.26	2.3	3.45	3.28	1.35	5.45
Electric breakdown field (E_C) (10^7 V m^{-1})	3.0	4.0	32.0	30.0	22.0	50.0	50.0	5.0	100.0
Relative dielectric constant (ε_r)	11.9	13.1	9.66	9.7	9.72	8.9	9.7	12.5	5.5
Electron mobility (μ_n) (m^2 $V^{-1}s^{-1}$)	0.15	0.85	0.04	0.10	0.08	0.125	0.100	0.54	0.22
Hole mobility (μ_p) (m^2 $V^{-1}s^{-1}$)	0.04	0.03	0.01	0.011	0.004	0.085	0.035	0.02	0.085
Saturated drift velocity of electrons (v_{sn}) (10^5 ms^{-1})	1.0	1.2	2.0	2.0	2.0	2.5	2.0	1.5	2.7
Thermal conductivity (K) (Wm^{-1} K^{-1})	150.0	46.0	490.0	490.0	450.0	225.0	130.0	69.0	1200.0

sources are complex and bulky. QCL, on the other hand, has the advantage of small size, though they require low temperature operation to directly generate THz. Thus, it seems that there is lack of availability of small-sized suitable THz source to serve a useful purpose. So, the development of high-power, low-cost, and compact semiconductor sources in THz regime has attracted the recent attention of researchers working in this field. Although reports of WBG IMPATTs in the MM-wave region are available in published literature [24–30], detailed and accurate investigations on the high-frequency characteristics of IMPATT diodes at THz region are scarcely available [31]. This prompted the author to study the prospects of IMPATT diodes at THz region. The unique material properties (Table 6.2) of WBG α-SiC (4H-SiC and 6H-SiC) and GaN (WZ and ZB), e.g., high critical electric field (E_C), high saturation velocity of carriers ($v_{sn,\ sp}$), and high thermal conductivity (K), all combined, make these materials ideal for realizing smaller transit times, an essential criteria for developing THz devices based on such materials. The author has thus made a detailed investigation on the relative merits and demerits of several WBG materials, such as 4H-SiC, 6H-SiC, WZ-GaN, and ZB-GaN, for developing small-sized THz IMPATT oscillators. Since all these semiconductors have different material parameters, separate studies on devices made from each of them are therefore necessary to evaluate the impact of the different polytypes of WBG semiconductors on IMPATT devices.

No experimental results on THz IMPATT diodes are available in recent literature. Only one theoretical analysis by Reklaitis et al. [31] on GaN-based IMPATT diode at around 0.7 THz predicted that GaN material has potential for developing high-frequency IMPATTs. However, at higher THz (>1.0 THz) region, the performances of GaN-based IMPATT devices have not been investigated till now. SiC IMPATTs as promising THz source have also not yet been studied by any researcher. A unique feature of this dissertation is that the author has made a timely approach to the simulation of WBG semiconductor-based IMPATT diodes for operation in the THz regime. In addition to WBG semiconductor-based IMPATT devices, considerable experimental and theoretical researches are being carried out to explore the high-frequency properties of another III-V compound, InP (indium phosphide) [46–49].

Compared with the III-V compound GaAs, the material parameters of InP are highly suitable for developing high-power MM-wave IMPATT devices. The material parameters, as shown in Table 6.2, reveal that although InP has a lower electron mobility compared with GaAs, the electron exhibits a higher saturation velocity (1.5×10^5 vs. 1.0×10^5 m s^{-1}). This fact is one of the main reasons for investigating the potential of InP-based IMPATTs as MM-wave sources. Under high electric fields, MM-wave and THz devices are expected to have shorter transit times resulting in higher frequency operation. Moreover, a higher value of carrier saturation velocity enhances the output power level of the devices. Although these properties are encouraging, experimental success in the fabrication of InP IMPATT diodes has been limited by the lack of established fabrication technologies. However, recently, with the advent of molecular beam epitaxy and metalorganic chemical vapor deposition techniques, the technological limitations in realizing InP-based IMPATT devices have been overcome significantly. Based on these improved technologies, one can expect fabrication of InP-based high-frequency IMPATTs. Keeping this in view, the author has simulated the DC and high-frequency properties of InP IMPATT diodes for operation at MM-wave window frequencies. Their performances are compared with those of Si and WBG semiconductor-based IMPATTs. Further, the prospects of InP IMPATT as THz sources have not been reported yet. Thus, the author has also undertaken the simulation of the properties of InP-based THz IMPATT diodes. This dissertation thus not only deals with the studies of SiC and GaN IMPATT diodes but also presents new results showing the prospect of InP as a material for THz IMPATT devices.

Scientists started looking into the "Terahertz-Gap" region toward the end of the 20th century. Various techniques have been developed by the scientific community to generate and detect THz waves. These systems can be categorized in three domains which are thermal, optical, and electronic-based systems.

Thermal Terahertz Systems

Blackbody radiator is a thermal-based THz source with radiated power ~ nano-watt. Since it can radiate up to the infrared region, characterization setup, for instance, is problematic. THz filters are required for this type of sources [50]. Among others, bolometers, pyroelectric devices, and Golay cell are thermal-based detectors [51,52]. They convert the incoming THz radiation into a thermal energy. A thermally dependent electric device is normally used to sense the temperature variation of the absorbing material. These devices can be very wide-band and very sensitive, but, having large time constants due to thermal dissipation, they are often cooled at cryogenic temperatures under very low pressure.

Optical Terahertz Systems

THz source development based on optical systems is wide, and they can be divided into two categories: continuous wave (CW) and pulsed sources. In the CW category, CO_2 optically pumped gas lasers are one of the high-power sources that could deliver a power of several hundreds of milli-watt that is available for laboratory experiments [52]. Based on the rotational frequency of pressure gas excited with a high-power laser source, the device can produce considerable power. As a consequence, the THz frequencies are discrete lines and can be selected by changing the low pressure gas. Thermal detectors are usually used with such sources to control the beam shape and the excitation modes. The photomixer is another CW source with an output power of about few nano-watts at THz frequencies [53]. It is based on the mixing product of two lasers running at different frequencies. As a result, the intermediate frequency of the mixing product is continuously tunable which is very useful in spectroscopy application. The photomixers can also be used as detectors by making use of the same mixing principle. The QCL is an optical-based THz source and can be CW or pulsed [54]. In a QCL, electrons are injected into a periodic structure of a biased superlattice [55]. The injected electrons undergo intersubband transitions in a cascade process resulting in an emission of a photon at THz frequencies. QCL sources can deliver power ~ few milli-watts, but they require cooling at cryogenic temperatures. Another pulsed source is the time-domain systems (TDSs). They are based on very short pulsed lasers in the order of few picoseconds [56]. With this technique, a wide-band THz pulse can be generated in a very short time. Photoconductive sampling and electrooptical sampling detectors are usually used for such system. Photoconductive dipole antennas have been used to produce broadband THz pulses up to about 1 THz. The most common use of the generation method, in medical applications, employs optical rectification, whereby the high-frequency oscillations of a femtosecond laser pulse are rectified by an optical crystal, leaving only the envelope of the laser signal which is a THz pulse [57].

Electronic Terahertz System

Backward wave oscillators and gyrotrons are high-power T-ray sources [58]. They are capable of delivering THz power in watt level. However, they require a strong magnetic field to operate. Nowadays, solid-state Gunn or tunnel diodes are dominating the THz market [59]. They are relatively compact in comparison to the previous technologies and are capable of delivering high power at >1 THz regime. Very recently, the development of a flexible and wearable THz scanner based on carbon nanotubes is reported [60]. The research team has achieved room temperature THz detection over a broad frequency band ranging from 0.14 to 39 THz and developed a portable THz scanner. RTD oscillators with a patch antenna were fabricated using an InGaAs/InAlAs/AlAs triple barrier structure. On the other side, Schottky barrier diode detectors with a log-periodic antenna were fabricated by thin-film technology on a Si substrate. Both devices can operate above 1 THz at room temperature [61–64]. Another research group has fabricated THz detectors in a low-cost 130 nm silicon CMOS technology. They have shown that the detectors consisting of an nMOS FET as rectifying element and an integrated bow-tie coupling antenna could achieve a record responsivity above 5 kV/W and a noise equivalent power below 10 pW/Hz in the important atmospheric window around 300 GHz and at room temperature. They have further demonstrated that the same detectors are efficient for imaging in a very wide frequency range from ~0.27 THz up to 1.05 THz [65]. Tera-Sense Company has developed a patent-protected technology for making a new generation of semiconductor detector arrays for THz imaging. The detector has good sensitivity compared with other available detectors working in THz range (0.1–0.5) THz. Tera-Sense detectors have an advantage with their low cost and ease of fabrication in large quantities in the form of 2D arrays. The detector arrays are scalable in the number of pixels. With the use of Tera-Sense imaging chips, an extremely compact and sensitive THz camera can be produced [66]. In addition to mammography, some more breast imaging modalities are used routinely [67]. Breast magnetic resonance imaging (MRI) is frequently used in breast cancer management especially to determine the extent of disease. 18F-fluorodeoxyglucose PET is increasingly used in staging advanced or recurrent breast cancer and in monitoring response to therapy. Though MRS and optical breast cancer imaging are not yet in routine clinical use, increasingly compelling data in patients will likely lead to more clinical use in the near future [67].

THZ IMAGING—AN OVERVIEW

Microwave and MM-wave imaging is used extensively for dielectric bodies. The comparatively larger wavelength is beneficial for penetration through optically opaque medium including wood, ceramic, plastics, concrete, fog, soil, clothing, as well as living tissues. MM-wave and microwave imaging has so far been largely used in medical diagnosis for imaging of isolated organ. With the advent of technology, these imaging techniques are used for bones, brain, and breast imaging. Most of the exciting developments happened in last two decades. However, clinical trials with patients are still under progress. In 1970, first experiment of microwave imaging of kidney was done by Larsen and Jacobi [68,69]. The generated images, 2D in nature, were sufficiently good to show various tissues. The imaged organ had been scanned in a plane perpendicular to both source and receiving antennae. The signals appeared as a function of x and y coordinate relative to the reference point on the organ plane. In a typical microwave scanning photograph of breast imaging, data acquisition is done by "Raster scanning technique." Larsen and Jacobi (1970) faced some fundamental challenges during the experiment related to the interaction issues between microwave field and living tissue. These issues could be dealt with during the installation of data acquisition apparatus and development of imaging algorithm. The basic principal of such microwave/millimeter (MM) wave imaging is to transfer the desired signal into human tissues and subsequently analyze changes in the back scattered ray. The changes appear due to the difference of electrical properties of tissues. If this variation is within the limit, then there is no question of concern. However, if the variation of scattered signal is beyond certain normal limit, then further investigation should be done for identifying any unwanted tumor cell within the organ under test. Usually tumor cell exhibits higher dielectric constant compared with its normal tissue counterpart. In case of standard microwave/MM-wave imaging, transmitting and receiving antennae along with sensors are implemented in the full system. The transmitting antennae sense MM-wave/microwave signal through the organ and the scattered signal (or in some cases the transmitted signals) from the organ under test is collected by the receiving antennae. The general properties of the antennae include directive power radiation, high gain and compact size, ability to transmit a good bandwidth of frequencies, higher efficiencies, and compatible penetration through human tissues. The available MM-wave antennae have some conducive properties such as high data rate, low interference, cost-effective design, robust application possibilities, and high precision values. Various electrical properties of living tissues, including muscle, fat, skin, and brain, are different from those of air. In lower MM-wave region, the relative permittivity of skin is 30 and specific conductivity is almost 3S m^{-2}, and thus skin acts as shielding layer against lower microwave or MM-wave radiation. Fat and muscle subsequent layers are responsible for rejection of the incident power by means of reflection and dissipation in form of conversion into heat energy. The electrical characteristics of tissues depend strongly on frequency. It is because of significant amount of water in living tissue. From experimental observation, it is found that relative permittivity of distil water is 90 at 1 GHz while with increasing frequency to 10 GHz it gets reduced to 50. Higher and lower permittivity of a given tissue is strongly associated with its relative water content. On the other hand, conductivity of a cell depends on variety of dissolved elements like sugar and salt. At higher MM-wave frequencies, the conductivity is influenced by water relaxation. In case of microwave imaging, the antenna along with the organ under test is immersed in coupling liquid. The liquid can be water or more sophisticated type liquid for getting optimal energy coupling. In this process, the antennae array are fitted within the tank filled with the liquid and the object is kept inside the tank. The body/organ of various dimensions can be accommodated in this setup. Most of the available proof-of-concept setups use these options. This technique has some disadvantages as well, those include spill over, reflection, and loss. Moreover, the maintenance of the system is to some extent problematic due to the immersed antennae into the liquid. Chances of patient contamination are also there. This problem can be addressed by designing microwave antennae with a different approach by coupling the power directly with the tissue. In this case, the power wastage is minimum and better sensitivity can be achieved. In microwave measurement, sensitivity is defined as the ability of the instrument to identify/detect the weakest signal against the noise background. Also better sensitivity means the ability of the system to detect low-dimensional and low-contrast objects. Tissues have significant conductivity; this results in significant signal attenuation and low-penetration depth. If a certain amount of microwave power can penetrate though the skin and tissue, it attenuates a 10 GHz signal by $> 80°$. This makes microwave unsuitable for deep body tumor within liver, brain, or kidney. Also in case of breast cancer imaging, the microwave system should be highly sensitive to identify signal that has been reduced by 100° than the initial signal. Considering the noise factor, this is indeed a challenge. The image quality of the scanning system is also another parameter of concern. Resolution limit is defined as the smallest distance in between two tiny but detectable objects in the image. If the objects are very close to each other and the in-between distance is smaller in comparison to the system resolution, that will appear as a single object. A typical resolution in a 3 T MRI system for breast image is 1 mm. The resolution depends upon diffraction limits. Diffraction limit is linked with far-field measurement and approximately one-quarter of the incident wavelength. In this way, diffraction limit is related to microwave frequency radiation. Thus, shorter the wavelength, smaller the capture size of the image and hence better resolution.

Over the last decades, biomedical imaging technologies have been developed for getting internal information of the human body. Computed tomography, ultrasound, X-ray mammography, and MRI are the most frequently used radiological diagnostic tools for detecting abnormalities in tissue level [70–73]. X-ray mammography, though a useful technique in screening breast malignancy, produces in between 10% and 30% false-negative diagnosis and more than 5% false-positive diagnosis. In addition to that mammography uses ionizing radiation X-ray which is harmful for cell/tissue. Additionally, mammography procedure requires uncomfortable compression of the breast organ for examination and thus younger women show less interest to go through this procedure. Deep-lying malignant tissues are also difficult to detect in X-ray mammography. Such procedure has serious limitation with radiation risk, many false negatives occur since tumors are frequently located in the upper outer side of the breasts where the scans do not reach. So, alternative methods are required. T-rays are neither energetic enough to break chemical bonds nor do they ionize molecules/atoms; therefore, T-ray imaging is harmless for living organisms, unlike to high-energy photons such as X-rays and UV rays that may induce cancer. Besides, low-energy T-ray imaging has potential ability to scan deep into tissues in such cases where X-rays either fail to reach or are potentially threatening as has been mentioned above. Thus, this safe T-ray imaging technique has opened up infinite opportunities in biomedical research. THz imaging systems are expected to detect the early stage of cancer before it is visible or can be detected by any other means of identification. As a matter of fact, refractive index, absorption coefficient, and dielectric properties of the malignant tissues are higher than those of normal tissues due to higher water content and structural changes due to carcinoma. Hence, T-ray imaging is a safer and better method for breast tumor screening and timely retention. Till date, a concise report on the state-of-the art of availability and applicability of T-ray in biomedical imaging is not as such available. Therefore, the current chapter proceeds with such an aim. By analyzing the T-ray generated thermographs, it would be easy and accurate to distinguish healthy tissue and soft tissue basal cell carcinoma in breast/colon, and this will play significant role in mapping the exact margin of tumor. As is widely accepted, the proliferation of the THz applications into everyday life has been hindered by the lack of compact, portable, high-power, cost-effective, room temperature sources and sensitive and fast THz detectors. Currently, T-ray imaging technology has been encountering obstacles such as the use of bulky and expensive equipment, the necessity for cryogenic cooling, and slow read out speed. Hence, research should be aimed at overcoming the said obstacle in T-ray imaging technology by designing and developing a suitable active source able to target and detect breast tumors by THz procedure.

The above review clearly reflects the limitations of available imaging systems and the importance of THz imaging for reliable identification of in situ malignancy. However, for biomedical applications, compact room temperature sources are required. The suitability of ATT diodes are already established and briefly outlined earlier. Therefore, future research could be focused on developing THz radiation using ATT oscillator technology. Various technological advancements are required for its real-time on-chip development for biomedical applications. Harmonic analysis and power generation, structural changes in active region, and nanoscale fabrication of devices are some of the proposed technology that could be incorporated in developing high-power, high-frequency devices for biomedical imaging. However, substantial research has already been done exploring the promising IMPATT oscillators for THz technology using a wide range of efficient materials [74–80]. Such research has subsequently revealed the needs of fabrication friendly semiconductors for preventing this IMPATT technology from entering into saturation. Therefore, the following section will give some futuristic idea on technological advancements that could be incorporated in the development of IMPATT oscillator for medical imaging.

Proposed New Technology

Strain is an inevitable outcome of any composite structure which consists of various materials having different lattice and thermoelastic constants. All most all semiconductor devices are an ensemble of a wide range of materials, namely metals, insulators (oxides), and semiconductors. Moreover, for nanostructures a suitable substrate is always required for subsequent fabrication steps to follow, e.g., ultrathin films lying atop of buried oxide. The above-mentioned film forms the channel of the device. The lattice constants of the film and the substrate are obviously different from each other; this in turn induces a lattice mismatch strain in the thin film, since such film is being physically supported by the substrate. In this context, it deserves mention that the nanoscale dimensions of the film amplify the impact of the induced strain, whereas the counter strain in the underlying substrate is negligible and vanishes rapidly with depth. Such lattice mismatch strain is coupled with the thermal strain induced by the mismatch of thermal and elastic constants of the materials constituting the film and the substrate. By elastic constant, the fundamental material parameters such as Young's modulus and Poisson's ratio are meant. On the other hand, thermal constant means linear or multidimensional thermal expansion coefficients of the concerned materials. Subsequent steps involved in the fabrication process flow require such ensemble of various materials as in a semiconductor device, to go through various temperature cycles. This implies expansion and contraction of the various materials to different extents which in turn results in a subsequent tension or compression of the semiconductor channel depending on the mismatch of thermoelastic parameters. As a consequence, the combined effect of lattice and thermoelastic mismatch induces inherent strain to various extents in various portions of the device. The lattice mismatch-induced strain in a concerned material A due to any other misfitting material B can be estimated from a fundamental strain, $\varepsilon_{ij}^{lattice-mismatch}$, which has been shown in Eq. (6.1). However, several intricacies, modifications, and very subtle analysis are required depending on the geometric structure of the strained layer as well as the stressor constituting the specific device.

$$\varepsilon_{ij}^{lattice-mismatch} = \frac{\left(L_{ij}^{B} - L_{ij}^{A}\right)}{L_{ij}^{A}} \tag{6.1}$$

Here, $L_{ij}^{A(B)}$ is the lattice constant of material A (or B), i and j represent dimensions (i.e., directions depending on orientation of the lattice of the two relevant materials). On the other hand, the strain induced due to the mismatch of thermal expansion coefficients and other such thermal parameters between materials A and B can be expressed as follows:

$$\varepsilon_{ij}^{thermal-mismatch} = \Delta\alpha\Delta T\left(\delta_{ij}^{A} - \delta_{ij}^{B}\right) \tag{6.2}$$

Here, $\Delta\alpha$ is the cumulative mismatch of thermal expansion coefficients, and it will be n-dimensional depending on the nature of induced strain, which has been described in details in the subsequent sections of this chapter. ΔT is the temperature variation which has induced the mismatch of expansion (or contraction) between the two relevant materials, A and B, which are in contact with each other.

$$S_{ijmn} = D_{ijmn}\varepsilon_{ij}^{Total} \quad (6.3)$$

S_{ijmn} and D_{ijmn} are the resultant stress and dimension as well as direction-dependent elastic parameters. However, such involuntary strain inherently induced in the portion of the semiconductor constituting the channel/active region of the device can be quite concerning, since strain can remarkably alter device performance by affecting carrier mobility. Strain alters the dispersion curvature in case of electrons and the band warping for the holes. As is known effective mass is given by

$$m^* = \frac{\left(\frac{h}{2\pi}\right)^2}{\frac{d^2E}{dk^2}} \quad (6.4)$$

Therefore, it is evident from Eq. (6.1) that the dispersion curvature is inversely proportional to effective mass. Again electron mobility is related to effective mass as follows:

$$\mu = \frac{e\tau}{m^*} \quad (6.5)$$

Therefore, altering the dispersion curvature which is what strain specifically does, the carrier mobility can be significantly changed. In this context, it deserves mention that strain can be classified into two principal categories namely (A) uniaxial and (B) in-plane biaxial, based on its orientation. The nature of strain which acts along a specific axis of the three-dimensional structure that is supposed to be under strain is termed uniaxial if the respective amounts of strain along the two remaining dimensions are negligible compared with the principal axis of strain. On the other hand, if the amounts of strain acting along both of the two dimensions of a plane along the device are comparable in magnitude and compatible in nature, then this can be termed as in-plane biaxial strain. This again can be of two types: (A) equi-biaxial and simply (B) biaxial. This categorization is based on the magnitudes of strains of identical nature that are acting along each of the two axes of the concerned plane. If the amounts of strain along both axes are almost equal, then the complete strain profile along the plane can be termed as an equi-biaxial one. Otherwise, if the strains along the two axes are of the same nature but appreciably varying in magnitude, then it is simply biaxial.

Usually an inherent strain which is involuntarily induced into the semiconductor constituting the active region of a composite device, as has been explained above, is biaxial and very rarely uniaxial or even equi-biaxial in nature. However, study reveals such a strain profile of somewhat irregular nature affects the dispersion curve in such ways as to increase the carrier effective mass and so in turn retard the corresponding mobility [81]. Therefore, an involuntary incorporation of such inherent strain has up till recently thought of as undesirable since it generally has an adverse effect on device performance due to a degraded mobility. This has evoked current research to engineer such inherently induced strain incorporated along the channel region of the device by adjusting the dimensions of various portions of the device depending on its geometry [82–89]. A judicious choice of relevant materials involved in the fabrication of the device, such as the buried oxide or gate insulator and the metal or poly-Si sort of gate material etc, serves as another important tool for such strain engineering. Since this completely new approach of strain engineering is absolutely device-specific, in the sense that it depends solely on the device geometry, its dimensions, required materials, temperature variations involved in the fabrication process, etc., this is process-induced strain engineering. Such process-induced strain engineering has been recently applied to a wide range of devices, including ultrathin body (UTB) MOSFETs, nanowire FETs, vertical ATT devices, etc. In this context, it deserves mention that the semiconductor used in all such strain-engineered devices is Si. It has been reported long back by both the research community and industry that Si has reached saturation due to its low mobility. However, Si has its own fundamental advantages, most importantly its ease of fabrication. Though researchers have been proposing various striking advancements in the field of semiconductor devices using III-V, II-VI, or other advanced materials, yet extremely complex technologies are required to fabricate such advanced semiconductor devices at a large scale. Besides, the standard process flows and technologies on which the industry is currently based on are compatible to Si. Hence, despite the ample promises of the advanced semiconductor materials, Si still remains the reliable material. As has been already mentioned, strain engineering can increase the mobility of Si by tampering the dispersion curve depending on the required nature of strain. Such strain-induced mobility boosting can allow further use of Si in high-frequency devices, by overcoming its basic shortcoming. It has already been shown that process-induced strain is capable of remarkably increasing carrier mobility in Si, even for holes and of course electrons. Such mobility enhancement scheme has been recently proved to be successful for UTB MOSFETs and various other classes of FETs. Therefore, process-induced strain is a promising candidate and its introduction to ATT devices can further extend their applicability as high-frequency sources, detectors, and sensors. Current research has shown that incorporation of strain engineering in the active region of a Si-based vertical SDR ATT diode can immensely reduce the transit time for avalanche operation and, therefore, result in a Si-based ATT diode which operates in sub-MM range.

REFERENCES

[1] A. Crocker, H.A. Gebbie, M.F. Kimmitt, L.E.S. Mathias, Nature 201 (1964) 250.

[2] T.Y. Chang, T.J. Bridges, Optics Communications 1 (1970) 423.

[3] K.J. Button, D.R. Cohn, M. von Ortenberg, B. Lax, E. Mollwo, R. Helbig, Physical Review Letters 28 (1972) 1637.

[4] K.H. Yang, P.L. Richards, Y.R. Shen, Applied Physics Letters 19 (1971) 320.

[5] Y.R. Shen, Progress in Quantum Electronics 4 (1976) 207.

[6] P.L. Richards, Journal of the Optical Society of America 54 (1964) 1474.

[7] K. Sakai, T. Fukui, Y. Tsunawaki, H. Yoshinaga, Japanese Journal of Applied Physics 8 (1969) 1046.

[8] G.A. Mourou, K.E. Meyer, Applied Physics Letters 45 (1984) 492.

[9] P.R. Smith, D.H. Auston, M.C. Nuss, IEEE Journal of Quantum Electronics 24 (1988) 255.

[10] Fattinger, D. Grischkowsky, Applied Physics Letters 54 (1989) 490.

[11] M. van Exter, D. Grischkowsky, IEEE Transactions on Microwave Theory and Techniques 38 (1990) 1684.

[12] B.S. Williams, Nature Photonics 1 (2007) 517.

[13] G.T. Liu, Q.J. Wang, Recent Developments of Terahertz Quantum Cascade Lasers, IEEE Journal of Selected Topics in Quantum Electronics 23 (4) (2017), 1200118, p. 1–18, https://doi.org/10.1109/JSTQE.2016.2625982.

[14] K. O, IEEE Journal of Solid-State Circuits 45 (2010) 1554.

[15] M. Urteaga, Z. Griffith, M. Seo, J. Hacker, M.J.W. Rodwell, SAVE Proceedings.

[16] IEEE 105 (2017) 1051.

[17] B.B. Hu, M.C. Nuss, Optics Letters 20 (1995) 1716.

[18] J.T. Kindt, C.A. Schmuttenmaer, Journal of Physical Chemistry 100 (1996) 10373.

[19] C. Ronne, P.-O. Astraand, S.R. Keiding, Physical Review Letters 82 (1999) 2888.

[20] J. Boyd, A. Briskman, V. Colvin, D. Mittleman, Physical Review Letters 87 (2001) 147401.

[21] A.G. Markelz, A. Roitberg, E.J. Heilweil, Chemical Physics Letters 320 (2000) 42.

[22] M. Brucherseifer, M. Nagel, P.H. Bolivar, H. Kurz, A. Bosserhoff, R. Buttner, Applied Physics Letters 77 (2000) 4049.

[23] M. Koch, Terahertz-technology: Quo Vadis, Photonik International (2006) 1–5 (Originally published in German in Photonik, 4/2005.

[24] L. Yuan, M.R. Melloch Jr., J.A. Cooper, K.J. Webb, Silicon Carbide IMPATT oscillators for high power microwave and millimeter-wave generation, IEEE/Cornell Conf. Advanced Concepts in High Speed Semiconductor Devices and Circuit, Ithaca, NY, August 7–9, 2000.

[25] S. Ono, M. Arai, C. Kimura, Demonstration of high power X-band oscillation in p^+ n– n^+ 4H SiC IMPATT diodes with guard-ring termination, Materials Science Forum 483–485 (2005) 981–984.

[26] K. Vassilevski, A. Zorenko, et al., 4H-SiC IMPATT diode fabrication and testing, in: Tech. Digest of Int. Conf. on SiC and Related Materials- ICSCRM, Tsukuba, Japan, 2001, p. 713.

[27] I. Mehdi, G.I. Haddad, R.K. Mains, Microwave and millimeter-wave power generation in silicon carbide avalanche devices, Journal of Applied Physics 64 (3) (1988) 1533–1540.

[28] J.H. Zhao, et al., Monte Carlo simulation of 4H-SiC IMPATT diode, Semiconductor Science and Technology 15 (2000) 1093–1100.

[29] S.R. Pattanaik, G.N. Dash, J.K. Mishra, Prospects of 6H-SiC for operation as an IMPATTdiode at 140 GHz, Semiconductor Science and Technology 20 (2005) 299–304.

[30] A.K. Panda, D. Pavlidis, E. Alekseev, DC and high frequency characteristics of GaN based IMPATTs, IEEE Transactions on Electron Devices 48 (4) (April 2001) 820.

[31] A. Reklaitis, L. Reggiani, Monte Carlo study of hot carrier transport in bulk wurtzite GaN and modeling of a near terahertz impact avalanche transit time diode, Journal of Applied Physics 95 (12) (June 2004) 7925–7935.

[32] R.J. Trew, High frequency solid state electronic devices, IEEE Transactions on Electron Devices 52 (5) (2005) 638–649.

[33] Y. Gurbuz, et al., Diamond semiconductor technology for RF device applications, Solid-State Electronics 49 (2005) 1055–1070.

[34] P.G. Neudeck, R.S. Okojie, L.-Y. Chen, High-temperature electronics – a role for wide bandgap semiconductors, Proceedings of the IEEE 90 (2002) 1065–1076.

[35] V.V. Buniatyan, V.M. Aroutiounian, Wide gap semiconductor microwave devices, Journal of Physics D Applied Physics 40 (2007) 6355–6385.

[36] C.A. Schmuttenmaer, Exploring dynamics in the far-infrared with terahertz spectroscopy, Chemical Reviews 104 (2004) 1759.

[37] E.C. Camus, et al., Polarization-sensitive terahertz detection by multi contact photoconductive receivers, Applied Physics Letters 86 (2005) 254102.

[38] Y.C. Shen, T. Lo, P.F. Taday, B.E. Cole, W.R. Tribe, M.C. Kemp, Detection and identification of explosives using terahertz pulsed spectroscopic imaging, Applied Physics Letters 86 (2005) 241116.

[39] L. Senesac, T.G. Thundat, Nanosensors for trace explosive detection, Materials Today 11 (3) (2008) 28.

[40] T. Kiwa, et al., Chemical sensing plate with a laser-terahertz monitoring system, Applied Optics 47 (2008) 3324.

[41] E.C. Camus, M.B. Johnston, Conformational changes of photoactive yellow protein monitored by terahertz spectroscopy, Chemical Physics Letters 455 (2008) 289.

[42] R.M. Woodward, B.E. Cole, V.P. Wallace, R.J. Pye, D.D. Arnone, E.H. Linfield, M. Pepper, Terahertz pulse imaging in reflection geometry of human skin cancer and skin tissue, Physics in Medicine and Biology 47 (2002) 3853.

[43] J. Kolodzey, T.N. Adam, R.T. Troeger, P.C. Lv, S.K. Ray, G. Looney, A. Rosen, M.S. Kagan, I.N. Yassievich, Proc. Tropical Meeting on Silicon Monolithic Integrated Circuits in RF Systems, 9th – 11th April 2003 Germany.

[44] A. Sharma, A. Singh, Rectangular microstirp patch antenna design at THz frequency for short distance wireless communication systems, Journal of Infrared, Millimeter and Terahertz Waves 30 (2009) 1–7.

[45] K. Maki, C. Otani, Terahertz beam steering and frequency tuning by using the spatial dispersion of ultrafast laser pulses, Optics Express 16 (2008) 10158.

[46] J.J. Berenz, F.B. Frank, T.L. Hiert, Ion-implanted p^+ n junction indium-phosphide impatt diodes, Electronics Letters 14 (1978) 683.

[47] H. Eisele, C.C. Chen, G.O. Munns, G.I. Haddad, The Potential of InP IMPATT Diodes as High Power Millimeter-Wave Sources: First Experimental Results, IEEE MTTs Digest, 1996, pp. 529–532.

[48] R. Mukherjee, J.P. Banerjee, Avalanche and drift layer contributions to the negative resistance of millimeter wave p^+ n n^+ InP IMPATT diode for different current densities, International Journal of Electronics 76 (1994) 589–600.

[49] Y. Nemirovsky, A. Svetlitza, I. Brouk, S. Stolyarova, Nanometric cmos soi-nems transistor for uncooled thz sensing, IEEE Transactions on Electron Devices 60 (5) (2013) 1575–1583, 2.

[50] B. Karasik, A. Sergeev, D. Prober, Nanobolometers for THz photon detection, IEEE Transactions on Terahertz Science and Technology 1 (1) (September 2011) 97–111.

[51] T. Klaassen, N. Hovenier, J. Fischer, G. Jakob, A. Poglitsch, O. Sternberg, Terahertz calorimetry: an absolute power meter for terahertz radiation and the absorptivity of the herschel space observatory telescope mirrorcoating, in: Cof. on Integrated Optoelectronic Devices, 2004, pp. 159–167, 2.

[52] V. Gorobets, B. Kuntsevich, V. Petukhov, Terahertz gas laser, in: Int. Conf. on Infrared, Millimeter, and Terahertz Waves, 2006, pp. 218–220.

[53] E. Brown, K. McIntosh, K. Nichols, C. Dennis, Photomixing up to 3.8 THz in low-temperature grown GaAs, Applied Physics Letters 66 (3) (1995) 285–287, 3.

[54] B.S. Williams, Terahertz quantum-cascade lasers, Nature Photonics 1 (9) (2007) 517–525.

[55] G. Gallerano, S. Biedronet al., Overview of terahertz radiation sources, in: Proceedings of the FEL Conference, 2004, pp. 216–221.

[56] M. Tonouchi, Cutting-edge terahertz technology, Nature Photonics 1 (2) (2007) 97–105, 3.

[57] S. Mickan, D. Abbott, J. Munch, X.-C. Zhang, T. van Doorn, Analysis of system trade-offs for terahertz imaging, Microelectronics Journal (2000) 503–514.

[58] J.H. Booske, J. Dobbs, C.D. Joyee, J. Perk, R.J. Tompk, Vacuum Electronic high-power THz sources, IEEE Transactions on Terahertz Science and Technology 1 (No. 1) (September 2011) 54.

[59] J.L. Hesler, T. Crowe, High-power Solid-State Terahertz Sources, SPIE Newsroom, 2015, https://doi.org/10.1117/2.1201507.005859.

[60] D. Suzuki, S. Oda, Y. Kawano, A flexible and wearable terahertz scanner, Nature Photonics 10 (2016) 809–813.

[61] S. Suzuki, M. Asada, A. Teranishi, H. Sugiyama, H. Yokoyama, Fundamental oscillation of resonant tunneling diodes above 1 THz at room temperature, Applied Physics Letters 97 (2010) 242102.

[62] H. Kanaya, H. Shibayama, R. Sogabe, S. Suzuki, M. Asada, Fundamental oscillation up to 1.31 THz in resonant tunneling diodes with thin well and barriers, Applied Physics Express 5 (2012) 124101.

[63] Y. Koyama, R. Sekiguchi, T. Ouchi, Oscillations up to 1.40 THz from resonant tunneling diode based oscillators with integrated patch antenna, Applied Physics Express (2013) 064102.

[64] InP-based planar-antenna-integrated Schottky-barrier diode for millimeter- and sub-millimeter-wave detection, Japanese Journal of Applied Physics 47 (2008) 6256.

[65] F. Schuster, D. Coquillat, H. Videlier, M. Sakowicz, F. Teppe, L. Dussopt, B. Giffard, T. Skotnicki, W. Knap, Broadband terahertz imaging with highly sensitive silicon CMOS detectors, Optics Express 19 (2011) 7827.

[66] Tera-Sense, US Patent, High-Speed Giga-Terahertz Imaging Device and Method, (US 20130161514 A).

[67] S. Holfvind, B.M. Geller, J. Skelli, P.M. Vacek, Sensitivity and specificity of mammographic screening aspractised in Vermont and Norway, in: L.E. Larsen, J.H. Jacobi (Eds.), British Journal of Radiology, Medical Applications of Microwave Imaging, vol. 85, IEEE Press, 2012, p. 1020, 1986.

[68] L.E. Larsen, J.H. Jacobi, "Microwave interrogation of dielectric targets—part I: by scattering parameters, Medical Physics 5 (6) (1978) 500–508.

[69] N.K. Nikolova, Microwave imaging for breast cancer, IEEE Microwave Magazine 12 (7) (2011) 78–94.

[70] D.M. Sheen, D.L. McMakin, T.E. Hall, Near field imaging at microwave and millimeter wave frequencies, in: Proceedings of the IEEE MTT-S International Microwave Symposium (IMS '07), June 2007, pp. 1693–1696.

[71] D.M. Sheen, D.L. McMakin, T.E. Hall, Three-dimensional millimeter-wave imaging for concealed weapon detection, IEEE Transactions on Microwave Theory and Techniques 49 (9) (2001) 1581–1592.

[72] D. Sheen, D. McMakin, T. Hall, Near-field three-dimensional radar imaging techniques and applications, Applied Optics 49 (19) (2010) E83–E93.

[73] J. Detlefsen, A. Dallinger, S. Schelkshorn, Effective reconstruction approaches to millimeter-wave imaging of humans, in: Proceedings of the 28th General Assembly of International Union of Radio Science, 2005, pp. 23–29.

[74] M. Mukherjee, N. Mazumder, S.K. Roy, K. Goswami, GaN IMPATT diode: a photo-sensitive high power terahertz source, Semiconductor Science and Technology 22 (12) (October 2007) 1258–1260, https://doi.org/10.1088/0268-1242/22/12/003.

[75] M. Mukherjee, S.K. Roy, Optically modulated III–V nitride-based top-mounted and flip-chip IMPATT oscillators at terahertz regime: studies on the shift of avalanche transit time phase delay due to photo generated carriers, IEEE Transactions on Electron Devices 56 (7) (June 2009) 1411–1417, https://doi.org/10.1109/TED.2009.2021441.

[76] A. Kundu, S. Adhikari, A. Das, M.R. Kanjilal, M. Mukherjee, Design and characterization of asymmetrical super-lattice Si/4H-SiC pin photo diode array: a potential opto-sensor for future applications in bio-medical domain, Microsystem Technologies (September 2018), https://doi.org/10.1007/s00542-018-4119-4.

[77] M. Mukherjee, N. Mazumder, S.K. Roy, Photosensitivity analysis of gallium nitride and silicon carbide terahertz IMPATT oscillators: comparison of theoretical reliability and study on experimental feasibility, IEEE Transactions on Device and Materials Reliability 8 (3) (September 2008) 608–620, https://doi.org/10.1109/TDMR.2008.2002358.

[78] A. Kundu, M.R. Kanjilal, M. Mukherjee, III–V super-lattice SPST/SPMT pin switches for THz communication: theoretical reliability and experimental feasibility studies, Microsystem Technologies (July 2018), https://doi.org/10.1007/s00542-018-4053-5.

[79] A. Kundu, M.R. Kanjilal, M. Mukherjee, Cubic versus hexagonal SiC vertical pin SPST/SPDT/SPMT switches for MMW communication systems: a modified quantum drift-diffusion model for switching characteristics analysis, Microsystem Technologies: Micro- and Nanosystems Information Storage and Processing Systems (May 2019), https://doi.org/10.1007/s00542-019-04445-9. Springer Nature.

[80] M. Mukherjee, N. Majumder, Prospect of a β-Silicon based IMPATT oscillator for application in THz communication and growth of a β SiC p-n junction on a Ge modified Si(100) substrate of realize THz IMPATTs, Journal of Semiconductors 31 (12) (2010) 124001, https://doi.org/10.1088/1674-4926/31/12/124001.

[81] S.E. Thompson, G. Sun, Y.S. Choi, T. Nishida, Uniaxial process- induced strained-Si: extending the CMOS roadmap, IEEE Transactions on Electron Devices 53 (5) (May 2006) 1010–1020, https://doi.org/10.1109/TED.2006.872088.

[82] S. Chatterjee, M. Mukherjee, "Strain-Engineered asymmetrical superlattice $Si/Si_{1-x}Ge_x$ nano-ATT ⟨p++-n-n⁻-n++⟩ oscillator: enhanced photo-sensitivity in terahertz domain", IEEE Transactions on Electron Devices 66 (8) (July 2019) 3659–3667, https://doi.org/10.1109/TED.2019.2923108.

[83] S. Chatterjee, S. Sikdar, B.N. Chowdhury, S. Chattopadhyay, Investigation of the performance of strain-engineered silicon nanowire field effect transistors (ε-Si-NWFET) on IOS substrates, Journal of Applied Physics 125 (2019) 082506, https://doi.org/10.1063/1.5051310.

[84] S. Chatterjee, S. Chattopadhyay, Fraction of insertion of the channel-fin as performance booster in strain-engineered p-FinFET devices with insulator-on-silicon (IOS) substrate, IEEE Transactions on Electron Devices 65 (2) (2018) 411–418, https://doi.org/10.1109/TED.2017.2781264.

[85] S. Chatterjee, S. Chattopadhyay, Analytical modeling of the lattice and thermo-elastic coefficient mismatch-induced stress into silicon nanowires horizontally embedded on insulator-on-silicon substrates, Superlattices and Microstructures 101 (Jan. 2017) 384–396, https://doi.org/10.1016/j.spmi.2016.12.001.

[86] S. Chatterjee, S. Chattopadhyay, Modeling and estimation of process-induced stress in the nanowire field-effect-transistors (NW-FETs) on insulator-on-silicon substrates with high-k gate-dielectrics, Superlattices and Microstructures 98 (Oct. 2016) 194–202, https://doi.org/10.1016/j.spmi.2016.08.022.

[87] S. Chatterjee, B.N. Chowdhury, A. Das, S. Chattopadhyay, Estimation of step-by-step induced stress in a sequential process integration of nano-scale sosmosfets with high-*k* gate dielectrics, Semiconductor Science and Technology 28 (Nov. 2013) 125011, https://doi.org/10.1088/0268-1242/28/12/125011.

[88] S. Chatterjee, Process-induced-strain maximisation of nanoscale silicon-on-sapphire high-k gate-dielectric mosfets by adjusting device aspect ratio, 2nd IEEE International Conference on Emerging Electronics, Electron Device Society (Icee-2014), IISC, Bangalore.

[89] S. Chatterjee, S. Chattopadhyay, A. Bhattacharyya, Process-induced strain engineering in the silicon-on-sapphire (SOS) fin field effect transistor (finfet) channels, Proc. of 2015 6th International Conference on Computers and Devices for Communication (CODEC) Institute of Radio Physics & Electronics, University Of Calcutta.

CHAPTER 7

A Framework Development on Big Data Analytics for Terahertz Healthcare

DEBASHIS DAS, MTECH • CHINMAY CHAKRABORTY, PHD • SOURAV BANERJEE, PHD

INTRODUCTION

Healthcare information mainly includes radiology images, 3D imaging, personal medical information, signals or sensor readings, genomic expression, etc., which consume a volume of around 150 exabytes (EB), followed by a regular increment of 1.2–2.4 EB per annum [3]. These data show as well effective variations to be engaged in big data analytics. The information generated from healthcare traditionally is static, the speed of accumulation takes a big leap with digital monitoring of health conditions. With the evolution of big data, two "V's" come under the spotlight: veracity and value [4].

Big data analysts are attempting to make use of the tremendous sum of data to reach a conclusion which progresses not as it were their choice making capacity but benefit, efficiency and control to peep into the past to look upon the longer term to create it much more great and effective [5]. Numerous analysts have characterized big data utilizing the concept of V's, which may vary from three to five depending on how they see the big data and how they are utilizing the big data. The fundamental definition of huge information is clarified by utilizing the three V's, volume (how big the volume of data is, which can be in petabytes), velocity (how quick the data is produced and overseen), and variety (the diverse designs of the data that can be processed together) [1]. Most of the countries uses open healthcare frameworks for storing electronic records with progressive therapeutic imaging media. Big data provides an awesome opportunity for disease transmission experts, clinicians, and medical approach specialists to form data-driven judgments that will, in the long run, direct patient care.

The healthcare industry is one of the world's largest industries in development [6]. There is a change happening, from disease-centric to patient-centric and from volume-based to value-based healthcare, around the world. To supply viable patient-centered care, it is fundamental to oversee and analyze a tremendous amount of health information. The administrative information are not adequate to analyze big data, as the assortment and volume of information sources have expanded since 2000. There is a requirement for new and imaginative huge information devices and advances that can meet and surpass the capacity to oversee healthcare data. Big data frameworks are collecting large amounts of medical information from different healthcare establishments and overseeing, analyzing, and visualizing the data for viable choice making.

These days, there is an expanding request for more data by clinicians regarding their healthcare alternatives or choices, and they need support in their health decision-making [6]. The big data will offer assistance to patients by supplying them with up-to-date information to help them make the best choices and comply with their therapeutic treatment. Nowadays, information quality relates to the quality of patient care. This move to value-based installments compares with a focus on patient-centric care. Healthcare experts and health insurance providers must work together to provide individualized care that is productive, is straightforward in billing, and make strides in patient satisfaction [7].

Utilizing big data in healthcare can assist healthcare companies in supplying proactive care, adding to their understanding by continually observing imperative signs. Information from these screens can be analyzed in real time, and if a patient's condition changes, a care supplier can be alerted instantly. Doctors can pick up valuable bits of knowledge and make lifesaving choices by comparing real-time occasions with machine learning algorithms. The healthcare industry is encountering [7] a major information change due to the rising notoriety of progressive analytics and big data advances.

Terahertz Biomedical and Healthcare Technologies. https://doi.org/10.1016/B978-0-12-818556-8.00007-0

The utilization of big data in healthcare is allowing different players in this division to better outcomes [2]. Therapeutic information envelops diverse healing centers from different territorial or geological areas. They incorporate a few authoritative frameworks. This requires the utilization of new instruments that can offer assistance to information suppliers and information clients to collaborate with each other.

Terahertz (THz) imaging (around 1012 Hz) is a well-suited method for medical image analysis purposes. THz reflection imaging is nonionizing and has potential as medical imaging; however, there is currently no consensus on the optimum imaging parameters to apply and the procedure for data analysis. From the foregoing contemplations, THz innovation offers the guarantee of overcoming the aforementioned insufficiencies by actualizing a self-cross-checking procedure.

Big Data in Healthcare

The important role that big data play in healthcare [8] includes a part for positive and additionally lifesaving results. Big data alludes to the endless amounts of data made by the digitization of everything, which gets solidified and analyzed by particular advances. With regard to healthcare, it will utilize particular health data of a populace (or of a specific person) and possibly offer assistance to avoid scourges, remedy infection, minimize costs, etc.

At present, we live longer, and treatment frameworks have changed, and many of these changes are specifically driven by information. Specialists are trying to identify the patients vital sign in the help of this tool with minimal cost. In fact, for a long time gathering gigantic sums of information for restorative use has been expensive and time consuming. With today's always improving advances, it becomes less demanding, not, as it were, to gather such information, but to change over it into important basic experiences that can then be utilized to supply superior care. The healthcare analytics utilizes data-driven discoveries to foresee and illuminate an issue, sometimes early as well as late, but also to survey strategies and medicines faster, keep much better track of stock, and involve patients more in their health maintenance and enable them with the devices to do so.

Importance of Big Data Analysis in Healthcare

The quality of healthcare [9] can be expanded in view of the following:

Patient-centric services: to supply quicker alleviation to the patients by giving evidence-based pharmaceuticals, identifying illnesses at the early stages based on the accessible clinical information, minimizing sedative dosages to dodge side effects, and giving proficient medications based on hereditary makeup.

Early disease identification: foreseeing viral infections before spread based on a live investigation. This may be recognized by analyzing the social logs of the patients suffering from a malady in a specific geo-location. This makes a difference so that healthcare experts to reduce casualties by taking fundamental preventive measures.

Hospital quality monitoring: The patients health monitoring tool has been developed for predicting the disease status in a timely manner The periodic patient status monitoring tool was developed for predicting the disease status in a timely manner [10].

Advancement of treatment methods: customized case treatment monitors the impact of pharmaceuticals ceaselessly, and based on the investigation, the dose of medicine can be changed for speedier help. This method is used to observe imperative signs for supplying proactive care to patients. Making an examination of the information created by patients who up to now had endured the same symptoms helps the specialist to supply viable drugs to new patients.

Big Data Analysis Tools in Healthcare

Health information volume is anticipated to develop drastically for a long time ahead. Despite the fact that benefit is not and ought to not be an essential help, it is critical for healthcare organizations to secure the accessible apparatuses, foundation, and procedures to use big data viably or else risk losing possibly millions of dollars in income and benefits. Fig. 7.1 shows the analysis process of big data in healthcare [11].

To be precise, big data are large volumes of high-speed, complex, and variable information that require progressive strategies and advances to empower the capture, capacity, dispersion, administration, and examination of the information. Big data envelop these types of characteristics as assortment, veracity, and speed, especially for healthcare.

Existing expository strategies could be connected to the tremendous sum of available (but right now unanalyzed) disease-related health and therapeutic information to reach a more profound comprehension of results, which at that point can be connected to healthcare. In a perfect world, person and populace data would illuminate each doctor and patient amid the decision-making process and offer assistance in deciding the best-fitting treatment alternative for that specific case. Fig. 7.2 shows that various sources are used for collecting big data to apply in healthcare

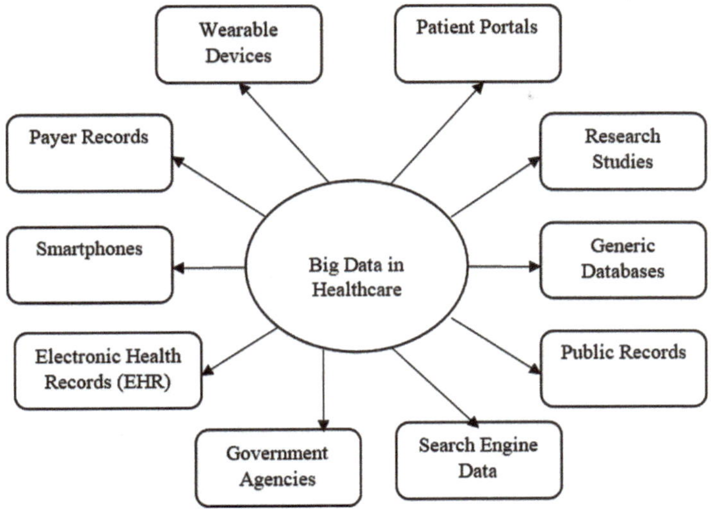

FIG. 7.1 Big data in the healthcare analysis process.

[12]. Depending on whether the information is organized or unstructured, a few information designs such as an input big data analytics stage can be entered. Within the healthcare system, these are, of course, noteworthy downsides, and so the trade-offs must be tended to. Moreover, these platforms/tools require an unusual amount of programming abilities that the commonplace end user in healthcare may not possess. Fig. 7.3 [13,14] shows a conceptual architecture of big data analytics.

Moreover, considering the later development of big data analytics in healthcare, management issues [15] involving possession, protection, security, and guidelines have to be tended to:

1. The Hadoop Distributed File System (HDFS): This allows for basic capacity for the cluster of Hadoop. It isolates the information into little parts and disperses it over the different nodes.
2. MapReduce: This provides the interface for subtask dissemination and yield collection. When errors

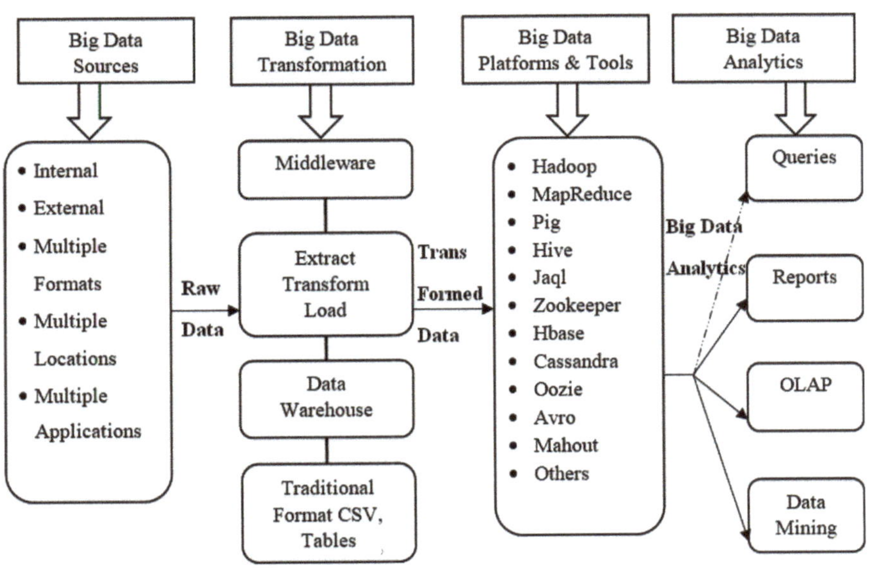

FIG. 7.2 Sources of big data in healthcare. *CSV*, comma separated values; *OLAP*, Online Analytical Processing.

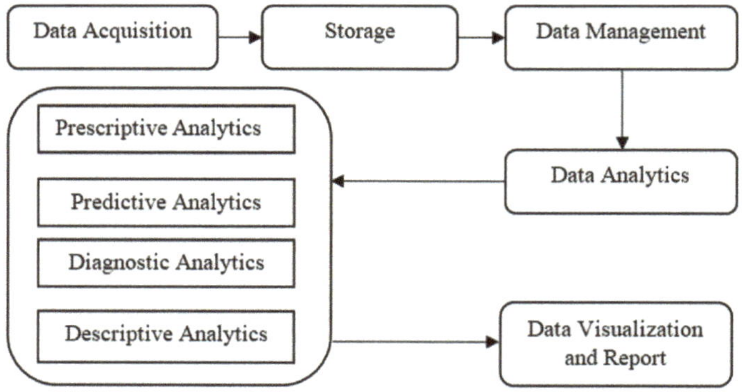

FIG. 7.3 Conceptual architecture of big data analytics.

are made, MapReduce tracks each server/node preparation.

3. Pig and Pig Latin: The language of Pig programming is designed to absorb all kinds of information (organized/unstructured, etc.). It consists of two key modules: the dialect itself, called Pig Latin, and the runtime adaptation that executes the Pig Latin code.
4. Hive: The Hive might be a runtime Hadoop back engineering that uses the Hadoop stage to leverage structured query language (SQL). It allows SQL software engineers to create Hive query language articulations with common SQL explanations.
5. Jaql: Jaql can be a useful, explanatory query language outlined to prepare expansive information sets. To encourage parallel processing, Jaql changes over "'high-level' questions into 'low-level' queries" comprising MapReduce assignments.
6. Zookeeper: Zookeeper permits a centralized foundation with different administrations, providing synchronization across a server cluster. Applications of big data analytics use these administrations to manage large clusters in parallel.
7. HBase: HBase is a column-oriented framework for managing databases that sit on the HDFS beat. The non-SQL approach is used for it.
8. Cassandra: Cassandra is a disseminated database framework. It is assigned as a top-level venture to handle large data disseminated across numerous servers of utilities. It also gives a reliable advantage without a specific failure point and can be a non-SQL framework.
9. Oozie: Oozie is an open-source venture that streamlines between assignments the workflow and coordination.
10. Lucene: This is widely used to analyze/search content and has been included in a few open-source ventures. Its scope includes ordering full text and seeking to use libraries within a Java application.
11. Avro: This encourages the administration of information serialization. Extra valuable features are versioning and adaptation control.
12. Mahout: Mahout is another Apache venture whose goal is to create free applications of conveyed and versatile machine learning calculations that support Hadoop's big data analytics.

Terahertz Technology

THz electromagnetic waves include the range between microwaves and the optical infrared band within the 0.1–10 THz recurrence run [16]. They speak to a large parcel of the electromagnetic range and have a wide range of applications. THz radiation can enter lean layers up to a few millimeters of nonmetallic substances such as clothing, plastics, and ceramics. Since its disclosure in 1895, radiographic imaging using X-rays has been the essential symptomatic imaging innovation used within dentistry. Whatever it may be, it is ionizing radiation with a few impediments to our health and has inalienable restrictions, such as differentiating anatomical structures and delicate tissue. THz waves are not ionizing at all, like X beams, and therefore do not pose a danger to life forms.

A novel method for therapeutic imaging is THz imaging [17]. It uses nonionizing radiation and can be used safely to image various types of tissue, such as typical cells and tumors; it is believed that the difference between tissue types is due to contrasts in water assimilation, protein thickness, or cellular structure. However, in the field of restorative conclusion, THz imaging is still relatively modern. The ideal strategies are still being decided for the use of the various information angles recorded by THz frameworks. This includes the use of "intelligent" information examination strategies to optimize THz imaging for cancer determination and the most valuable parameters and strategy for examination.

Role of Big Data in Terahertz Healthcare

THz imaging and backscatter X-ray are the most promising technologies. This innovation can be used for security screening, semiconductor evaluation, nutritional evaluation, pharmaceutical examination, and 2D and 3D imaging, including for therapeutic determination within the ranges of tooth structure, skin cancer, and tumors.

THz reflection imaging (at ~0.1–10 THz/1012 Hz frequencies) is nonionizing and has potential as a therapeutic imaging method; however, there is no agreement as of this writing on the ideal imaging parameters to be used and the information examination strategy. This may hold back the strategy's progress. This chapter describes the use of various brilliant research strategies to select important image parameters and optimize the handling of THz information in ex vivo colon cancer testing. Decision trees were used to detect critical parameters and neural systems, and vector bolsters were used to classify THz information as typical or irregular tests.

A few extracted breast tissue tests were imaged and time-domain beat parameters were used to evaluate tissue contrasts. The measurement and shape of tumor districts in the THz pictures [16] were compared with the comparative area of histology. The creators found a great relationship for the tumor area and shape compared with the histology. In addition, for the tissue that contained tumor, the retention coefficient and refractive file were found to be higher compared with those of typical tissue. These reflections illustrate the potential of THz pulsed imaging (TPI) to illustrate both obtrusive breast carcinomas and ductal carcinoma in situ and to stimulate forward thinking. Both THz pulsed spectroscopy (TPS) and TPI [16] are capable of investigating atomic frameworks with low-frequency torsional and vibrational movements. These solid vibrations can provide insight into the basic flow of polymorphs and hydrates of crystalline materials that has many applications in pharmaceutical science. The water assimilation range shows a very solid, wide top centered at 5.6 THz. The impact of this assimilation top, which amplifies the range of recurrence used in TPI and TPS, makes these strategies extremely sensitive to the concentration of water. THz reflective pulsed imaging was used in vivo to reflect on human skin. The creators explored human tissue crisply extracted using a broadband TPI framework with frequencies of approximately 0.5–2.5 THz. For skin, fat tissue, striated muscle, veins, and nerves, the refractive file and direct assimilation coefficient were found to be diverse. The difference between basal cell carcinoma and typical tissue in THz images of skin cancer was observed in the expansion.

Understanding the Concept of V's in Healthcare

Volume, velocity, and variety are all imperative for big data analytics in healthcare, but there are more V words to honestly think about, too. Within the healthcare domain, big data have rapidly become basic for almost every operational and clinical errand, including populace health administration, quality benchmarking, income cycle administration, prescient analytics, and clinical choice bolster. Information researchers and tech writers both appreciate designs, and few are more satisfying to both callings than the alliterative properties of huge information described by the numerous V's. Initially, there were the big three—volume, velocity, and variety—presented by Gartner examiner Doug Laney back in 2001. "Big data" has been a standard buzzword for some time. What are the three, four, ten [18] (or more) most critical big data V's, and how can healthcare organizations apply these standards to their clinical and financial activities?

Volume (how much data are there?): Big data is, no question, well ... big. Most of the information is temporary—gushed music or movie images that rarely have ever been analyzed for experiences—but by the end of the decade, more than 35% of the world's information resources could be valuable for analytics if properly labeled and curated. Not at all like the latest Netflix fling, information about healthcare tends to be on the value side. Clinical notes, claims information, laboratory results, quality arrangements, therapeutic gadget information, and imaging results are informative and have actually become more valuable when combined in new ways to create brand-neutral experiences.

Velocity (how quickly are the data being created, moved, or accessed?): Healthcare data accounts for a highly respectable portion of the information spreading throughout the world, and the figures will continue to rise as the Web of Things, therapeutic gadgets, genomic testing, machine learning, natural language processing (NLP), and other new methods of information generation and handling progress.

Variety (how many different types of sources are there?): Sorting may be the zest of life, but it may also be a small amount for healthcare organizations to deal with in some cases. Significant information comes in all shapes and sizes, and routine intelligence says the richer the bits of knowledge are, the more data you can crush together. Information technology (IT) tragically though for the pharmaceutical industry, the erratic improvement in within a significant period of time has provided many suppliers with information walls that are impossible to break through. Basically, information sets cannot be compared when held in partitioned areas or in contradictory designs, limiting the bits of knowledge providers can collect around their patients or operations. Health IT designers are beginning to solve the problem by enrolling application programming interface assistance and new measures such as Fast Healthcare Interoperability Resources, both of which also make it much easier to vault over marketplaces and simply raise the remaining assortment.

Veracity (can we trust the data?): It is difficult to confirm the veracity of a dataset, but suppliers cannot use bits of knowledge that will be inferred from information that is deficient, one-sided, or filled with commotion. Information management and its close relative data management are key techniques to be used by healthcare organizations to ensure that their information is clean and complete, standardized.

Validity (are the data accurate and correct?): The validity of information could be a fundamental concern for clinicians and analysts, comparable to veracity. A set of data may be complete, but does it tell the client what it means? Are the values being adjusted? Is it up to date? Were the data created using logical conventions and strategies acknowledged? Who is careful to curate and manage the information? Healthcare datasets should incorporate accurate metadata representing when, how, and by whom the information was produced. Metadata make a difference in ensuring that researchers get it to one another, and that their analytics can be repeated so that future information researchers can investigate the information and find what they are looking for.

Viability (are the data relevant to the case at hand?): Many prominent analytical undertakings are focused on recognizing inventive factors to enumerate certain patient behaviors or clinical outcomes, and this will undoubtedly be a continuous operation as more datasets become available.

Volatility (how often do the data change?): Healthcare information is rapidly changing—at the moment in a few cases—which raises the questions of how long the information is important, which chronic measurements should be incorporated in an investigation, and how long the information can be stored? As the volume of information proceeds to develop on a day-by-day basis, these choices will become progressively imperative. Datasets with a higher turnover rate and less relevance to analytics may be more qualified for a reuse container than those that remain stable and reusable for exceptionally long periods of time, such as the genomic test of a patient.

Vulnerability (can we keep the data secure?): Speaking of HIPAA, information helplessness in the wake of various ransomware assaults and a depressingly long reiteration of information breaches have skyrocketed up the list of needs. For the healthcare industry, security is the best knowledge, especially as capacity moves into the cloud and information begins to travel between organizations as a result of progress made in interoperability. Organizations concerned with information impotence should ensure that their employees are prepared to keep data private and secure and that their business accomplices have signed HIPAA Business Associate Agreements to maintain compliance with the strict protection and security rules of healthcare.

Visualization (how can the data be presented to the user?): Designers should consider visualizations that use recognizable colors and chart designs to highlight key experiences without overpowering the viewer, rather than black-and-white printouts on punctured printer paper from 1977. Sifting information will naturally help to avoid overloading data and may help moderate burnout feelings among exhausted clinicians. Another alternative to announcing monetary, operational, or clinical measurements to end users is intuitive dashboards. New online image recognition tools are becoming well known for imaging open health concerns or innovation appropriation rates on a neighborhood and national scale, while a variety of new apps for desktops, tablets, and indeed smartphones are giving customers ways to more definitely connect with information than they ever have before.

Value (can these data produce a meaningful return on investment?): The goal is to extricate some kind of appreciation from the data at hand. Whether this appreciation comes in the form of better results, progressed trade efficiencies, or smarter key decision-making, healthcare organizations cannot disregard the huge question of nearly all big data: what has it done for me lately?

Many healthcare organizations are still in the early stages of obtaining the skills that will enable them to achieve these goals, and generating actionable insights that can be linked to real-world issues could be a complicated and challenging task. More V's having large information analytics unfurls in healthcare, but there is the value will remain the primary vital metric to screen during any and all data-driven choice making. Fig. 7.4 [18] shows that there are a lot of big data, which also applies to health data.

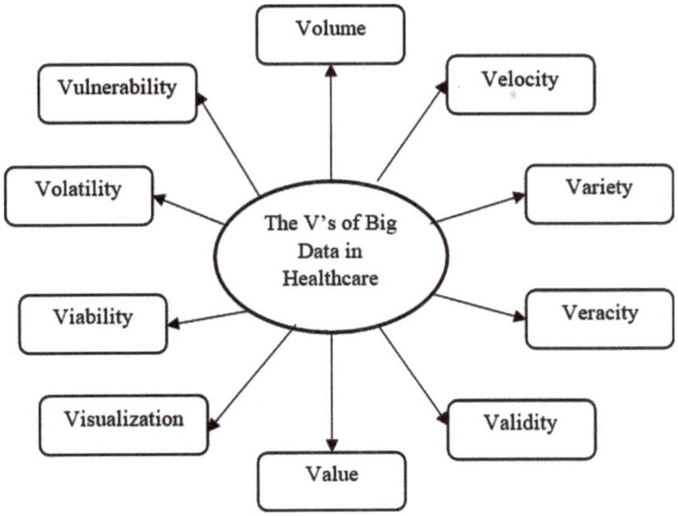

FIG. 7.4 The many V's of big data, which also apply to health data.

TECHNIQUES FOR BIG DATA ANALYSIS

The biggest distinction between conventional health analysis and big data health analytics is the execution of computer programming [19]. Within the conventional framework, the healthcare industry depends on other businesses for big data investigation. Numerous healthcare shareholders believe in data innovation because of its significant outcomes: their working frameworks are useful and they can handle the information in standardized shapes. There is a desire for a strategy that combines different information sources. Fig. 7.5 shows the types of data analysis techniques [20]. A number of conceptual approaches can be utilized to recognize inconsistencies in endless sums of information from diverse datasets. The systems accessible for the analysis of healthcare information are discussed next.

Data analysis [20] may be used for reviewing, cleansing, changing, and modeling information with the objective of finding valuable data, informing conclusions, and supporting decision-making. Information examination has numerous features and approaches, including different strategies beneath a variety of names while being utilized totally differently in commerce, science, and social science spaces. Essential sorts of data analysis are as follows: (1) quantitative analysis, (2) qualitative analysis, (3) statistical analysis, (4) visual analysis, (5) data mining, (6) machine learning, and (7) semantic analysis.

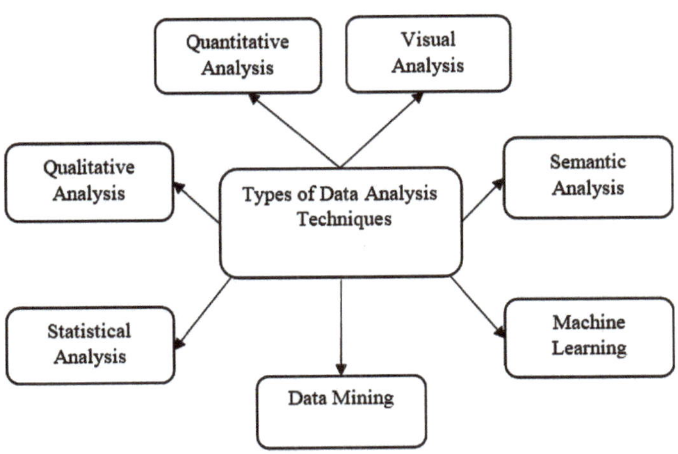

FIG. 7.5 Data analysis techniques.

Quantitative Analysis

Quantitative analysis is an information investigation method that centers on quantifying the designs and relationships found within the information. This strategy includes analyzing a huge number of perceptions from a dataset. Since the test estimate is large, the results can be connected in a generalized way to the whole dataset. For illustration, a quantitative examination of ice cream sales may find that a 5-degree increment in temperature increases ice cream sales by 15%. The yield of the quantitative investigation is numerical in nature. This result can be utilized for numerical comparisons. The yield of the subjective examination could be portrayed as a relationship using words, as appears in Fig. 7.6 [20].

Qualitative Analysis

The rest of this information is subjective and is, subsequently, not as effortlessly measured. This work, included in subjective information collection, is less characterized and more troublesome to oversee. In any case, measures are as of this writing being taken by companies to create uses for quantitative information in other ways. It is imperative not to generalize the information you discover but to attempt as best you can to consider the information in terms of the setting from which it was collected. In cases done right, subjective information can make a gigantic difference in your business's victory [21].

The subjective investigation is an information investigation strategy that centers on portraying different information qualities utilizing words. It includes analyzing a small test in more prominent profundity compared with a quantitative information examination. The results of this analysis cannot be generalized to a whole dataset due to the small test measure. They moreover cannot be measured numerically or utilized for numerical comparisons. For example,

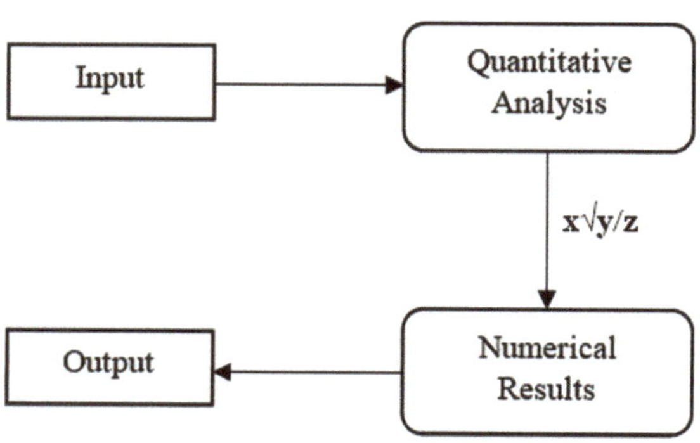

FIG. 7.6 The output of the quantitative analysis is numerical in nature.

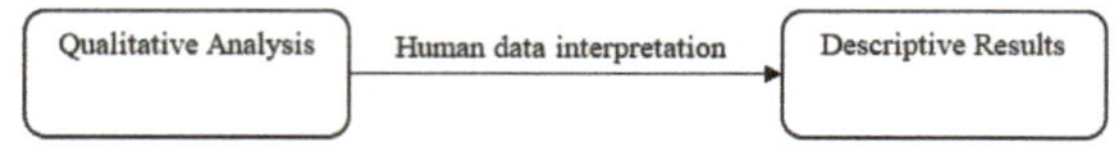

FIG. 7.7 Qualitative results are descriptive in nature and not generalizable to the entire dataset.

an examination of ice cream sales may reveal that May's sales figures were not as high as June's. The examination results state, as it were, that the figures were "not as high as" and do not give a numerical distinction. The yield of the subjective examination could be portrayed as a relationship using words, as appears in Fig. 7.7 [20].

Statistical Analysis

Factual investigations based on scientific equations are used for analyzing information. This examination is most usually quantitative, but can be subjective, too. This sort of investigation is commonly utilized to depict datasets by means of summarization, such as giving the mean, middle, or mode of measurements related to the dataset. It can moreover be utilized to gather designs and connections inside the dataset, such as relapse and relationship. There are three sorts of factual examination, which are described next.

A/B testing

A/B testing [22], also known as part or bucket testing, compares two adaptations of a component to decide which adaptation is predominant based on a predefined metric. The component can be a run of things. A/B testing may be a way to compare two forms of a single variable, usually by testing a subject's reaction to variation A against variation B, and deciding which of the two variations is more successful. For illustration, it can be substantial, such as a web page, or an offer for an item or benefit, such as bargains on electronic devices. The current form of the component is called the control adaptation, whereas the altered form is called the treatment. Both forms are subjected to a test at the same time. The perceptions are recorded to decide which adaptation is more effective. A/B testing comparison is shown in Fig. 7.8 [23].

Correlation

The correlation is an examination utilized to decide whether two factors are related to each other. In case they are found to be related, the next step is to decide what their relationship is. For such cases, the value of variable A increases at whatever point the value of B increases. We may be fascinated to find how closely variables A and B are related, which implies we may also need to analyze the degree to which variable B

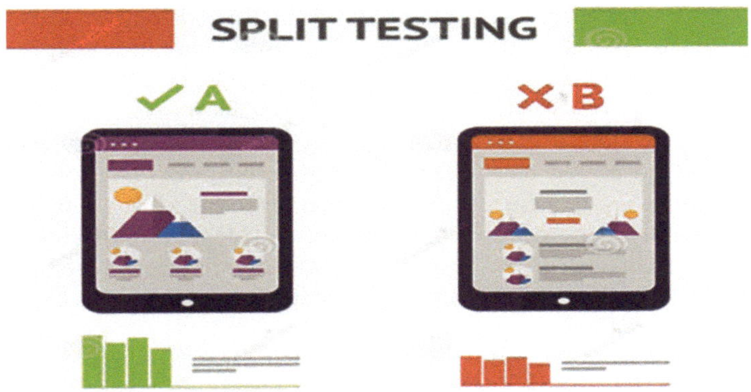

FIG. 7.8 A/B testing.

increases in connection to variable A's increase. The utilization of the correlation makes a difference in creating an understanding of a dataset and discovering connections that can help in clarifying a phenomenon. A correlation is hence commonly utilized for information mining where the recognizable proof of connections between factors in a dataset leads to the disclosure of designs and peculiarities. This may uncover the nature of the dataset or the cause of the phenomenon. When two factors are considered to be related they are adjusted based on a direct relationship. This implies that when one variable changes, the other variable changes relatively and continually. The correlation is communicated as a decimal number between -1 and $+1$, which is known as the correlation coefficient. This makes a difference in creating an understanding of a dataset and discovering connections that can help in clarifying the phenomenon.

Regression

The investigation method of relapse investigates how a subordinate variable is related to an autonomous variable inside a dataset. As a test situation, it may offer assistance in deciding the sort of relationship that exists between "temperature" (the autonomous variable) and "edit abdicate" (the subordinate variable). Applying this procedure makes a difference in deciding how the value of the subordinate variable (edit abdicate) changes in connection to changes within the value of the free variable (temperature). Direct relapse speaks to a steady rate of change and nonlinear relapse speaks to a variable rate of change. Another thing is that more than one free variable can be tried at the same time. Regression can offer assistance to empower an improved understanding of what a phenomenon is and why it happened. It can be utilized to form expectations of the approximate values of the subordinate variable.

Visual Analysis

The visual investigation may be a framework of information investigation that includes the realistic representation of information to empower or improve its visual recognition. People can understand and draw conclusions from illustrations more rapidly than from content; visual analysis acts as a disclosure apparatus within the field of big data. It makes a difference in distinguishing and highlighting hidden design relationships and irregularities. This segment portrays the following sorts of visual analysis.

Heat maps

The heat map is one of the fundamental components of visual analysis. By and large, how can one outwardly distinguish any design related to carbon outflows over a huge number of cities around the world? Fundamentally, green is utilized to highlight the finest-performing districts, whereas red is utilized to highlight most exceedingly the bad-performing districts. For illustration, in an arrangement to identify the top- and worst-selling districts for sales, the sales information is plotted in a heat map.

Time series plots

Time series plots permit the examination of information that is recorded over intermittent periods of time. This sort of examination makes use of a time series, which is a time-ordered collection of values recorded over standard time periods. It moreover makes a difference in revealing design inside information that is time dependent. Once distinguished, the design can be extrapolated for future expectations. Time series analyses are ordinarily utilized for estimation by identifying long-term patterns, regular intermittent designs, and unpredictable short-term varieties within the dataset. Not at all like other sorts of investigations, time arrangement examination continuously incorporates time as a comparison variable, and the information collected is continuously time dependent.

Network graphs

Network analysis is a method that centers on analyzing connections between substances inside the network. A network graph portrays an interconnected collection of substances (individuals, items, etc.). Substances may be associated with one another straightforwardly or by implication. There are specialized varieties of arranging analysis, including course optimization, social network analysis, and spread forecast (such as the spread of an infection).

Spatial data mapping

Spatial data examination is analyzing location-based information in an arrangement to reveal diverse geographic connections and designs between substances. Spatial data examination is centered on analyzing location-based information in an arrangement to reveal diverse geographic connections and designs between substances. With the ever-increasing accessibility of location-based information, such as sensor and social media information, spatial information can be analyzed to pick up area experiences. The application of spatial information examination incorporates operations and coordination optimization, natural sciences, and foundation arranging. Fundamentally, areas are extracted from the user's social media messages, and personalized offers are conveyed in real-time based on the nearness of the client to the store.

Data Mining

Data mining shapes the premise for prescient analytics and commerce insights. It also is known as information disclosure, and is a specialized type of data analysis that targets expansive datasets. It involves extracting covered up or obscure designs within the information with the purpose of distinguishing already obscure designs. In connection to big data analysis, data mining, by and large, refers to robotized, software-based procedures that filter through big datasets to recognize designs and patterns.

Machine Learning

People are great at spotting designs and connections inside information. Shockingly, we cannot handle expansive sums of information exceptionally rapidly. Machines, on the other hand, are exceptionally capable of processing huge sums of information rapidly, but only in the event that they know how. If human information can be combined with the handling speed of machines, machines will be able to handle expansive sums of information without requiring much human mediation. This machine learning method is utilized to recognize peculiarities, anomalies, and deviations that can be profitable, such as openings, or unfavorable, such as dangers [24]. Machine learning and its relationship to information mining are investigated through the scope of the following sorts of machine learning strategies.

Classification

Classification is a supervised learning strategy by which information is classified into pertinent, already learned categories. Classification comprises two steps: in the first step, the framework is built, processing information that is already categorized or labeled, so that it can create an understanding of the distinctive categories, and in the second step the framework is fed uncategorized but comparable information for classification, and based on the understanding it created from the processed information, the calculation will classify the unlabeled information. A common application of this method is the sifting of email spam. Note that classification can be performed for two or more categories.

Clustering

Clustering is an unsupervised learning method (no earlier learning of categories) by which information is separated into diverse bunches (verifiably produced based on gathering) so that the information in each bunch has comparable properties (decided depending on the sort of calculation). Clustering is by and large utilized in information mining to induce an understanding of the properties of a given dataset. After creating this understanding, classification can be utilized to create much better expectations from comparable new or inconspicuous information. It also can be connected to the categorization of obscure archives and personalized promotion campaigns by gathering together clients with comparable behavior.

Outlier detection

Outlier detection is the method of finding data that are altogether distinctive from or conflicting with the rest of the information inside a given dataset. The calculation center finds irregular values. It can be based on either directed or unsupervised learning. Outlier detection is utilized in network data analysis, sensor data analysis, outlier detection, and therapeutic conclusion. For example, in an arrangement to discover whether an exchange is likely to be false, a bank's IT group builds a system utilizing an outlier detection method that is based on supervised learning. After the framework is prepared, obscure exchanges are fed into the outlier detection calculation to anticipate whether they are false.

Filtering

Filtering is the computerized method of finding pertinent things from a pool of things. Things can be sifted either based on a user's own behavior or by coordinating the behavior of numerous clients. For the most part, this method has been connected through two approaches:

Collaborative filtering: Collaborative filtering is a thing sifting method based on the collaboration, or blending, of a user's past behavior with the behaviors of others. A target user's past behavior, including his or her likes, appraisals, buying history, and more, is collaborated with the behavior of comparable clients. Based on the closeness of the user's behavior, things are filtered for the target client. It is exclusively based on the closeness to the user's behavior. It requires a huge sum of client behavior information to precisely channel things.

Content-based filtering: Content-based filtering is a thing filtering method centered on the similitude between clients and things. A client profile is made based on that user's past behavior. The similitude is recognized between the client profile and the properties of different things, leading to things being filtered for the client. Opposite to collaborative sifting, content-based filtering is exclusively committed to the client's inclinations and does not require information from other clients.

Semantic Analysis

Semantic analysis is a part of the speech information that can carry diverse implications in completely different settings, but whose meaning is defined within a complete sentence, even when organized in completely different ways. In arranging for machines to extricate important data, content and discourse information ought to be recognized by the machine in the same way as people do.

There are the following types of semantic analysis methods.

Natural language processing

NLP is "the capacity of machines to get it and decipher human dialect the way it is composed or spoken." The objective of NLP is to make computers/machines as clever as human beings in understanding language. Rather than hard coding the desired learning rules, machine learning is connected to create the computer's understanding of the natural language. In brief, the more learning information the computer has, the more accurately it can translate human content and speech. Big data come from data put away in big organizations as well as ventures. Illustrations include the data of representatives, company buying, sales records, commerce exchanges, past records of organizations, social media, etc.

Text analytics

Unstructured text is for the most part much more troublesome to analyze and look at in comparison to organized content. Text analysis is the specialized examination of content through the application of data mining. Machine learning and NLP methods are used to extricate value/insights from unstructured text utilizing semantic rules and organization. As the number of digitized archives, emails, social media posts, and log records increases, businesses have an expanding need to use any value that can be extracted from these types of semistructured and unstructured information. Text analysis steps are shown in Fig. 7.9 [20].

Sentiment analysis

Sentiment analysis is a specialized type of content analysis that centers on deciding the predisposition or feelings of people. This type of examination decides the state of mind of the creator of the content by analyzing the content inside the setting of the common dialect. These data can be coordinated into the decision-making method. Common applications for sentiment analysis incorporate distinguishing client fulfillment or disappointment early, gauging item success or disappointment, and spotting unused patterns.

THE SIGNIFICANCE OF BIG DATA ANALYSIS IN TERAHERTZ HEALTHCARE MANAGEMENT

By digitizing, combining, and using massive information successfully, healthcare organizations, ranging from single-clinician workplaces and multiprovider clinics to large-scale healing center systems and responsible care organizations, are achieving critical benefits [15]. Positive effects have included identifying diseases at an earlier stage, when they can be treated more effortlessly and effectively; monitoring the health of individuals and populations; and more rapidly and effectively recognizing fraud in healthcare.

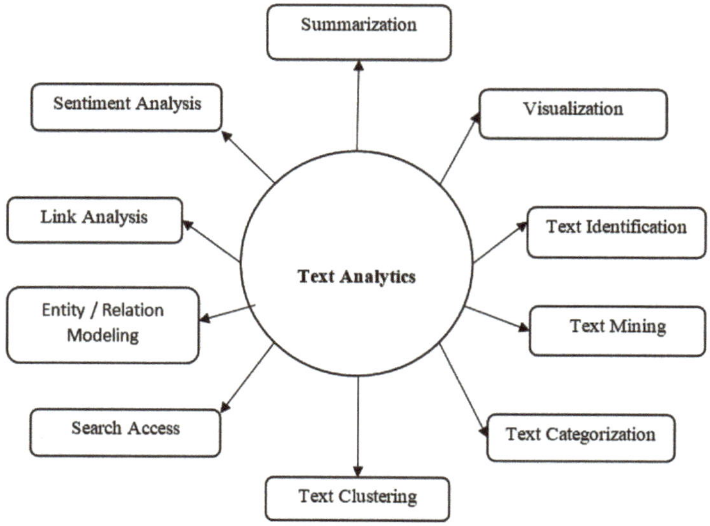

FIG. 7.9 Text analytics techniques.

Clinical Operations

Comparative adequacy investigates ways of analyzing and treating patients that are more clinically relevant and cost-effective.

Research and Development

- More focused drug and gadget research and development pipeline in a faster way;
- Statistical tools or heuristics for advancing the clinical trial plan and patient enlistment to better coordinate medicines for individual patients, thus reducing disappointment in the trial and speeding up the use of modern medicines;
- Analysis of clinical studies and case records to recognize follow-up signs and to detect unfavorable impacts.

Public Health

- Analysis of infection patterns and disease episodes and the power train to also make progress toward the open observation of health and velocity reaction;
- Speedier progression of more accurate immunization focus, e.g., selection of annual influenza strains;
- Transforming large amounts of information into important data that can be used to recognize needs, provide administration, and anticipate and prevent emergencies, especially for the benefit of populations.

Evidence-based medicine: Compare, and analyze a variety of organized and unorganized data, electronic medical records (EMRs) data, monetary and logistical information, medical information, and phenotypic information, to coordinate with results of medicines, anticipate patients at risk for deadly disease or hospitalization, and also provide constructive care.

Genomic analytics: Make gene mutation sampling much more productive and cost effective and prepare a portion of the normal restorative care choice for the genomic investigation and the development of the case therapeutic record.

Preadjudication fraud analysis: Quickly analyze the enormous number of claims to reduce fraud, waste, and misreporting.

Device/remote monitoring: Capture and analyze huge amounts of fast-moving data from in-hospital and in-house gadgets in real time for security observation and unfavorable opportunity forecasting.

Patient profile analytics: Apply statistical models mostly to online case profiles (e.g., division or prescient designing) to distinguish for illustration those patients at risk of contracting a particular disease (e.g., diabetes) who would benefit from preventive care, proactive care, or lifestyle changes [13,14]. Concurring with the study conducted by Health Catalyst [25], a whopping 90% of the respondents conceded that analytics is likely to be either "extremely important" or "very important" to their organization within a few years. And the respondents moreover appraised the significance of healthcare patterns and the part played by analytics in them. Analytics is hence becoming exceptionally pivotal in following distinctive sorts of healthcare patterns. Progressive analytics touches each perspective of healthcare computer program frameworks, including clinical, operational, and monetary divisions. Analysis of healthcare big data also contributes to more noteworthy understanding of cohorts that are at most noteworthy risk for sickness, subsequently allowing a proactive approach to anticipation. By bringing monetary and clinical information together, it can highlight the efficiency and viability of treatment plans.

THz imaging of human tissue with the focus of recognizing irregular zones is not, however, in broad standard use. This may be due to the fact that there is as of this writing no standardized information investigation technique that permits a basic clinically valuable result to be decided. There are contrasts both within and between patients in the boundaries between ordinary and irregular tissue. Different analysts have recommended different information parameters, both in time and in recurrence spaces, to produce and decipher THz imaging, and this lack of an agreement does not advance THz assistance as a valuable therapeutic imaging methodology.It seeks to discover a standardized information analysis strategy for THz imaging output for this disease.

Healthcare organizations have started to receive advances like PACS (picture archiving and communication system) imaging frameworks and EMRs that endeavor to create the sense of the gigantic information that streams through the framework (both organized and unstructured). There are genome analyzers and other analytics apparatuses that are advertised to offer assistance in understanding the truths and dispense with unwanted/useless points of interest to extract only what is required. The conclusion of this can be superior clinical results for understanding. THz imaging [26] is a modern method with numerous potential applications. It employs a nonionizing radiation scheme to get both recurrence and time-space data.

Data analytics is another case of a developing innovation to handle big data with noteworthy suggestions for healthcare settings. Such devices look at designs inside large and complicated datasets to pick up information and bits of knowledge. It is becoming a fundamental tool for health organizations to provide better administration of healthcare and to reduce costs. There are numerous and critical clinical applications of prescient analytics, as exceptionally individualized predictions of understanding results are conceivable. For illustration, one can predict of patients with a high chance of heart attack, which case is likely to be readmitted after surgery or whether a case will remain longer than normal after surgery. The information gathered through the use of prescient health and pharmaceutical analytics will alter the manner in which medicine is practiced while improving our ability to avoid and treat critical diseases [27]. Big data, assists in the recognition of fraud in healthcare, particularly in healthcare insurance claims [28]. It is possible to detect false claims and irregularities. This will make it easier for companies to protect against misfortune. Big data are used in healthcare to recognize and address therapeutic problems before they become unmanageable. Healthcare experts can lower the chance and overcome the problem with the data from big data.

Big data can provide much benefit to medical care through database management, electronic therapy records, and data analysis. In addition, the presence of big data will allow a program or mediation to be improved or adjusted to better target the health issue [29]. It will empower the prompt initiation of clinical trials. Big data will provide a clearer picture of both the type of population and its therapeutic problem. The design of dispersion or disease data will allow for the rapid improvement of an intercession program as well as focusing as early as possible on the influenced group. The industry is changing, and big data are beginning to convert it, like every other one—but there is still some work to be done. The sector gradually receives the advances that will push it into the future, which will make a difference in making better-informed choices, moving forward, etc. In a nutshell, here is a short list of the examples [8] we have gone over in this chapter. The healthcare data analytics provides the following areas: (1) predict patients monitory status, (2) use electronic health records, (3) use instant care real-time alert, (4) improve patients engagement with their own health, (5) use health data for better informed strategic planning, (6) extensive vaccine research, (7) use predictive analytics, (8) eliminate scams or improve the security of data, (9) practice telemedicine, (10) fully integrate clinical imaging with a wider treatment, and (11) avoid excessive visits to the emergency room.

RECENT WORK

A written audit was carried out to identify blogs about the use of big data in healthcare coverage. The following search terms were used: "big health care data," "big data medicine," and "clinical big data." With PubMed, Google Researcher, Science Coordinate, and Web of Information, as well as Google, the search terms were used to find both peer-reviewed writing and skilled diary articles aimed at the usefulness and application of big data in healthcare settings. The essential list included articles distributed for a long time in the final five. Auxiliary references from more seasoned articles were used to allow full discussion of differentiated issues in essential articles later on. Sonnati [30] proposes to analyze healthcare utilizing big data analytics particularly for any given geographic area and the accessible information. It is noticed that sometimes digitization is necessary in hospital systems, as a large sum of health data is created in connection with a case health record to its genome examination to keep track of these data its ability to use big data and its analytics [31]. In 2015, Sathiyavathi [32] said that, because of the digital technology of medical information, specialists can create in-depth experiences that can really automate diagnostic frameworks, automate care in the first place, strengthen physician-patient connections, reduce costs, and achieve progress. In 2014, Wullianallur Raghupathi et al. [15] explained in their own paper also that big data analytics now has the power to turn modern advances into clinical and other information stores and make choices. In 2014, Kumar and Manjula [33] stated that achieving better results at a lower level of cost is vital to healthcare and can be accomplished by executing HDFS and MapReduce to reveal data in large health datasets. The earlier distributed work on colon cancer THz imaging at the time of writing is that of Reid et al. [11], whose information is reanalyzed in the current investigation. These are not transcribed here, but in their publication the full points of interest can be found.

Senthilkumar et al. [6] investigates the forms and applications of big data in the management of health care. They also examined the search methodology and the steps that were presented in the writing survey of articles dealing with big data in healthcare and the method of managing big data in healthcare. Sim et al. [34] said THz imaging was used to diagnose oral cancer using seven oral tissues from four patients. THz imaging at 20°C seemed better than at room temperature to distinguish between cancer tissue and ordinary mucosa. Cancer tumor recognized by THz waveform deeper than 1.2 mm from the tissue surface. Healthcare organizations have put into several databases, groups, and frameworks a sufficient sum of value-based information. Many other sets of raw data, such as completely nontraditional, far less structured data from Internet articles, social media sites, call centers, chatting sessions, Skype calls, email, pressure sensors, photographs, and computerized pictures, can also be extracted as well by choice. Big healthcare data are added to the following [31]:

Traditional enterprise data, such as value-based data from protections, patient affirmations, research facility test records, etc.

Health and medical devices data, such as computerized tomography scanners, life-enhancing frameworks, information on telemetry and telemedicine.

Social media data related to streams of patient criticism, Twitter or Facebook blogs, MySpace, and TuDiabetes

Medical science research: genome investigations, clinical and value-based investigations of drug analysis, random information like arrangements for health, medication, clinical trials, etc.

LIMITATIONS OF EXISTING WORK

By evaluating big data types of cases, our research gave a better real understanding of just how big data analysis can be used by healthcare organizations as a means of changing IT to gain trade value. The main impediment to this thinking is the source of information. The main challenge in the health industry is that it still usually lags in IT selection behind other businesses, which is one of the biggest difficulties in finding cases. Despite efforts to discover cases from various sources, the greater part of the cases identified for this study came from merchants. There is a potential predisposition [35] in this situation, as sellers usually advertise their "success" stories, as it were. It is possible to assist and provide superior disclosure by collecting and analyzing essential data. Because of the increasing number of healthcare organizations that embrace big data analytics, the test outline for gathering essential information becomes larger. Analysis of the effect of large-scale data analytics capabilities on the execution of healthcare organizations with a quantitative review strategy based on essential information can shed a variety of light. In addition, however, there are a few major impediments to be attended to. Big data's advantages are unquestionable, but too many restrictions have to be examined [36].

Weighted Averages for Actuarial Tools

Big data should help them advance their actuarial models to a point. Be that as it may, some impediments exist. Tod Emerick and David Toomey of Protections Thought Authority [36] focus on not usually disseminating unstructured healthcare data. This means that in their models, statisticians cannot use weighted midpoints. Instead, for distinctive subgroups, they must be seen at information sets. It has been observed that numerous big data extraction devices are not yet ready to analyze data at such a granular level.

Difficulty Assessing Doctor Performance

Insurers, the Medicaid and Medicare Administration, and other statisticians monitor the execution of distinctive specialists in their systems carefully. Unfortunately, they have exceptionally uncertain techniques. The problem is that specialists regularly refer their colleagues to their highest risk patients to advance their claim win rate.

Data Availability and Reliability

Big data necessitate reliable sets of information point by point. This implies that healthcare providers need to obtain as much data as possible on their patients. They should also carefully examine it, as errors can weaken their entire healthcare toolkit. Specifically, social media is often questionable as patients are less likely to double check what they place on their profiles. They may actually intentionally post incorrect data to adorn their curriculum vitae or see their companions as being more engaging. But the awesome constraining calculations [37] in tackling all of this information/feedstock is not a "big data problem," or even a "messy data problem." In a place where there are tons of possibly valuable information to look at, we do not make it available in ways that individuals really need to utilize it. Either the information is not simple or instinctive to get at or it simply is not enlightening. Organic frameworks are truly complex, versatile frameworks with numerous moving parts, which we have, as it were, only started to scratch the surface of understanding.

FUTURE RESEARCH SCOPES

As officials in commerce and mechanical divisions pronounce their big data activities to have been fruitful and transformational, the viewpoint for healthcare is indeed more energizing. The following are a couple of areas where big data is ordained to change healthcare. Machine learning, depends on big data, is as of this writing making a difference for doctors to move forward in understanding care. Machine learning with the help of big data analytics provides caregivers the capacity to upgrade patient care. THz imagery is in its early stage of development, but it has tremendous potential in the future to be a profitable imaging method. Since 2010, THz imaging applications in biomedical areas have drawn wide-ranging interest, and image strategies and hypothetical examination proceed to empower applications to still be fully explored. As an advance work, the big data characteristics give a fitting premise to utilize promising computer program stages for the improvement of applications that can handle big data in pharmaceutical and healthcare. The open-source disseminated information handling stages are Apache, Hadoop, MapReduce, which utilizes massively parallel processing (MPP). These applications ought to empower the use of information mining procedures to this heterogeneous and complex information to reveal covered-up designs and novel knowledge from the data. The complete huge potential of big data in healthcare can be opened up to the sharing of data between organizations. The entire concept of the values of the Learning Health Framework center can serve as a guiding concept for advancing efforts to collect information on healthcare that would be used to acknowledge all the many openings outlined in this chapter. We in this way anticipate that future investigations ought to take an expository workforce into thought within the big data analytics system.

CONCLUSIONS

Proficiency is in this manner at the heart of the plan, and information analytics has a vital seat at the table. Big data is only starting to revolutionize healthcare and move the industry forward on numerous fronts. The changes in medicine, innovation, and financing that big data in healthcare guarantees offer arrangements that make strides in understanding the care and drive value in healthcare organizations. The improvement of methods that utilize THz waves for applications in pharmaceuticals is developing quickly with the advancement of the instrument. THz imaging has the potential to be utilized in evaluating a few structures. The commitment of this investigation is to create proposals for the THz imaging technique and data analysis, ideally making a difference in bringing it closer to being a clinically valuable innovation. The big data in healthcare provides security, productive dealing with huge volumes of restorative imaging data, and preventing inappropriate use of health data or inability to defend medical data, and consideration of unstructured clinical notes within the right setting, extricating possibly valuable data. Big data analytics plays an important role in pharmaceuticals and healthcare sector It may be an exceptionally promising method of coordination of, investigating, and analyzing an expansive sum of complex heterogeneous data with diverse natures: biomedical information, exploratory information, e-health records, and social media data. Integrating the assorted data helps big data analytics to interlace a few areas, such as bioinformatics, radiology, therapeutic imaging, 3D imaging, sensor informatics, restorative informatics, health informatics, and computational biomedicine.

REFERENCES

[1] P. Zikopoulos, C. Eaton, D. deRoos, T. Deutsch, G. Lapis, Understanding Big Data: Analytics for Enterprise Class Hadoop and Streaming Data, McGraw-Hill Osborne Media, 2011.

[2] R. Nambiar, R. Bhardwaj, A. Sethi, R. Vargheese, A look at challenges and opportunities of big data analytics in healthcare, in: Big Data, 2013 IEEE International Conference, IEEE, 2013, pp. 17–22.

[3] V. Galloro, Prime numbers, Modern Healthcare 38 (2008) 14–16.

[4] V. Ganjir, B.K. Sarkar, R. Kumar, Big data analytics for healthcare, International Journal of Research in Engineering, Technology, and Science 6 (2016) 1–6.

[5] P. Vashisht, V. Gupta, Big data analytics techniques: a survey, in: 2015 International Conference on Green Computing and Internet of Things (ICGCIoT), Noida, 2015, pp. 264–269, https://doi.org/10.1109/ICGCIoT.2015.7380470.

[6] S.A. Senthilkumar, B.K. Rai, A.A. Meshram, A. Gunasekaran, S. Chandrakumarmangalam, Big data in healthcare management: a review of literature, American Journal of Theoretical and Applied Business 4 (2) (2018) 57–69, https://doi.org/10.11648/j.ajtab.20180402.14.

[7] C.A. Alexander, L. Wang, Big data in healthcare: a new frontier in personalized medicine, Open Access Journal of Translational Medicine & Research 1 (2017) 0005.

[8] M. Lebied, The Datapine Blog in Business Intelligence, 2018. Available from: https://www.datapine.com/blog/big-data-examples-in-healthcare/.

[9] J. Archenaa, E.A.M. Anita, A survey of big data analytics in healthcare and government, Procedia Computer Science 50 (2015) 408–413. Available from: https://doi.org/10.1016/j.procs.2015.04.02.

[10] C. Chinmay, G. Bharat, K.G. Soumya, Tele-wound technology network for assessment of chronic wounds, International Journal of Telemedicine and Clinical Practices 1 (4) (2016) 345–359.

[11] C.B. Reid, A. Fitzgerald, G. Reese, R. Goldin, P. Tekkis, P.S. O'Kelly, Terahertz pulsed imaging of freshly excised human colonic tissues, Physics in Medicine and Biology 56 (14) (2011) 4333–4353.

[12] NEJM Catalyst, Healthcare Big Data and the Promise of Value-Based Care, 2018. Available from: https://catalyst.nejm.org/big-data-healthcare/.

[13] IBM, Large Gene Interaction Analytics at University at Buffalo, SUNY, 2012. Available from: http://public.dhe.ibm.com/common/ssi/ecm/en/imc14675usen/IMC14675USEN.PDF.

[14] IBM, IBM Big Data Platform for healthcare. Solutions Brief, 2012. Available from: http://public.dhe.ibm.com/common/ssi/ecm/en/ims14398usen/IMS14398USEN.PDF.

[15] W. Raghupathi, V. Raghupathi, Big data analytics in healthcare: promise and potential, Health Information Science and Systems 2 (3) (2014), https://doi.org/10.1186/2047-2501-2-3.

[16] K. Yetimoglu, N.O. Kamburoglu, Applications of terahertz imaging in medicine, OMICS Journal of Radiology 3 (2014), https://doi.org/10.4172/2167-7964.1000e127.

[17] L.H. Eadie, C.B. Reid, A.J. Fitzgerald, V.P. Wallace, Optimizing multi-dimensional terahertz imaging analysis for colon cancer diagnosis, Expert Systems with Applications 40 (6) (2013) 2043–2050. Available from: https://doi.org/10.1016/j.eswa.2012.10.019.

[18] J. Bresnick, Understanding the many V's of healthcare big data analytics, Source: Thinkstock, Health IT Analytics (2017). Available from: https://healthitanalytics.com/news/understanding-the-many-vs-of-healthcare-big-data-analytics.

[19] S. Kumar, M. Singh, Big data analytics for healthcare industry: impact, applications, and tools, in: Big Data Mining and Analytics, vol. 2 (1), 2019, pp. 48–57, https://doi.org/10.26599/BDMA.2018.9020031.

[20] P. Buhler, W. Khattak, T. Erl, Big Data Fundamentals: Concepts, Drivers & Techniques, Ch. 8, Prentice Hall, 2016, ISBN 9780134291185, p. 24.

[21] ICS, Taking the Qualitative Approach With Big Data, 2019. Available from: https://www.ics.ie/news/view/1652.

[22] J. Hanington, The ABCs of A/B Testing, Salesforce, Pardot, 2012. Available from: https://www.pardot.com/blog/abcs-ab-testing/.

[23] A. Fokina, Flat AB Split Testing. Isolated Vector Illustration. Results Comparing Two Web Site Pages, Graphics. Wireframe of Mobile Site on Your Tablet, 2018. Available from: https://www.dreamstime.com/stock-illustration-flat-ab-split-testing-isolated-vector-illustration-results-comparing-two-web-site-pages-graphics-wireframe-mobile-site-your-image67645948.

[24] C. Chakraborty, B. Gupta, S.K. Ghosh, D. Das, C. Chakraborty, Telemedicine supported chronic wound tissue prediction using different classification approach, Journal of Medical Systems 40 (3) (2016) 1–12.

[25] S. Menon, Importance of Advanced Analytics in Healthcare, CABOT, 2018. Available from: https://www.cabotsolutions.com/importance-of-advanced-analytics-in-healthcarE.

[26] V. Wallace, E. MacPherson, K.T. Chan, Y.T. Zhang, A.T. Ahuja, W.H. Cheung, Medical Applications of Terahertz Imaging, The Shun Hing Institute of Advanced Engineering, 2004. Available from: http://www.ee.cuhk.edu.hk/∼emma/SHIAEmma.htm.

[27] H. Alharthi, Healthcare predictive analytics: an overview with a focus on Saudi Arabia, Journal of Infection and Public Health 11 (6) (2018) 749–756.

[28] Insurance Nexus, The Role of Data and Analytics in Insurance Fraud Detection, 2016. Available from: https://www.insurancenexus.com/fraud/role-data-and-analytics insurance-fraud-detection.

[29] Q.K. Fatt, A. Ramadas, The usefulness and challenges of big data in healthcare, Journal of Healthcare Communications 3 (2) (2018).

[30] R. Sonnati, Improving healthcare using big data analytics, International Journal of Scientific & Technology Research, Directory of Open Access Journals 4 (8) (2015) 142–146 (5).

[31] M. Ojha, K. Mathur, Proposed application of big data analytics in healthcare at Maharaja Yeshwantrao Hospital, in: 2016 3rd MEC International Conference on Big Data and Smart City (ICBDSC), Muscat, 2016, pp. 1–7, https://doi.org/10.1109/ICBDSC.2016.7460340.

[32] R. Sathiyavathi, A survey: big data analytics on healthcare system, Contemporary Engineering Sciences 8 (3) (2015) 121–125. HIKARI Ltd. Available from: www.m-hikari.com.

[33] M. Kumar, R. Manjula, Big data analytics in rural health care - a step towards Svasth Bharath, International Journal of Computer Science and Information Technologies 5 (6) (2014) 7172–7178. ISDN: 0975-6946.

[34] Y.C. Sim, J.Y. Park, K.M. Ahn, C. Park, J.H. Son, Terahertz imaging of excised oral cancer at frozen temperature, Biomedical Optics Express 4 (2013) 1413–1421.

[35] Y. Wang, L. Kung, T.A. Byrd, Big data analytics: understanding its capabilities and potential benefits for healthcare organizations, Technological Forecasting and Social Change 126 (2018) 3–13.

[36] L. Diaz, What are the limitations of big data in healthcare? HealthWorksCollective (2017). Available from: https://www.healthworkscollective.com/limitations-big-data-in-healthcare/.

[37] C. Leaf, The Real Limitations of Big Data, 2017. Available from: http://fortune.com/2017/08/02/big-data-healthcare-limits/.

CHAPTER 8

Medical Imaging, Artificial Intelligence, Internet of Things, Wearable Devices in Terahertz Healthcare Technologies

AMIT BANERJEE, PHD • CHINMAY CHAKRABORTY, PHD • MEGHA RATHI, SR., PHD

INTRODUCTION

There has been a keen interest in the exploration of new-generation thermal detectors for surveillance applications, such as night vision cameras, etc. However, improvements in infrared (thermal) detectors due to advancements in the semiconductor device processing technologies and innovation of new materials have opened up many new frontiers [1]. Terahertz (THz; ~300 GHz to 3 THz) technology is based on thermal radiation, and has some exceptional advantages for various applications. The electromagnetic spectrum's ~1 THz frequency region can be applied to remote nondestructive testing and sensing for homeland security. Shorter wavelengths (millimeter waves) cannot penetrate deeper interiors of matter, whereas THz wave yields can penetrate materials and provide high-resolution imaging. Also, THz waves do not ionize, nor do they trigger detrimental reactions in tissue, because of low photon energies. Among various applications are high-speed mobile and wireless communications; conservational, ecological, and environmental observation and real-time monitoring; security and surveillance related to remote examination of materials for possibility of explosives, poisons, weapons, and ammunition; biomedical and healthcare applications and diagnosis (screening and imaging of perished or decayed teeth, diagnosis of cancerous cells in skin and possibility of tumors, analysis of proteins, genes, DNA, etc.); drug delivery [2,3]; T-ray vision for night goggles or looking through walls [4–6]; defects in substances; materials for inspection of imperfections, e.g., in food for the presence of foreign substances [7]; etc. Furthermore, THz spectra can be used for radio telescopes and remote-sensing investigations of interstellar materials and the chemical composition and atmospheres of remote planets [8,9]. Although some key innovations in the THz domain have taken place since 2010, mainly in powerful sources [10], uncooled detectors [11–13], and real-time imaging [14,15], fundamental problems need to be addressed for commercial applications of these systems to replace solid-state devices and for further incorporation in advanced and flexible electronics [16–20]. The THz field is emerging toward an interdisciplinary approach driven by the needs of commercial systems for day-to-day usage, and hence the study of new-generation powerful THz sources, sensitive and fast detectors, and efficient optical elements has become a matter of prime importance.

This chapter deals with the emerging advances in THz systems in the interface of artificial intelligence (AI), the Internet of Things (IoT), and wearable devices that are expected to revolutionize many fields, as described earlier, particularly the biomedical and healthcare industry. A detailed review of theoretical, methodological, and empirical work dealing with the state of the art of experimental and technological implementation of AI, the IoT, and wearable devices in THz biomedical and healthcare technologies will help in comprehensive understanding for anyone venturing toward medical applications of THz, covering a vast audience from basic science to engineering and technology experts and learners. Here, emerging methods for medical data evaluation and diagnosis of diseases, including trends in the IoT, wearable technologies, machine learning, and big data analytics, are reported. To begin with, a few of the key areas of interest in THz biomedical and healthcare technologies are outlined: (1) THz medical imaging: currently medical imaging is done mostly with X-rays, ultrasound, computed tomography

Terahertz Biomedical and Healthcare Technologies. https://doi.org/10.1016/B978-0-12-818556-8.00008-2

scans, magnetic resonance imaging (MRI), and a few other technologies. However, emerging technologies are in development for improved imaging, which are mostly various forms of electromagnetic imaging techniques, like THz or infrared imagining or thermography. These could be efficiently combined with medical AI, the IoT, and virtual reality, to provide the ease of real-time and accurate views, and may help in image-guided surgeries, high-resolution and multidimensional imaging, etc. (2) Telemedicine: telemedicine combines various interdisciplinary areas, including informatics, medicine, materials science, telecommunications, AI, virtual presence, computer engineering, and robotics, enhancing the depth and understanding of diagnostic and medical information at an affordable cost. The importance of robotics and AI in IoT-based healthcare technology, mainly for remote patient monitoring, medical information technology, medical data analysis and accurate diagnosis with proper decision-making technology, and enabling telerobotic surgeries based on the Internet of Robotic Things (IoRT), will be discussed here. (3) Wearable devices and the IoT: recently commercially available wearable and IoT devices have become quite commonly visible and come combined with mobile applications and data management and analysis tools. However, the application of these devices may extend to the biomedical and healthcare industry far beyond tracking steps or heart rate, as they are capable of comprehensive health data collection with the use of various types of sensors in the same device and can serve as a fancy-looking smart watch or simple jewelry or any other wearable attachment that combines mobile applications. Standard protocols of machine intelligence use the collected data, seeking out possible anomalies and preventive predictions of major health risks.

Background of Terahertz Biomedical and Healthcare Technologies

In 2018, the global THz market was ~$318.6 million and estimated to exceed ~$906.2 million by 2024 [21]. Electromagnetic waves like THz play an integral role in multisensor applications that vary between millimeter wave and infrared. Few important types of sources and detectors of THz are electronic sources, lasers, electro-optical sources and bolometers, Golay cells, pyroelectric and heterodyne mix receivers, respectively [22]. The THz laser is planned by scholars at the Massachusetts Institute of Technology to achieve specific targets, such as tight beam pattern, high constant power, and broad electric frequency tuning. The Internet of Multimedia Nano-Things (IoMNT), with major research challenges and THz channel modeling for nano-thing communication, has been presented [23]. The multiple device components (nanocameras, nanoprocessors, scalar nanosensors, nanophones, nanomemories, power nanosystems, nanoantennas, and nanotransceivers) have been considered. THz technology is a nondestructive method, which has progressed drastically in biomedical research, such as in medical diagnosis and testing. This technology is used to detect hidden objects using nonionizing radiation. THz is mainly focused on imaging, spectroscopy, and communication technology. THz enhances technological growth tremendously in various areas, including informatics, medicine, materials science, astronomy, AI, military and security, computer engineering, and robotics. An AI-integrated THz technology enhances healthcare performance. The aim of this chapter is to discuss the significant role of robotics and AI in IoT-based healthcare technology. Here, the main focus is on four major applications: remote patient monitoring, medical information technology, medical data analysis, and accurate diagnosis with proper decision-making technology. The main contributions of THz technology are in main categories, such as quality control, operation, preventive healthcare, and nondestructive evaluation. Here, telerobotic surgery and the importance of the IoRT are discussed with reference to recent literature. The Internet of Nano-Things (IoNT) has some significance in THz technology by giving reliable and safe information exchange among nanonetworks and nanodevices. New security schemes are required to protect the IoNT infrastructure. Josep and Ian [24] proposed the IoMNT in the THz band for defense, biomedical, industrial, and environmental fields. They mentioned various components of nano-things, as follows: nanocameras, nanoprocessors, nanophones, scalar nanosensors, nanomemories, power nanosystems, nanoantennas, and nanotransceivers.

Fig. 8.1 depicts the various applications of THz for health monitoring. THz is based on cross-disciplinary and fusion technology. This technology provides better services, like biosensors, biomedical sensing/imaging, atmosphere monitoring, hazards detection, ultrafast nanodevices, ultrawideband wireless communication, semiconductors, optical devices, and military uses (small-scale radar).

Giuseppe et al. [25] discussed the role of nanoscale wireless communications in healthcare applications. The channel capacity and the transmission ranges have been analyzed in human tissues. This model enhances IoNT-enabled intrabody communication systems. Elayan et al. [26] introduced a number of

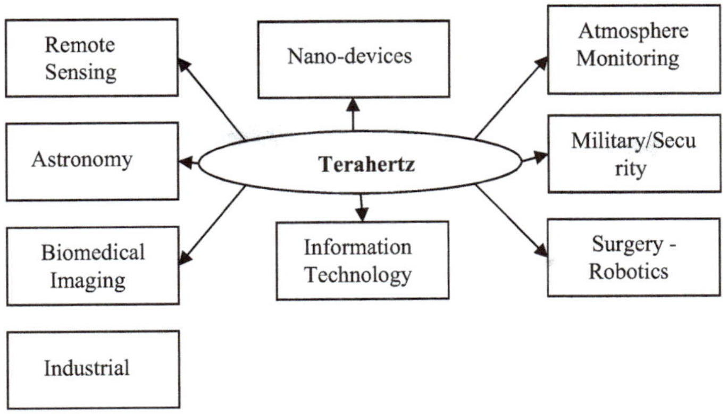

FIG. 8.1 Role of terahertz technology in various applications.

opportunities for THz wireless link deployment. It enhances the communication requirements with high data rates and satisfies user demand. The following characteristics of THz are as follows: band 100 GHz–10 THz, short/medium range, point-to-multipoint network topology, thermal noise source, robust weather conditions, and high security. Hadeel et al. [27] developed a channel model by analyzing the link budget between nanodevices working in the human body. This is used to predict the optical bioelectromagnetic propagation and THz effect. They briefly discussed the role of THz in communication technologies, THz transmitters, and receivers.

TERAHERTZ SPECTROSCOPY AND MEDICAL IMAGING

The subject of THz spectroscopy and medical imaging is important for the implementation of AI, the IoT, and wearable devices, as these tools or devices use the data or information collected from spectroscopic or imaging or a host of other sensors for application in THz healthcare technologies. The different types of frequency bands can be used for biomedical imaging platforms. The THz technology frequency band provides short waves that measure cell size. This technology is used to distinguish between different cells that are affected or not. The cancerous tissue can be detected using THz technology. This technology is employed in various healthcare applications, like skin cancer; burn and wound inspection; dentistry; biopsy; blood, breath, and brain imaging; dental imaging; endoscopy; breast cancer; arthritis; osteoarthritis; multispectral THz colonoscopy; full-body scanning; and cancer imaging [22]. THz imaging enhances the signal-to-noise ratio, spatial resolution, and sensitivity. THz can identify various cancer types by DNA analysis even in their early stage. This technology is used only to detect cancer [28]. THz cameras are having a good impact in healthcare. This noninvasive method provides high-resolution micrometer-scale imaging. THz wavelengths vary between microwaves and infrared. The emitted light from this region can be used in different biomedical applications. THz medical imaging is useful in effectively distinguishing tumorous, cancerous, and abnormal tissue from normal and healthy tissue. This light, unlike X-rays, does not affect the skin tissue because it does not bear much energy (0.41–41 meV). THz can be applied to gather real-time imaging during surgical operations. THz imaging systems give better visualization and high medical data security. The systems currently used for THz medical imaging fall into the following main categories: (1) pulsed THz imaging and (2) continuous-wave THz imaging. Eva et al. [29] discussed the use of a robotic arm (IRB 120 from ABB) for free-form surface using THz imaging principles. Also, the sensor head position on the surface has been measured. Andreas and Michael [30] surveyed THz medical imaging in the nanotechnology field. The performance metrics (higher sensitivity and good resolution) are achievable in nano techniques. The advantages and limitations of THz imaging have been broadly discussed. Sigfrid et al. [31] measured the breast cancer margin using time-domain spectroscopy (TDS). They also observed that THz breast specimen images can precisely distinguish between breast carcinoma, standard fibroglandular, and fat or adipose tissue. The advantages of THz imaging are that it can penetrate clothing and has low radiation. Jinsong et al. [32] identified concealed items using a deep learning technique and measured performance on a real-time basis effectively and efficiently.

The THz region of the electromagnetic spectrum, along with its applications, is shown in Fig. 8.2. The "THz gap" is defined by the absence of sensitive detectors and powerful, reliable sources that can function between electronics and photonics, at least until lately, after several discoveries like ultrafast lasers and modern THz TDS techniques. These have helped harness this wavelength for various applications, including in biomedical science [33].

Yang et al. have reported extensively on biomedical results from THz TDS and medical imaging [33]. The usefulness of the THz spectrum in biomedical and healthcare usage is described in Table 8.1 [33]. THz can couple with intra/intermolecular domain vibrations, like hydrogen bonds, van der Waals, or hydrophobic interactions, which can be used for biomedical information extraction. For biomedical applications considering detection and signal processing, THz biomedical technologies may include the following categories: (1) THz spectroscopy and (2) THz imaging (or medical imaging in the current context). However, a host of other macroscopic and molecular applications are also available [34].

2.1 Terahertz Spectroscopy for Biomedical Applications

It is immensely important to build up a comprehensive database for THz spectroscopy for biomolecule recognition, as the same will be useful for medical applications with the help of various devices, sensors, and computing tools. THz spectroscopy has been used for characterization and hence fingerprinting of various biomolecules and biomaterials. By identifying low-frequency biomolecular motions, molecular vibrations, and rotations that overlap in the THz frequency range, biomolecules can be identified and associated with their distinctive spectral fingerprints. THz spectroscopy can be used for identifying biomolecule hydration shells, couplings, etc. [33]. Some useful examples of THz spectroscopy for possible biomedical applications have been discussed [33] and are described in Fig. 8.3.

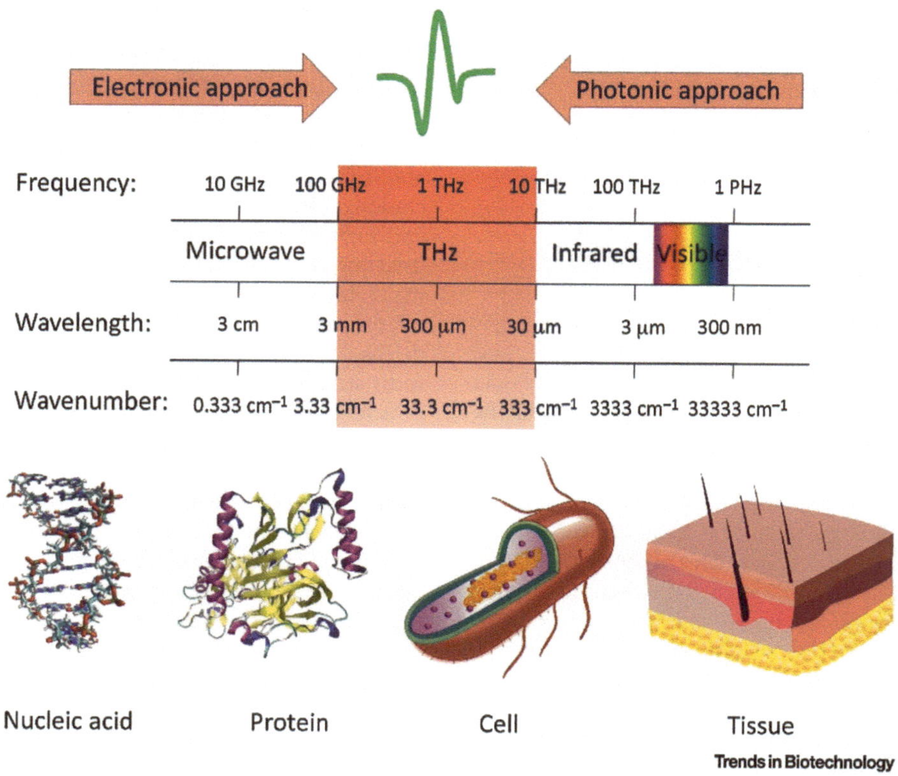

FIG. 8.2 Terahertz (THz) spectrum, including the so-called "THz gap." The application of THz technology has been extended in the detection of various biomaterials, biomolecules, nucleic acids, and proteins at the cellular level and in tissues. (Reproduced with permission from X. Yang, X. Zhao, K. Yang, Y. Liu, Y. Liu, W. Fu, Y. Luo, Biomedical applications of terahertz spectroscopy and imaging, Trends in Biotechnology 34 (10) (2016) 810–824.)

TABLE 8.1
Terahertz Spectrum for Biomedical and Healthcare Technology.

Spectral fingerprint The photon energy of the THz wave largely coincides with energy levels corresponding to low-frequency motions, such as the vibration, rotation, and translation of the molecular skeleton. These molecule-specific motions identify biomolecules by measuring their characteristic spectral signatures in the THz range.
Transparency of materials comprising nonpolar molecules Materials such as paper and plastic, which are opaque to visible and near-infrared waves, may be transparent in the THz range. This property enables the detection of hazardous substances without opening packages, because THz radiation can easily penetrate common packing materials.
Strong absorption by water Polar molecules, such as water, exhibit strong absorption in the THz range. Specifically, the THz absorption coefficient of water at 1 THz is approximately 220 cm^{-1} at room temperature, exceeding that of common biomolecules. Normal tissues and cancer tissues can be accurately differentiated because their water contents are different. Moreover, THz radiation has the potential to rapidly assess the living state of bacteria (live or dead) according to their different hydration levels.
Excellent time and spatial resolution THz radiation interrogates characteristic frequency features with spatial resolution of several micrometers by near-field spectroscopic modalities and reveals time-resolved dynamics on the subpicosecond to picosecond timescales. Thus, THz spectroscopy permits time-resolved investigations of the collective vibration modes of biomolecules in solution with unprecedented sensing capability.
Noninvasive and nonionizing properties The low-energy photons of THz radiation (i.e., 1−10 meV) make it suitable for medical imaging because the noninvasive imaging modality can be applied for in vivo real-time diagnosis without causing ionization damage, unlike X-rays. Moreover, THz wavelengths are longer than infrared and visible light, and scattering losses in biological tissues are negligible.

THz, terahertz.
Reproduced with permission from X. Yang, X. Zhao, K. Yang, Y. Liu, Y. Liu, W. Fu, Y. Luo, Biomedical applications of terahertz spectroscopy and imaging, Trends in Biotechnology 34 (10) (2016) 810–824.

2.2 Terahertz Medical Imaging

THz could be extremely useful for medical imaging, considering that intrinsic properties and morphological information can combined in an image-spectrum merging modality, from which amplitude-phase information can be found synchronously [33]. THz medical imaging can differentiate tumor cells with higher resolution and sensitivity, in a nonionizing manner and hence without harmful radiation health hazard, compared with X-rays. The THz medical imaging technique has a penetration depth of a few hundred micrometers, for intraoperative imaging and identification of distinctive molecular fingerprints, and the advantage of miniaturized instruments, which may be superior to MRI. Various advantages and limitations of THz medical imaging and schemes of signal and sensitivity enhancement are reported by Yang et al. [33]. It was found that various factors in sample tissues can alter THz medical imaging crucially, e.g., (1) water content: tumorous, unhealthy, diseased tissues contain higher interstitial water (due to abundant vascularity or tissue edema) and alter THz absorption results, and they seem different from healthy tissues; (2) alterations in cellular structure in tissues: microenvironmental variations in cellular structure and morphology, deterioration, and compositional variations alter THz image contrast compared with a perfectly healthy tissue; and (3) contrast-enhancing agents: a few elements (e.g., glycerol, targeted gold nanorods, consumption of tryptophan) help in artificial contrast enhancements [33]. Also, absorption of water and higher temperature enhance sensitivity of THz molecular imaging. The THz imaging contrast can be further improved by altering the design of the THz imaging system on a case-by-case basis. The status of THz medical imaging for 5 years has been described by Yang et al. [33] and is shown in Table 8.2. This shows the effectiveness of THz imaging for different types of tissues, including in vitro imaging applied in digestive, integumentary, respiratory, and nervous systems, with comparison to pathological biopsy for reference.

As is evident from Table 8.2, THz in vitro imaging can be used for biomedical identification and may complement pathological diagnostics. Some examples of THz medical imaging are given in Fig. 8.4 [33]. It is important to note that pretreatment processes like

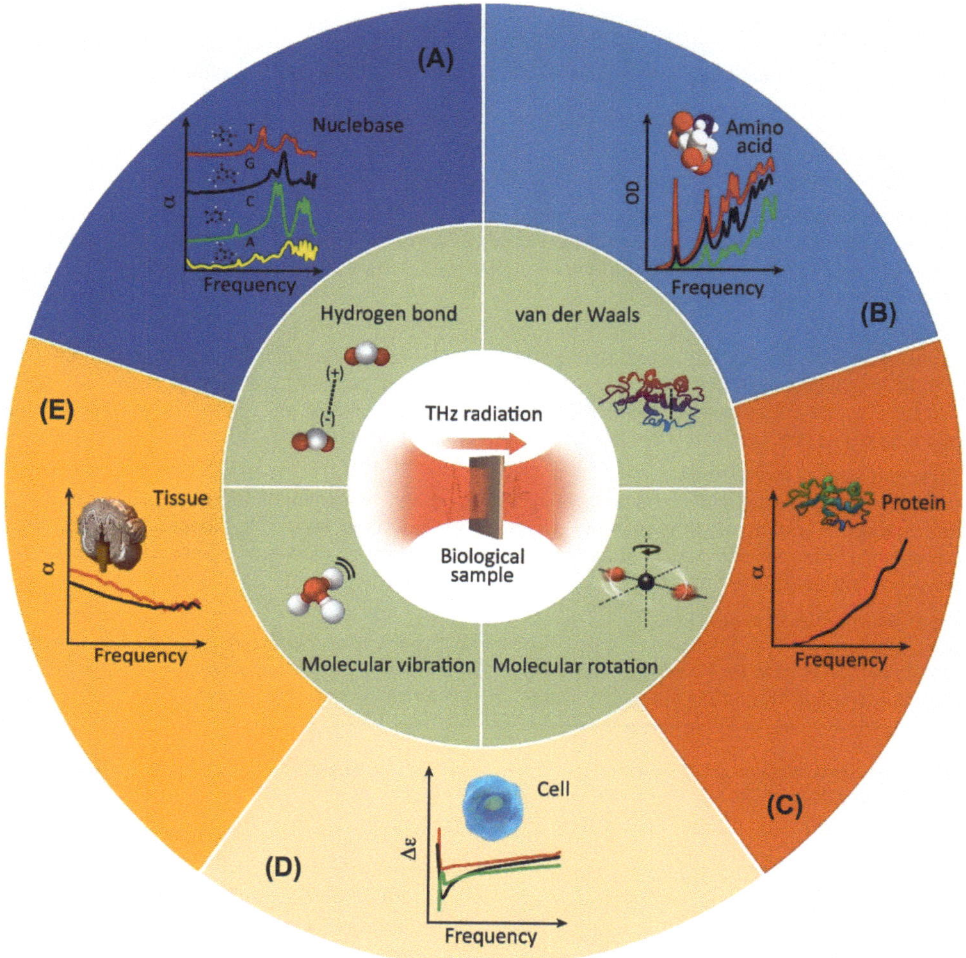

FIG. 8.3 Terahertz (THz) spectroscopy for possible biomedical applications. THz can couple with low-frequency molecular rotations and vibrations of biomaterials, hydrogen bonds, weak interactions, and van der Waals interactions that are in the THz range, and hence THz may be used for biomolecular probing, e.g., **(A)** THz absorption (absorption coefficient α) for nucleobases adenosine (*A*), cytosine (*C*), guanine (*G*), and threonine (*T*) at 10 K. **(B)** Optical density (*OD*) with THz of L-glutamic acid (at various concentrations: 0.314 [*green*], 0.585 [*black*], and 0.837 mol L^{-1} [*red*]), found to be linearly proportional to the concentration with notable and distinct peaks at 1.22, 2.03, 2.46, 2.68, 2.80, and 3.24 THz. **(C)** THz absorption coefficient (α) for lysozyme (HEWL, egg white) solution (*red*) and HEWL + triacetylglucosamine solution (*black*) at 270 K. **(D)** Comparison of complex dielectric constants of distilled water and cultured human cancer cells, including DLD-1 (*red*), HEK293 (*black*), and HeLa (*green*). **(E)** Comparison of absorption coefficient (α) of paraffin-embedded brain gliomas (*red*) and normal tissues (*black*) shows α for glioma tissue higher than for normal tissue below 1 THz; however, these differences are not notable at higher frequencies. (Reproduced with permission from Reproduced with permission from X. Yang, X. Zhao, K. Yang, Y. Liu, Y. Liu, W. Fu, Y. Luo, Biomedical applications of terahertz spectroscopy and imaging, Trends in Biotechnology 34 (10) (2016) 810–824.)

formalin fixation, paraffin sections, or dehydrated samples can be used to overcome the absorption loss from water in tissues. The THz identification of cancerous tissue in the middle of normal fibrous and adipose tissues (fat) is possible as it looks darker owing to structural variations. The in vivo THz imaging is used on skin tissues (epidermal), considering the low penetration depth of THz waves, and also it is good to note that water absorption in human skin or tissue may dominate the shape of variable-angle ellipsometry or polarized

TABLE 8.2
Effectiveness of THz Biomedical Imaging in THz Imaging for Different Types of Tissues for 5

Anatomical System/Animal Model	Tissue	Specimen Source	Instrumentation	Spatial Resolution (μm)	Year	References
Digestive system	Mouth neoplasms: mucoepidermoid and SCC	Frozen section	TPI reflection system	250[b]	2013	[34]
	Colonic neoplasm	Paraffin section	CW THz imaging system	500	2016	[35]
		Formalin fixation	CW THz endoscopic system	100[b]	2014	[36]
		Frozen section	THz near-field imaging system	220	2015	[37]
		Freshly excised	CW THz imaging system	600	2013	[38]
		Freshly excised	Portable TPI reflection system	—[e]	2011	[39]
	Stomach neoplasms: EGC	Freshly excised	TPI reflection system	500[b]	2015	[40]
	Liver neoplasm	Frozen section	THz near-field imaging system	240	2013	[41]
	Liver neoplasm: hepatocellular carcinoma	Frozen section	THz in-line digital holography system	158	2015	[42]
	Pancreatic neoplasm: IDC	Paraffin section	TPI reflection system	500[c]	2010	[43]
Integumentary system	Skin neoplasms: BCC and SCC	Freshly excised	CW THz imaging system, polarized light imaging system	100[b]	2014	[44]
	Skin neoplasm: nonmelanoma	Frozen section	CW THz imaging system	390	2011	[45]
Reproductive system	Breast neoplasm: IDC	Paraffin section	TPI reflection system	50[b]	2015	[46]
	Breast neoplasm: IDC and papillary tumor	Frozen section	THz near-field imaging system	240	2011	[47]
	Breast neoplasm	Freshly excised/ formalin fixation	CW THz imaging system	1000[c]	2013	[48]
	Uterine cervical neoplasm: SCC	Freshly excised	TPI reflection system	500[b]	2011	[49]
Respiratory system	Lung neoplasm: SCC	Paraffin section	TPI reflection system	500[c]	2010	[43]
Motor system	Normal skeleton	Air dried	THz computed tomography system	2700	2012	[50]

Continued

TABLE 8.2
Effectiveness of THz Biomedical Imaging in THz Imaging for Different Types of Tissues for 5

Anatomical System/Animal Model	Tissue	Specimen Source	Instrumentation	Spatial Resolution (μm)	Year	References
Swine	Normal skin, subdermal fat, and muscle	Freshly excised	THz QCL interferometry imaging system	50	2014	[51]
	Normal cornea	Freshly excised (immersed in polyethylene glycol solution)	TPI reflection system	1200[c]	2011	[52]
Rat	Normal gastrointestinal tract	Freshly excised	TPI reflection system	250[b]	2014	[53]
	Breast neoplasm (xenograft)	Freshly excised	TPI transmission system	1100[d]	2011	[54]
	Glioblastoma	Freshly excised	TPI reflection system	—	2014	[55]
	Liver cirrhosis	Freshly excised/ formalin fixation	TPI reflection system	—	2010	[56]
	Normal skin	Burn	TPI reflection system	—	2012	[57]
	Normal vessels in ear	In vivo	THz near-field imaging system	500	2015	[58]
Rabbit	Cartilage	Formalin fixation	TPI reflection system	—	2010	[59]
	Normal cornea	In vivo	TPI reflection system	1000[c]	2015	[60]

[a] Abbreviations: *BCC*, basal cell carcinoma; *CW*, continuous wave; *EGC*, early gastric carcinoma; *IDC*, infiltrating ductal carcinoma; *QCL*, quantum cascading laser; *SCC*, squamous cell carcinoma; *TPI*, terahertz pulsed imaging.
[b] Scanning resolution.
[c] Spot size.
[d] Lateral resolution.
[e] —, not given.

Reproduced with permission from Reproduced with permission from X. Yang, X. Zhao, K. Yang, Y. Liu, Y. Liu, W. Fu, Y. Luo, Biomedical applications of terahertz spectroscopy and imaging, Trends in Biotechnology 34 (10) (2016) 810–824.

reflectometry in the THz spectrum [33]. The quantitative study of water content in blood vessels and corneal tissues by the THz in vivo imaging modality can be useful for blood monitoring [33] and could be further extended to tracing drugs and computed tomography in blood or various kinds of tissues, bones, and skeletons [33], with possible application of this technique and the prospect of clinical adoption in the near future.

2.3 Limitations and Biological Effects of Terahertz

The medical imaging application of THz is currently only in its beginning, due to poor diffraction-limited spatial resolution and investigations, sample preparations, operating procedures (slice thickness, water content, storage conditions, instrumentation, etc.), and measurements with THz that are yet to be standardized; and reliable databases should be established for reproducible and reliable results for possible clinical adoption [33]. Also, there is a need for comprehensive understanding and development of endoscopic surgery instruments, transceivers, and instrumentation for molecular imaging modalities based on THz for superior image quality and enhanced brightness and contrast, for reduction of signal loss in aqueous environments, and for biomolecular fingerprinting at spatial resolution as low as few nanometers and with THz pulsed near-field microscopy for intraoperative diagnostics, real-time monitoring, and other critical information for prescribing medicine for practical applications.

Another issue to address, as with all other electromagnetic waves, is the health hazard and biological

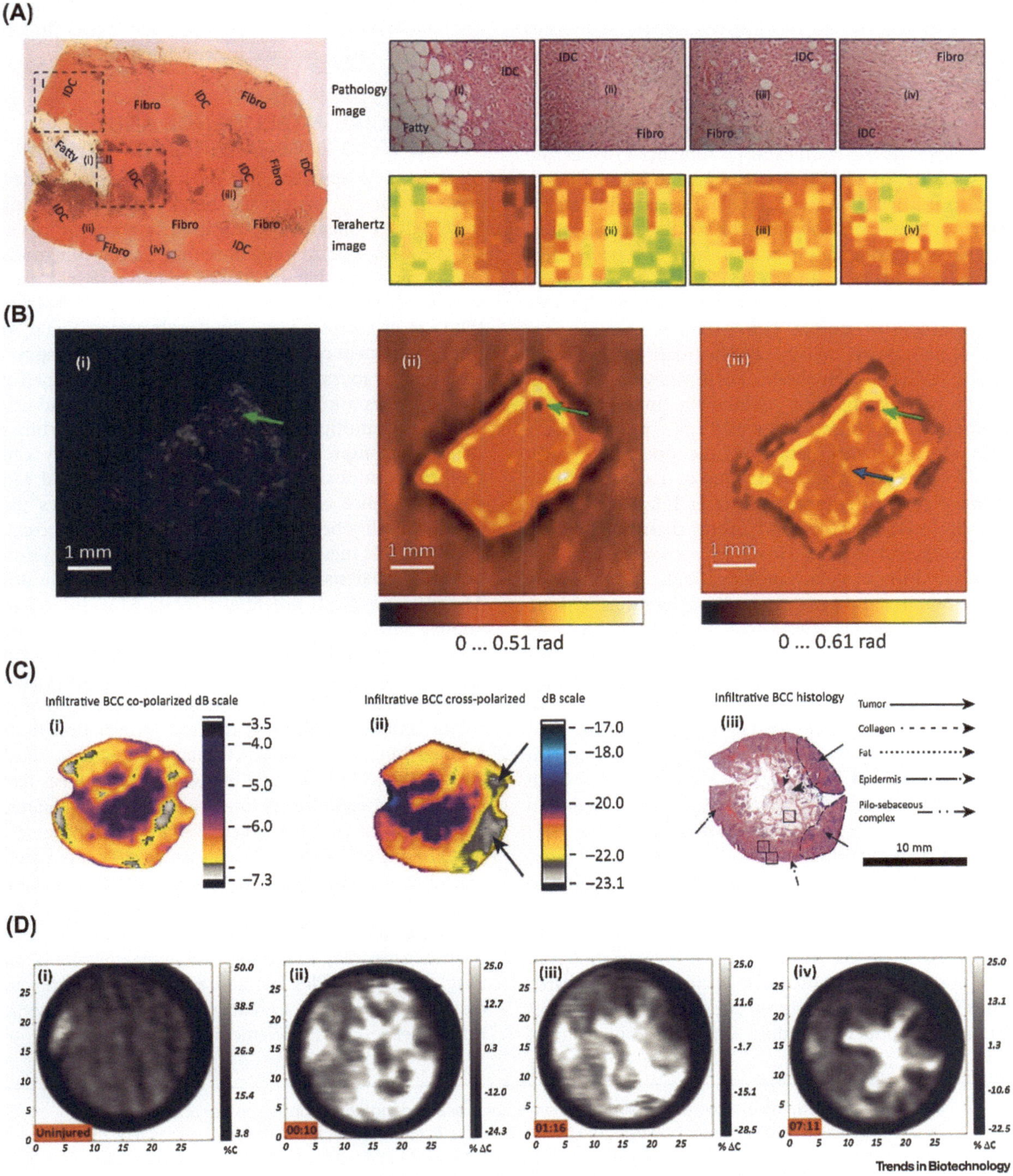

FIG. 8.4 Examples of terahertz (THz) medical imaging. **(A)** Selected locations of breast cancer tissue (i—iv) on THz frequency domain image at 1.5 THz, identified with undistinguishable or poorly distinguishable infiltrating ductal carcinoma (*IDC*), alongside pathology images, which show macroscopic distributions of IDC, fatty, and fibrous tissue. **(B)** Human hepatocellular carcinoma tissue, with THz holography. (i) Images of the carcinoma tissue; (ii) phase-shift distributions reconstructed from the normalized hologram; (iii) phase-shift distributions

concerns regarding exposure to THz, which has been a matter of anxiety for medical researchers and needs comprehensive study at the levels of organism, tissue, cell, and biomolecules to understand the possible health effects of exposure to THz for short and long periods of time. The THz biological effects depend on the THz power densities on exposed superficial tissues and cells. It is reported [33] that exposure to THz radiation at a low-power density (1.89 THz, 189.92 mW cm^{-2}) may not cause harm by inducing tissue damage, which is a likely outcome of exposure to high THz power densities (0.1–1.0 THz, 2000–14,000 mW cm^{-2}), with a damage threshold of 7160 mW cm^{-2}, which may vary from sample to sample. Other than temperature rise due to high power density of THz, tissue and cell damage or death has been observed in primary dermal fibroblasts in humans due to the thermal effects of continuous exposure to 84.8 mW cm^{-2} power density THz radiation [33]. However, the operating power used for THz pulses is several orders of magnitude lower in most medical scanners and laser THz TDS systems that are reported to cause harmful thermal effects in real biological studies. However, a concern for THz-induced biomolecular modifications, protein and DNA damage, and gene expression alterations with no recordable thermal effects was reported in low-level THz irradiation [33], which could be due to low-frequency collective biomolecular vibrations induced by THz. In general, there are contradicting reports citing no visible or negligible damages to DNA or genes at exposure to 2.3 THz, along with studies showing that DNA damages, if any, may be repaired [33], which makes these effects more or less inconclusive owing to our lack of comprehensive knowledge in the THz domain of nonthermal effects. There have been interesting reports [33] on the effects of THz irradiation at the organism level, citing behavioral alterations, increased depression in a mice, inflammatory responses, and perturbation of wound healing shown in case of mouse skin, which may indicate health hazards from THz radiation. However, due to the lack of systematic and reproducible studies, at present knowledge of the adverse biological effects of THz and their impact on human tissues is not complete and needs further studies to create a risk assessment database.

3 ARTIFICIAL INTELLIGENCE AND ROBOTICS IN TERAHERTZ HEALTHCARE

AI is used to enhance the capacity of a computer-enabled robotic system to handle data processing from a large database. Medical AI is mainly focused on the design of AI programs that execute diagnosis and recommend therapy. The AI system analyzes decision support methods for critical care and observes the level of acceptance by the health professionals. AI improves patient communication and enhances the system capacity to transfer and store big data in a superior way. AI plays a major role in THz healthcare and can collect the multiple technologies enabling machines to sense, comprehend, act, and learn, so they can perform administrative and clinical functions. AI can greatly enhance care delivery and also increases the interoperability between systems, patients and doctors, and electronic medical record (EMR) vendors. As per an Accenture analysis, when combined, key clinical health AI applications can potentially create $150 billion in annual savings for the US healthcare economy by 2026. The main challenges of THz are to expand system capabilities and improve the procedures to solve specific problems. AI in THz and telemedicine provides robust patient monitoring, medical information technology, intelligent assistance diagnosis, and medical data analysis. AI is broadly focused in many areas like (1) management information systems, (2) data streams, (3) rule-based (expert) systems, (4) data mining, (5) neural networks, (6) machine learning, (7) case-based reasoning, (8) data visualization, and (9) telerobotics. AI is used for various applications such as image recognition and interpretation, diagnostic assistance, biofield science, generating reminders and alerts, therapy planning, etc. AI provides fast and accurate diagnostics to reduce human errors, to reduce costs, to provide a virtual presence, and for telemedicine.

reconstructed from the extrapolated hologram. Here a small tissue perforation (top left corner of image shown by *green arrow*) is visible in (i–iii); however, the thin vertical line (fibrosis in the carcinoma tissue, shown by *blue arrow*) is evident only in (iii). **(C)** THz polarized reflectance images of infiltrative basal cell carcinoma (*BCC*) tissue. (i) THz copolarized reflectance image; (ii) THz cross-polarized reflectance image, (iii) H&E-stained histology image. Here low-reflectance areas (*solid arrow*) in the THz cross-polarized image are consistent with the size and shape of the tumor region. **(D)** THz features from skin burn of rat, where lighter areas indicate edematous response areas postburn due to the higher reflected signal from local water. Thus from (i) to (iv): THz images of unburned skin and burned skin after 10 min, >1 h, and >7 h, respectively. (Reproduced with permission from Reproduced with permission from X. Yang, X. Zhao, K. Yang, Y. Liu, Y. Liu, W. Fu, Y. Luo, Biomedical applications of terahertz spectroscopy and imaging, Trends in Biotechnology 34 (10) (2016) 810–824.)

AI is used in THz technologies to identify diagnostics and visualize the contrast and absorption. THz imaging technology has been recently applied in the clinical environment. Robotic technology, machine learning, and AI will offer the future development of IoT applications. Today, the emerging IoRT brings innovative convergence issues for better programming and understanding between various robotic/medical things for information exchange, good linkup, security, and configuration. AI will revolutionize all industries, but perhaps none so much as healthcare. Instead of looking at single molecules, it can analyze how entire networks of molecules work together to create a system and combine this knowledge with other disciplines to gain a better understanding and compare with available databases and then use that information to develop more effective treatments. Both biomedicine and machine learning could analyze data available in national health databases to identify potential complications, as well as effective protocols, using the intelligence gained via data. Telemedicine is used to process medical data for diagnosis, therapy, education, management, and remote consultation [61]. The most important types are as follows: teleconsultation, teleeducation, telemonitoring, and telesurgery—assistance in surgery given via video, i.e., robotic arms used to carry out remote surgical stages with good accuracy.

3.1 Robotics in Healthcare

Robotic technology has been widely applied in healthcare and resolves several health issues. This technology is superior in surgery compared with any other. The major features of robotic technology are as follows: (1) mobility, (2) programmability, (3) sensors, and (4) flexibility; it works in a range of programs to manipulate and transport materials in diverse ways. Machines have assisted humans for a long time. The robot is the best example of a machine device that is applied to minimize risk and burden and gives better surgical outcomes with low cost. Robotic technology in the medical domain plays an important role to promote good coordination between expert doctors and patients. It provides unique synergy between medicine, health science, and many subdisciplines of engineering. Robotic technology provides good diagnostics and maintains EMRs and medical history archives and digital imaging technologies. The aim of this section is to understand the current state of robotics in healthcare and the transitioning of electronic records that requires enhanced reliable security. Robotic technology enhances the healthcare system via real-time access whereby large volumes of data are processed through a reliable transmission path, like patient X-rays or digital scans. Fig. 8.5 presents the principles of robotic technology.

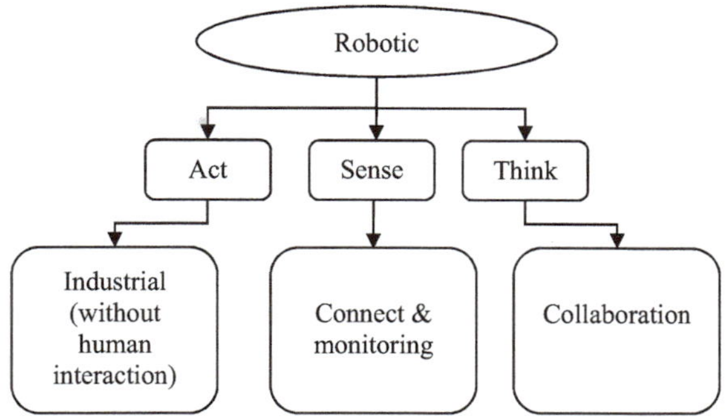

FIG. 8.5 Characteristics of the robotic approach.

Lars et al. [62] designed an inexpensive robotic tool, i.e., the Sister Kenny home therapy system, that gives observance support for home exercises, prescriptions, feedback, and communication between doctors. The home-based robotic tool gives good performance with the help of various wireless and wearable sensors for the biomedical field. Clinicians can simply monitor and prescribe concurrently to multiple patients who belong to different geographical locations. Anett et al. [63] improved movement predictions from measurements of brain activity, i.e., electroencephalogram, using robotic technology that provides more spontaneous human–machine communication. Yepes et al. [64] implemented an android-based mobile application (Asimov) for remote control of a KUKA KR6 via WiFi.

3.2 Telesurgery

Telesurgery has been done with robotic technology under remote control by a human operator. The doctor gives surgical procedure and treatment modalities to the remote patient. The robotic platform (da Vinci) has been developed to allow surgery at a distance from the bed with the robot and patient in the operation theater. It permits the doctors to operate in another room or building and also provides expert advice via teleconferencing, teleradiology, and telepathology. Ashrafian et al. [65] mentioned five important emerging dimensions for robotic surgeries, which are as follows: (1) technology that improves the precision of surgery and provides good results, (2) cost, (3) evidence that aids in the best robotic operation, (4) training—large datasets improve the system's accuracy—and (5) awareness, required for patients as well as society. Ayush et al. [66] mentioned various surgical robotic platforms, such as

(1) ROBODOC, (2) ORTHODOC, (3) da Vinci and ZEUS, (4) Acrobot, (5) PROBOT, (6) Minerva, (7) Pathfinder, (8) Renaissance, (9) RIO robotic arm, (10) iBlock, (11) NAVIO PFS, (12) Stanmore Sculptor, (13) AESOP, (14) Telelap ALF-X, (15) INNOMOTION, (16) Sensei X, (17) Niobe, (18) CyberKnife, (19) Novalis with TrueBeam STx, (20) AutoPulse, and (21) C-Leg (Ottobock). The lists of robot-assisted surgery can be categorized as follows: (1) thoracic, (2) urology, (3) vascular, (4) cardiac, (5) general, and (6) gynecology.

3.3 Applications

Amit et al. [67] discussed the latest trends of the IoT for healthcare technology for big data analysis. The various robotic applications are (1) surgical—robotic procedures; (2) physical therapy—range of motion, flexibility; (3) bionic prosthetics—replacement limbs, organs; (4) caregiver—patient interaction; (5) simulators—procedure planning, education; (6) pharmacy—compounding and dispensing; (7) logistics—materials handling, delivery. Robotics is mostly contributing to three important sections, i.e., surgeons, hospitals, and patients, which are shown in Table 8.3. The major limitations of robotic surgeries are as follows: (1) high purchase and maintenance cost; (2) requires a cultural shift in the hospital; (3) increased space in procedure and operating rooms, storage, and maintenance areas; (4) potential possibility of intraoperative mechanical failure; (5) steep learning curve; (6) lacks tactile and force feedback; (7) operation may take longer due to setup; (8) no additional insurance to offset higher costs; and (9) AI in healthcare.

3.4 Internet of Robotic Things

Robotic technology, autonomous functions, and the IoT jointly provide a good result in terms of the IoRT. The IoRT is the most demanding framework where intelligent devices can acquire sensor data from patients and process it to a cloud server in an intelligent way in terms of a proper decision-making unit. It makes faster decisions, proper visualization, data manipulation, data acquisition, analytics, and communication. Robotic technology is used for sensing, data collection, movement, manipulation, mobility, and intelligence that improves IoT services. Machine learning–integrated robotic technology provides better intelligence with the IoT, where several robots can be interconnected. The central processor controls robots via secure WiFi networks. AI-based IoT robotic technology will be associated with IoT applications to provide optimized outcomes over particular applications. The main feature of the IoT and robotics is the ability sense the data and interact with the network-enabled devices. This feature may be expanded and implemented in terms of "sense as a service" among various applications. The IoRT exchanges data streams in real-time computation mode via internal communication [69]. Chen et al. [70] proposed a cloud-enabled pillow robot for emotion sense and communication between patients through sensor robots. AI has been providing continuous support for making proper decisions in medical robotics. Concerns about robotic technologies have to do with lack of evidence and cost. Self-powered robot-assisted surgery gives better geometric accuracy. Doctors can use surgical robots to observe a soft-tissue model with 3D imagery. The limitation of robotic surgery is the lack of tactile feedback. Doctors are mostly dependent on haptic feedback, but robotic methods do not permit it. Currently, robots are controlled by humans, who are error prone, which is why there is a need to develop an automated AI-enabled robotic approach for better patient monitoring. Advanced intelligent

TABLE 8.3
Important Areas Covered by Robotic Technology [68].

Surgeons	Clinics	Patients
Enhanced patient care	Improved efficiency	Reduced hospital stay
Complex tasks allowed	Reduced costs	Reduced pain
True-life 3D vision	Reduced litigation	Faster recovery times
Increased dexterity	Marketing tool	Smaller incisions, resulting in reduced risk of infection, blood loss, and scarring
Better ergonomics		Autologous donation not required
Easy seated posture		
Less blood loss		
Smaller incisions		
Scalable motions		
Elimination of tremor		

microinstruments need to be designed that can offer accurate dimensions during operations effectively and efficiently. THz spectroscopy generates high-quality tissue images. THz helps to provide better imaging patterns. These images can be processed through the IoRT for better management and data visualization. Qiushuo et al. [71] introduced the latest advance in the field of THz technology for biomedical applications.

4 INTERNET OF THINGS AND WEARABLE DEVICES IN TERAHERTZ HEALTHCARE

4.1 Background and Driving Forces

The IoT is an innovative technology that is actually an amalgamation of digital, computing, and mechanical devices; unique objects; and people who are rendered with distinctive identifiers, and has the potential to transfer data without manual or human–computer interaction [72]. A module in the IoT can be a component like an implanted heart-monitoring chip or a biochip transponder in a farm animal or a built-in sensor in an automobile that alerts the driver when the tire pressure is low or any other human-made object that has the potential to transfer bytes or big data over the communication network [73]. Organizations utilize IoT technologies because of their efficiency, to better understand customers, to deliver better service to the customer and improve decision-making, which in turn will contribute to increasing the business. The concept of the IoT evolved after the merging of technologies like the Internet, microservices, wireless technology, and microelectromechanical systems [74]. Computational and information technology has been deployed by the convergence, enabling the data that are unstructured and at the same time machine generated to be analyzed for further improvements.

An IoT ecosystem is a mixture of smart devices that are enabled with the web and use advanced processors that are embedded, and it works on data extracted using sensors or any other means from the surroundings [75]. IoT devices often share the extracted data that they gather using sensors connecting through an IoT gateway or other means where the data are stored in the cloud-based server [76]. Sometimes, IoT devices also connect with other smart and advanced devices of similar type and then work on the knowledge they share between them. Most of the activity between devices works without any interference from humans, although devices can talk with people to take instructions or use the data.

Wearable devices play a significant role in tracking and assisting in day-to-day operations. For creating highly technocratic devices, sensors must be attached to body parts or to devices for data extraction. Theses smart integrated IoT devices permit doctors, patients, and everyone to live a happy and healthy life with a focus on preventive measures for severe disease [77]. In this modern era, these gadgets permit humans to gather real-time medical data for building quality systems.

4.2 Internet of Things in Healthcare

The IoT plays an important role in improving healthcare services. The healthcare sector these days is adopting new techniques and tools for offering quality health services with low cost [77]. Usage of the IoT in healthcare has tremendously increased in various domains, such as personalized healthcare system, treatment personalization, drug recommendation, diet recommendation, health insurance, etc. The IoT contribution to the health sector revolves around cases like telemedicine, remote monitoring, and online diagnosis, as a few basic main applications. Another important application is tracking daily activities and maintaining or supervising assets using IoT-enabled devices and radio-frequency identification [78]. Highly advanced and smart integrated techniques within the scope of health science need to be implemented, where the IoT can play a vital role in creating applications like real-time health monitoring systems, smart mobile applications for tracking daily activities of critical patients, advanced medicine systems, smart home automated health systems, personalized healthcare, etc. [79]. Medical procedures are time and cost consuming. Technology can upgrade the traditional hospital system to an advanced system in which everything is automated, from appointments to doctor consultations to paying bills, buying medicine, pathological reports, and many more. The Internet of Medical Things (IoMT) has an extensive applicability in health science or the health sector [80].

Smart IoT devices can easily connect with other advanced tools, techniques, devices, or the web and collect relevant data or information and then store the data in a cloud-based or any server for further decision-making or analysis. This is surely going to make a good impression in healthcare [81]. IoT devices and sensors can be used in assisting daily life operations in the health industry that can be backtracked to the use of real-time observation, advanced sensing devices, and medical equipment incorporation as well as work and employee trackers, wearable biometric sensors, blood sugar checkers, health sensors, insulin monitors, health suppliers, and smart beds, to name a few examples [82]. It would be very interesting to imagine what the future of industries, especially the health industry, could be if the IoT were brought into the trending industries and integrated in. Consider a real-time scenario in which a patient consults with a health specialist and is notified about the availability for consultation for future dates because their calendars were linked together. In another real-time example, if the patient got stuck on his way due to a traffic jam, a text message would automatically be sent to the health specialist notifying him about the late arrival. Internet-connected technologies will make every aspect of care ideal and will transfigure the manner in which real activities have been organized. To convert raw data into valuable information: medical quantification is going to be the future, because medical science that is quantifiable can assuredly be superior to that which is not [83]. Therefore, it is wise to take the edge of quantified medical science.

4.3 A Study of Wearable and Smart Devices in Healthcare

In a 2018 study [84], the authors proposed an integrated system using Raspberry Pi to monitor and supervise the health profile of persons in remote areas. The proposed model comprised advanced IoT devices like sensors, smartphones, and the Internet, which work in a connected network to record and track patient health data and information. The patient can manage his or her health from the comfort of home. The device predicts health status using the patient's blood pressure and heart rate. It would also alert the patient's family members and doctor with full medical information in case of an emergency.

In yet another work [85], a novel technique monitors the patient's posture. In the proposed research work, patient posture is monitored by employing an approach that utilizes the body weight of patient, which exerts pressure on a specifically drafted mattress. The authors utilized the computed pressure for examining the patient's position. Also, the proposed approach is validated using Cohen's coefficient with a value approximately equal to 0.866, which indicates higher prediction accuracy. The proposed research work also intends to reduce memory requirement and computational cost.

Another significant contribution [86] introduced a design that is an integration of 11073 IEEE service/DIM (domain information model) and CoAP (constrained application protocol) to apply on healthcare devices so that they can be used in IoT settings. They compared the performances of HTTP and 11073 DIM using CoAP. Performance evaluation was done relating to packet ampleness in one transaction, loss rate, and structure practicing JSON and XML. Results obtained described the fact that HTTP transmitted more packets compared with CoAP.

In another research work [87] the authors proposed an FPGA (field programmable gate array)-based computer-aided design algorithm for abnormality detection in kidney in ultrasound images. The data were first preprocessed, and then an ultrasound image of the region of interest in the kidney was segmented. A hybrid approach for classification works as a two-step process. In the first step the LUT lookup table technique is applied on the dataset, and in the second step a support vector machine is applied. An FPGA was used by the authors to implement the proposed hybrid approach. In another study [88], a data mining model was proposed, which helped in supervising autism patients using sensors. The proposed model also extracted sensor data, which were actually the brain signals of individual patients.

In a 2018 work [89], the authors implemented an algorithm to explore the advantages and use of big data analytics in healthcare. They had implemented a Naïve Bayesian and a J48 tree algorithm to predict the use of big data. The data were collected from the UCI website and the algorithm was implemented using Weka. The Naïve Bayesian provided accuracy of 95% and the J48 tree algorithm provided an accuracy of 100% for predictive analysis. In another paper [90], a novel approach was evaluated to check whether a dual-channel portable monitor could accurately predict and identify patients having OSA (obstructive sleep apnea). They compared the results of detecting OSA using a portable monitor in an unattended home setting with those of the laboratory polysomnography. In another novel work [91], the main emphasis was to create an automated tool to expand the trend of IoT applications in bioinformatics. In the health science domain, the proposed work focuses on tracking the health of patients by extracting and reading the measurements of heart rate. To extract heart rate value a smart sensor known as a smart health band is used, which precisely measures the value for heart rate. In case of an emergency, such as if the value exceeds a high range, an automatic message is dropped to family members or friends. Another contribution in this domain [92] proposed a technique to consistently observe the patient's physical condition with the aid of inertial measurement units. The study presented a meticulous and enhanced approach for sensing patient health activities. Table 8.4 summarizes the recent research work in the domain of the IoT in health and wearables.

TABLE 8.4
Integrated Summary of Recent Research Work in the Domain of the IoT in Wearables and Health Science.

Work	Objective	Methodology	Tools/Data	Contribution	Limitation
[84]	Smart health monitoring	Raspberry Pi	Raspberry Pi and GSM	The system can be used to accurately check the health status of any person	Can be improved using advanced artificial intelligence techniques
[85]	Sleep monitoring system	PCA for preprocessing, SVM for training	Data from Tactilus mattress, network of IoT devices connected by SSL	SVM gave 94.14% accuracy	Design optimization and physical monitoring problem
[86]	Healthcare communication system	ISO/IEEE 11073 and IHE PCD-01	IETF CoAP	CoAP uses fewer resources and has faster transaction rate than MQTT	Nil
[87]	Computer-aided abnormality detection for kidney	SVM with multilayer perceptron	Xilinx Kintex-7 board	FPGA-based CAD algorithm with accuracy of 98.14%	Using different ML algorithms may improve the results
[89]	To explore advantages of big data analytics in healthcare	Naïve Bayesian and J48 tree algorithm	Weka 3.8, kidney disease dataset from UCI website	Naïve Bayesian and J48 gave 95% and 100% accuracy	Other data mining algorithms may be compared on the given dataset for performance
[90]	Prediction of sleep apnea	Dual-channel portable monitor	PM and PSG	PM has specificity of 83%, while PSG has specificity of 100%	Data loss for present study from patient-related or technical failure
[93]	Smart watch–based platform for monitoring of fatigue	Cardiopulmonary care platform	PPG for heart rate	Device predicted accurate breathing cycles from PPG sensors	The device was unable to detect all the symptoms of an unhealthy fatigue

CAD, computer-aided design; *CoAP*, constrained application protocol; *IoT*, Internet of Things; *ML*, machine learning; *PSG*, polysomnograph; *SVM*, support vector machine; *UCI*, University of California at Irvine.

4.4 Opportunities for the Internet of Things in Healthcare

The healthcare industry is in a state of great anguish and the IoT has the ability to transform healthcare services in ways that cannot even be thought of. Healthcare services are costlier than ever, and with the aging of the global population, the number of diseases are on the rise. Nevertheless the evolving IoT technologies are to the rescue, as they have unparalleled benefits in this domain [94]. The IoT has countless utilizations in healthcare, from implementing smart sensors to remote or rural areas, to real-time health-monitoring systems designed for disabled persons or for outlying areas. IoT devices aid in every aspect of healthcare in providing quality services [95]. Listed below are some great applications of IoT in the health sector.

- Operation augmentation: The IoT has great applicability in surgical operations. Amalgamated with AI and machine learning, connected robotic devices have already been used for performing critical operations. It has been found that robotic surgery has refined vision and is more accurate, and such kind of surgical augmentation explores the limits of laparoscopy and operations that are slightly intrusive. Moving forward, all operational tasks can be altered into something in which interconnected devices continuously interact and describe one another's actions [96]. Linked devices and IoT applications minimize the tasks of health staffs before and after surgery. The patient's health condition can be monitored and connected to the personalized medical system and information regarding treatment and other contributing components can be assimilated before and after surgery.

- Data insights: The role of a data scientist can be tried by health professionals. Medical data are huge in size, and for collecting and analyzing data IoT applications are required for better processing. Behavioral, medical, environmental, and social data are collected for planning better health services [97]. Data are extracted using sensors and further processed by medical applications, wearable devices, and cloud solutions. Service providers can completely alter the system user have been used to utilize medical services. Data analysis has an impact on the healthcare industries, which actually analyze and process the huge medical records for effective decision-making.
- Drug management: The creation and management of medicines is a huge business and is one of the exceptional expenditures of the medical sector. IoT devices contribute to each and every aspect of the drug industry. Hospitals can implement systems that integrate effective approaches from the IoMT and other equipment linked to the IoMT platforms, which will have a positive impact on pharma inventory, reducing energy, and access to data repositories [98].
- Improved patient health: Consider the scenario in which smart wearables notify the patient of his or her heart rate, whether it is normal or not, or notify whether the patient has not been sustaining his or her good health or has been neglecting behavior in terms of his or her healthcare [78]. By upgrading the personal medical data of patients on the cloud server and then eliminating the need to input that into another device, the IoT ensures that every minute facet is taken into consideration and makes the most of the profitable and effective decisions of patients.
- Promotion of preventive care: Prevention these days is more important and is the area that needs more attention, as prevention is better than cure [99]. The universal access to real-time, high-dimensional medical data will reshape medical care units by assisting people to live healthier lives and prevent disease.
- Enhanced patient satisfaction and engagement: By streamlining operational workflow, we can enhance patient satisfaction by IoT-enabled devices for, e.g., discharge billing, and all other details that will be notified to family. It can enhance consultation of patients by allowing them to spend more time consulting with their doctors as it minimizes the requirement for direct patient–doctor interaction, since smart devices linked to the web are able to provide valuable information.
- Advanced care management: It can empower healthcare units to collect data and then correlate large numbers of data points on personal fitness from sensors, such as heart rate, pulse rate, sleep irregularity, and perspiration; sensor-fed information can provide alerts to patients and caretakers in an online monitoring system so that they receive event-triggered messages such as notification of raised heart beat, or any other abnormality.
- Advanced population health management: Advanced IoT devices empower suppliers to connect devices to supervise the growth of wearables, as the data extracted and collected by the devices will fill in the data that are, on other hand, overlooked in EMRs. Healthcare units can obtain insight-driven information and employ the IoT for real-time monitoring of persistent diseases.

4.5 Open Challenges

The IoT is widely accepted in building and creating smart models for different types of industries. But some challenges still exist that need researchers' attention [100]. Listed below are some challenges of the IoT that must be addressed while developing systems using it [101].

- Data security and privacy: Privacy and security are two of the most noteworthy warnings that the IoT produces. IoT devices extract, collect, and redirect data in real time. However, most of the IoT devices work without following any norms or protocols. In addition, the concept is still not clear with respect to data possession and its regulation. All these features make the data immensely vulnerable to cybercrime attacks, and thus present the prospect of compromising personal medical data of the patients as well as of the health experts. Cybercriminals can misuse the medical information to forge fake IDs of patients to buy medicines and other health devices that can be sold later. Hackers can easily file a fraudulent claim to the insurance companies in a patient's name.
- Integration of multiple devices and protocols: Assimilating multiple devices causes obstruction in the implementation of IoT-enabled medical devices in the healthcare sector. The main reason for this blockade is that the creators have not come to a standard point with respect to communication protocols and norms. So even if numerous devices are connected and attached; the dissimilarity in their communication protocol convolutes and acts as a barrier to the data aggregation process.

- Data overload and accuracy: Data aggregation is a tough job because of the utilization of various transmission norms and protocols. However, IoT gadgets are still able to store medical data on a large scale. Data collected by sensors or any other devices are used to gain insights within the data. The very large data size makes it difficult to gain important insights from the dataset and it can be very difficult for doctors to extract relevant patterns or information from it, which eventually influences the decision-making quality.

4.6 The Internet of Things in Sensor and Wearable Devices for Healthcare

Wearable and associated gadgets require an inordinate amount of commitment, especially for IoT-enabled medical applications. With these smart and advanced gadgets, we have continual access to relevant data rather than opting for recurring measurements of health-related data. The wearable device industry has extensively amplified over the past few years. The domain has been further split and classified into daily wear fitness and health applications [102]. These days industries are paying attention to modern gadgets that can be worn on disparate body parts. For the commoner, these electronic gadgets make daily routine activities much easier as now they get to know the human anatomy in a much easier way than going through the idioms. Wearable devices in today's era are one of the greatest effectual progressions in the technological sector because of the growth of sensor and wireless technology.

From the perspective of daily life operations, all sensors in wearable electronic devices are presumed to be adaptable to the human body as in to securely function on the body to extract relevant information. Sensors diverge from device to device [103]. A few smart sensors that are widespread in today's era and utilized in fitness and health tracker are the following.

- Gyroscope and accelerometer: These are devices used for navigation purposes and identify inclination and rotation. The gyroscope assists in estimating the angular momentum. Another electronic gadget that is generally used is the accelerometer, which records elementary human motion in all directions such as bending, inclination, and rotation of the body. For better tracking, to generate a 3D representation of human body movement, an accelerometer is often combined with a gyroscope. Fitness and daily tracking organizations uses both technologies to present 3D workout movements.
- Wearable electrodes: Wearable electrodes assist in tracking a person's heart rate in a manner such that electrodes are attached directly to body and continuously measure heart rate. The sensor typically consists of a photodiode and light-emitting diodes, both one side.
- Temperature sensor: Temperature sensors are used to measure body temperature. These sensors can be embedded in baby monitoring systems to continuously monitor the infant's temperature.
- Altimeter: An altimeter is one of the dominant sensors for wearable devices used by hikers and climbers. This electronic gadget measures the elevation while ascending. The aneroid barometer is the more advanced version of the normal barometer. A normal barometer measures pressure, while an altimeter measures elevation.
- Proximity sensor: For suggesting the proximity of an object, proximity sensors are used. The determined object differs from living objects to nonliving objects. However, when opting for a proximity sensor, it is required to know about the desired range of objects for detection and object distance. Applications include object detection, obstacle detection especially for visually impaired people, and many more.
- Biomechanical sensor: Biomechanical sensors have the capability to alter chemical elements in association with an electric signal. A biomechanical sensor employs the principle of chemical-resistive detection. Biochemical sensors are used in wearables to monitor alcohol intake in the human body and also to track daily lifestyle.

6 CONCLUSIONS

Impressive progress and great potential for application have been achieved in THz biomedical and biomolecular detection and tissue imaging, and in clinical applications. However, numerous challenges need to be addressed for widespread technological and commercially viable application in the medical sciences. THz systems are extremely costly at present, preventing usage of this technique in everyday healthcare. Also, improvement of accuracy, reproducibility of the analytical data with high and realistic real-time acquisition speed, enhanced signal-noise ratios, and portable, cost-effective, especially solid-state, higher power but safe and sophisticated systems with AI and the IoT will facilitate large-scale clinical applications of THz. Another issue is that most biological samples have water in them, with strong absorption in the THz waves, and sample pretreatments and new techniques like micro- and nanofluidics and ATR-mode THz spectroscopy can reduce the absorption loss for possible medical applications. Another complication is related to the lack of methodologies and proper computational modeling for data management and analysis and interpretation related to THz radiation for eventual application by machine learning, AI, and IoT and wearable devices in THz healthcare technologies. AI is mainly used in THz to make better decisions. From the trends of the emerging applications of the IoT and big data analytics in various fields discussed in the foregoing, it is very much evident that the future of the medical field will heavily count on the current research and methodologies developed for wide-scale application in real-life problems. However, it may be noted that even with extensive and sincere efforts in selecting the fields to discuss here, considering the massive volume of technical reports available on various technological advancements in the field, the readers are encouraged to study further and seek deeper insights into the specific fields of their interest. Currently, THz imaging has not been widely focused on due to the lack of enabling components, costly setup, and migration of software–hardware frameworks. The advanced THz technology will be a focus of mobile healthcare applications.

REFERENCES

[1] P. Martyniuk, J. Antoszewski, M. Martyniuk, L. Faraone, A. Rogalski1, New concepts in infrared photodetector designs, Applied Physics Reviews 1 (2014) 041102.

[2] R.M. Woodward, B.E. Cole, V.P. Wallace, R.J. Pye, D.D. Arnone, E.H. Linfield, M. Pepper, Terahertz pulse imaging in reflection geometry of human skin cancer and skin tissue, Physics in Medicine and Biology 47 (2002) 3853.

[3] M. Nagel, P.H. Bolivar, M. Brucherseifer, H. Kurz, A. Bosserhoff, R. Buttner, Integrated THz technology for label-free genetic diagnostics, Applied Physics Letters 80 (1) (2002) 154.

[4] N. Karpowicz, H. Zhong, C. Zhang, K.I. Lin, J.S. Hwang, J. Xu, X.C. Zhang, Compact continuous-wave subterahertz system for inspection applications, Applied Physics Letters 86 (5) (2005) 054105.

[5] K. Yamamoto, M. Yamaguchi, F. Miyamaru, M. Tani, M. Hangyo, Non-invasive inspection of c-4 explosive in mails by terahertz time-domain spectroscopy, Journal of Applied Physics 43 (3B) (2004) L414.

[6] K. Kawase, Y. Ogawa, Y. Watanabe, H. Inoue, Nondestructive terahertz imaging of illicit drugs using spectral fingerprints, Optics Express 11 (20) (2003) 2549.

[7] C. Joerdens, M. Koch, Detection of foreign bodies in chocolate with pulsed terahertz spectroscopy, Optical Engineering 47 (3) (2008) 037003.

[8] M. Tonouchi, Cutting-edge terahertz technology, Nature Photonics 1 (2007) 97.

[9] P.H. Siegel, Terahertz technology, IEEE Transactions on Microwave Theory and Techniques 50 (2002) 910.

[10] B.S. Williams, Terahertz quantum-cascade lasers, Nature Photonics 1 (2007) 517.

[11] F. Schuster, D. Coquillat, H. Videlier, M. Sakowicz, F. Teppe, L. Dussopt, B. Giffard, T. Skotnicki, W. Knap, Broadband terahertz imaging with highly sensitive silicon CMOS detectors, Optics Express 19 (2011) 7827.

[12] XinghanCai, et al., Sensitive room-temperature terahertz detection via the photothermoelectric effect in graphene, Nature Nanotechnology 9 (2014) 814.

[13] L. Liu, J.L. Hesler, H. Xu, A.W. Lichtenberger, R.M. Weikle, A broadband quasi-optical terahertz detector utilizing a zero bias Schottky diode, IEEE Microwave and Wireless Components Letters 20 (2010) 504.

[14] G.C. Trichopoulos, H.L. Mosbacker, D. Burdette, K. Sertel, A broadband focal plane array camera for real-time THz imaging applications, IEEE Transactions on Antennas and Propagation 61 (2013) 1733.

[15] C.M. Watts, D. Shrekenhamer, J. Montoya, G. Lipworth, J. Hunt, T. Sleasman, S. Krishna, D.R. Smith, W.J. Padilla, Terahertz compressive imaging with metamaterial spatial light modulators, Nature Photonics 8 (2014) 605.

[16] L. Liang, et al., Anomalous terahertz reflection and scattering by flexible and conformal coding metamaterials, Advanced Optical Materials 3 (10) (2015) 1311.

[17] D.B. But, C. Drexler, M.V. Sakhno, N. Dyakonova, O. Drachenko, F.F. Sizov, A. Gutin, S.D. Ganichev, W. Knap, Nonlinear photoresponse of field effect transistors terahertz detectors at high irradiation intensities, Journal of Applied Physics 115 (2014) 164514.

[18] X. Yang, A. Vorobiev, A. Generalov, M.A. Andersson, J. Stake, A flexible graphene terahertz detector", Journal of Applied Physics 111 (2017) 021102.

[19] X. Huang, T. Leng, M. Zhu, X. Zhang, J. Chen, K. Chang, M. Aqeeli, A.K. Geim, K.S. Novoselov, Z. Hu, Highly flexible and conductive printed graphene for wireless wearable communications applications, Scientific Reports 5 (2014) 18298.

[20] J. Noh, M. Jung, Y. Jung, C. Yeom, M. Pyo, G. Cho, Key issues with printed flexible thin film transistors and their application in disposable RF sensors, Proceedings of the IEEE 103 (2015) 554.

[21] T. Andy, Terahertz (THz) Technology Market Increasing Exigency with Top Key Players: Brainware Terahertz Information, Advantest Corporation, Hübner, 2019. Available from: https://newsexterior.com/terahertz-thz-technology-market-increasing-exigency-with-top-key-players-brainware-terahertz-information-advantest-corporation-hubner/17264/.

[22] A. Heidari, Terahertz technology in the future of health and medical applications, Springer Series in Bio-/Neuro-informatics 5 (2015) 663–670, https://doi.org/10.1007/978-3-319-12817-7_28.

[23] J.M. Jornet, I.F. Akyildiz, The Internet of multimedia nano-things in the Terahertz band, European Wireless (2012) 1–8, 978-3-8008-3426-9.

[24] M.J. Josep, F.A. Ian, The internet of multimedia nano-things in the terahertz band, European Wireless (2012) 18–20. https://bwn.ece.gatech.edu/papers/2012/c4.pdf.

[25] P. Giuseppe, Y. Ke, B. Gennaro, C. Nishtha, A.G. Luigi, A. Akram, Terahertz communications in human tissues at the nanoscale for healthcare applications, IEEE Transactions On Nanotechnology, Research Letters 14 (3) (2015) 1–3.

[26] H. Elayan, O. Amin, R.M. Shubair, M.-S. Alouini, Terahertz communication: the opportunities of wireless technology beyond 5G, in: 2018 International Conference on Advanced Communication Technologies and Networking (CommNet), 2018, Available from: https://doi.org/10.1109/commnet.2018.8360286.

[27] E. Hadeel, M.S. Raed, M.J. Josep, J. Pedram, Terahertz channel model and link budget analysis for intrabody nanoscale communication, IEEE Transactions on Nano-Bioscience 16 (6) (2017) 491–503.

[28] C. Hwayeong, Y. Hee-jin, H.L. Sang, A.K. Young, S. Joo-Hiuk, Terahertz molecular resonance of cancer DNA, Scientific Reports 6 (2016) 37103. https://www.nature.com/articles/srep37103.

[29] M.S. Eva, B. Yannick, J. Eric, H. Andreas, C.B. Jan, K. Martin, Robotic-based THz imaging system for free-form surfaces, in: IEEE, 42nd International Conference on Infrared, Millimeter, and Terahertz Waves (IRMMW-THz), 2017.

[30] S. Andreas, A.T. Michael, Nanotechnology-supported THz medical imaging, F1000Research (2013) 1–14.

[31] K. Sigfrid, Yngvessona, S.P. Benjamin, S. Paul, K. Patrick, G. Stephen, K. Andrew, K. Ashraf, Feasibility demonstration of frequency domain terahertz imaging in breast cancer margin determination, Proceedings of SPIE-The International Society for Optical Engineering 8221 (2012) 82210, https://doi.org/10.1117/12.907075.

[32] Z. Jinsong, X. Wenjie, X. Mengdao, S. Guangcai, Terahertz image detection with the improved faster region-based convolutional neural network, Sensors (2018) 1–19.

[33] X. Yang, X. Zhao, K. Yang, Y. Liu, Y. Liu, W. Fu, Y. Luo, Biomedical applications of terahertz spectroscopy and imaging, Trends in Biotechnology 34 (10) (2016) 810–824.

[34] Y.C. Sim, et al., Terahertz imaging of excised oral cancer at frozen temperature, Biomedical Optics Express 4 (2013) 1413–1421.

[35] F. Wahaia, et al., Terahertz absorption and reflection imaging of carcinoma-affected colon tissues embedded in paraffin, Journal of Molecular Structure 1107 (2016) 214–219.

[36] P. Doradla, et al., Single-channel prototype terahertz endoscopic system, Journal of Biomedical Optics 19 (2014) 080501.

[37] H. Chen, et al., Diagnose human colonic tissues by terahertz near-field imaging, Journal of Biomedical Optics 20 (2015) 036017.

[38] P. Doradla, et al., Detection of colon cancer by continuous-wave terahertz polarization imaging technique, Journal of Biomedical Optics 18 (2013) 090504.

[39] C.B. Reid, et al., Terahertz pulsed imaging of freshly excised human colonic tissues, Physics in Medicine and Biology 56 (2011) 4333–4353.

[40] Y. Bin Ji, et al., Feasibility of terahertz reflectometry for discrimination of human early gastric cancers, Biomedical Optics Express 6 (2015) 1398–1406.

[41] H. Chen, et al., The diagnosis of human liver cancer by using THz fiber-scanning near-field imaging, Chinese Physics Letters 30 (2013) 030702.

[42] L. Rong, et al., Terahertz in-line digital holography of human hepatocellular carcinoma tissue, Scientific Reports 5 (2015) 8445.

[43] M.A. Brun, et al., Terahertz imaging applied to cancer diagnosis, Physics in Medicine and Biology 55 (2010) 4615–4623.

[44] C.S. Joseph, et al., Imaging of ex vivo nonmelanoma skin cancers in the optical and terahertz spectral regions, Journal of Biophotonics 7 (2014) 295–303.

[45] C.S. Joseph, et al., Continuous wave terahertz transmission imaging of nonmelanoma skin cancers, Lasers in Surgery and Medicine 43 (2011) 457–462.

[46] T.C. Bowman, et al., Terahertz imaging of excised breast tumor tissue on paraffin sections, IEEE Transactions on Antennas and Propagation 63 (2015) 2088–2097.

[47] H. Chen, et al., Performance of THz fiber-scanning near-field microscopy to diagnose breast tumors, Optics Express 19 (2011) 19523–19531.

[48] B.S. Peter, et al., Development and testing of a single frequency terahertz imaging system for breast cancer detection, IEEE Transactions on Terahertz Science and Technology 3 (2013) 374–386.

[49] E. Jung, et al., Terahertz pulse imaging of micro-metastatic lymph nodes in early-stage cervical cancer patients, Journal of the Optical Society of Korea 15 (2011) 155–160.

[50] M. Bessou, et al., Three-dimensional terahertz computed tomography of human bones, Applied Optics 51 (2012) 6738–6744.

[51] Y.L. Lim, et al., High-contrast coherent terahertz imaging of porcine tissue via swept-frequency feedback interferometry, Biomedical Optics Express 5 (2014) 3981–3989.

[52] D.B. Bennett, et al., Terahertz sensing in corneal tissues, Journal of Biomedical Optics 16 (2011) 057003.

[53] Y.B. Ji, et al., Terahertz spectroscopic imaging and properties of gastrointestinal tract in a rat model, Biomedical Optics Express 5 (2014) 4162–4170.

[54] H. Chen, et al., High-sensitivity in vivo THz transmission imaging of early human breast cancer in a subcutaneous xenograft mouse model, Optics Express 19 (2011) 21552–21562.

[55] S.J. Oh, et al., Study of freshly excised brain tissues using terahertz imaging Biomed, Optics Express 5 (2014) 2837–2842.

[56] S. Sy, et al., Terahertz spectroscopy of liver cirrhosis: investigating the origin of contrast, Physics in Medicine and Biology 55 (2010) 7587–7596.

[57] P. Tewari, et al., In vivo terahertz imaging of rat skin burns, Journal of Biomedical Optics 17 (2012) 040503.

[58] T.-F. Tseng, et al., Near-field sub-THz transmission-type image system for vessel imaging in-vivo, Optics Express 23 (2015) 25058–25071.

[59] W.-C. Kan, et al., Terahertz pulsed imaging of knee cartilage, Biomedical Optics Express 1 (2010) 967–974.

[60] Z.D. Taylor, et al., THz and mm-wave sensing of corneal tissue water content: in vivo sensing and imaging results, IEEE Transactions on Terahertz Science and Technology 5 (2015) 184–196.

[61] C. Chinmay, B. Gupta, S.K. Ghosh, A review on telemedicine-based WBAN framework for patient monitoring, International Journal of Telemedicine and e-Health, Mary Ann Libert Inc. 19 (8) (2013) 619–626.

[62] I.E.O. Lars, V.R. Mary, W. Matthew, N. Daniel, A robotic home telehealth platform system for treatment adherence, social assistance and companionship – an overview, in: 31st Annual International Conference of the IEEE EMBS Minneapolis, Minnesota, 2009, pp. 6437–6440.

[63] S. Anett, W. Hendrik, S. Sirko, A.K. Elsa, Online movement prediction in a robotic application scenario, in: 6th Annual International IEEE EMBS Conference on Neural Engineering, 2013, pp. 41–44.

[64] J.C. Yepes, J.J. Yepes, V.J. Pérez, M.J. Betancur, J.R. Martínez, Asimov: Android based Mobile assistant for Robotic Teleoperation, PAN American health care exchanges (pahce), in: Conference, Workshops, and Exhibits. Cooperation/Linkages, 2015, pp. 1–6.

[65] H. Ashrafian, O. Clancy, V. Grover, A. Darzi, The evolution of robotic surgery: surgical and anesthetic aspects, British Journal of Anaesthesia 119 (S1) (2017) i72–i84.

[66] N. Ayush, N.K. Narula, K. Satyam, N. Ruchi, N. Jyoti, N. Arpi, Future prospects of artificial intelligence in robotics software, a healthcare perspective, International Journal of Applied Engineering Research 9 (22) (2014) 10271–10280.

[67] B. Amit, C. Chinmay, K. Anand, B. Debabrata, Emerging trends in IoT and big data analytics for biomedical and health care technologies, in: Elsevier: Handbook of Data Science Approaches for Biomedical Engineering, 2019, pp. 1–35, 9780128183182 (Chapter 5).

[68] T. Kush, Telemedicine and its Applications, 2018. Available from: http://www.authorstream.com/Presentation/kush20006-813622-telemedicine-its-applications/ (Accessed August).

[69] O. Vermesan, A. Bröring, E. Tragos, M. Serrano, D. Bacciu, S. Chessa, C. Gal-licchio, A. Micheli, M. Dragone, A. Saffiotti, P. Simoens, F. Cavallo, R. Bahr, Internet of robotic things: converging sensing/actuating, hypoconnectivity, artificial intelligence and IoT platforms, in: Cognitive Hyperconnected Digital Trans-formation: Internet of Things Intelligence Evolution, 2017, pp. 1–60.

[70] M. Chen, Y. Ma, Y. Hao, Y. Li, W. Di, Z. Yin, E. Song, Cp-robot: cloud-assisted pillow robot for emotion sensing and interaction, in: J. Wan, I. Humar, D. Zhang (Eds.), International Conference on Industrial IoT Technologies and Applications, Springer, Cham, 2016, pp. 81–93.

[71] S. Qiushuo, H. Yuezhi, L. Kai, F. Shuting, P.J.P. Edward, P.M. Emma, Recent advances in terahertz technology for biomedical applications, Quantitative Imaging in Medicine and Surgery 7 (3) (2017) 345–355.

[72] K. Ashton, That 'internet of things' thing, RFID Journal 22 (7) (2009) 97–114.

[73] L. Atzori, A. Iera, G. Morabito, The internet of things: a survey, Computer Networks 54 (15) (2010) 2787–2805.

[74] J. Gubbi, R. Buyya, S. Marusic, M. Palaniswami, Internet of Things (IoT): a vision, architectural elements, and future directions", Future Generation Computer Systems 29 (7) (2013) 1645–1660.

[75] L. Tan, N. Wang, Future internet: the internet of things, in: 2010 3rd International Conference on Advanced Computer Theory and Engineering (ICACTE), vol. 5, IEEE, Chengdu, China, 2010, p. 376.

[76] S. Tyagi, A. Agarwal, P. Maheshwari, A conceptual framework for IoT-based healthcare system using cloud computing, in: 2016 6th International Conference-Cloud System and Big Data Engineering (Confluence), IEEE, Noida, India, 2016, pp. 503–507.

[77] L. Catarinucci, D. De Donno, L. Mainetti, L. Palano, L. Patrono, M.L. Stefanizzi, L. Tarricone, An IoT-aware architecture for smart healthcare systems, IEEE Internet of Things Journal 2 (6) (2015) 515–526.

[78] B.M. Lee, J. Ouyang, Intelligent healthcare service by using collaborations between IoT personal health devices, International Journal of Bio-Science and Bio-Technology 6 (1) (2014) 155–164.

[79] N. Bui, M. Zorzi, Health care applications: a solution based on the internet of things, in: Proceedings of the 4th International Symposium on Applied Sciences in Biomedical and Communication Technologies, ACM, Barcelona, Spain, 2011, p. 131.

[80] D.V. Dimitrov, Medical internet of things and big data in healthcare, Healthcare Informatics Research 22 (3) (2016) 156–163.

[81] V. Sivaraman, H.H. Gharakheili, A. Vishwanath, R. Boreli, O. Mehani, Network-level security and privacy control for smart-home IoT devices, in: 2015 IEEE 11th International Conference on Wireless and Mobile Computing, Networking and Communications (WiMob), IEEE, Rome, Italy, 2015, pp. 163–167.

[82] P. Gope, T. Hwang, BSN-Care: a secure IoT-based modern healthcare system using body sensor network, IEEE Sensors Journal 16 (5) (2016) 1368–1376.

[83] C. Bhatt, N. Dey, A.S. Ashour (Eds.), Internet of Things and Big Data Technologies for Next Generation Healthcare, 2017.

[84] S. Banka, I. Madan, S.S. Saranya, Smart healthcare monitoring using IoT", International Journal of Applied Engineering Research 13 (15) (2018) 11984–11989.

[85] G. Matar, J.M. Lina, J. Carrier, A. Riley, G. Kaddoum, Internet of Things in sleep monitoring: an application for posture recognition using supervised learning, in: IEEE 18th International Conference on e-Health Networking, Applications and Services (Healthcom), IEEE, Munich, Germany, 2016, pp. 1–6.

[86] W. Li, C. Jung, J. Park, IoT healthcare communication system for IEEE 11073 PHD and IHE PCD-01 integration using CoAP, KSII Transactions on Internet & Information Systems 12 (4) (2018).

[87] K.D. Krishna, V. Akkala, R. Bharath, P. Rajalakshmi, A.M. Mohammed, FPGA based preliminary CAD for kidney on IoT enabled portable ultrasound imaging system, in: IEEE 16th International Conference on e-Health Networking, Applications and Services (Healthcom), IEEE, Bogotá, Colombia, 2014, pp. 257–261.

[88] K.S. Kumar, K. Bairavi, IoT based health monitoring system for autistic patients, in: Proceedings of the 3rdInternational Symposium on Big Data and Cloud Computing Challenges (ISBCC–16′), Springer, Cham, 2016, pp. 371–376.

[89] S. Al Mayahi, A. Al-Badi, A. Tarhini, Exploring the potential benefits of big data analytics in providing smart healthcare, in: International Conference for Emerging Technologies in Computing, Springer, Cham, Jaipur, 2018, pp. 247–258.

[90] L. Simpson, S. Mukherjee, M.N. Cooper, K.L. Ward, J.D. Lee, A.C. Fedson, J. Kirkness, Sex differences in the association of regional fat distribution with the severity of obstructive sleep apnea, Sleep 33 (4) (2010) 467–474.

[91] G.J. Joyia, R.M. Liaqat, A. Farooq, S. Rehman, Internet of Medical Things (IOMT): applications, benefits and future challenges in healthcare domain, Journal of Communication 12 (4) (2017) 240–247.

[92] V. Chandel, A. Sinharay, N. Ahmed, A. Ghose, Exploiting IMU sensors for IoT enabled health monitoring, in: Proceedings of the First Workshop on IoT-enabled Healthcare and Wellness Technologies and Systems, ACM, Singapore, 2016, pp. 21–22.

[93] S. Choudhary, H. Arbat, U. Patkar, An innovative study on artificial intelligence and robotics", International Journal of Innovative Research in Computer and Communication Engineering (2016) 2320–9801.

[94] F. Fernandez, G.C. Pallis, Opportunities and challenges of the Internet of Things for healthcare: systems engineering perspective, in: 4th International Conference on Wireless Mobile Communication and Healthcare-Transforming Healthcare through Innovations in Mobile and Wireless Technologies (MOBIHEALTH), IEEE, Athens, Greece, 2014, pp. 263–266.

[95] M. Elhoseny, G. Ramírez-González, O.M. Abu-Elnasr, S.A. Shawkat, N. Arunkumar, A. Farouk, Secure medical data transmission model for IoT-based healthcare systems, IEEE Access 6 (2018) 20596–20608.

[96] S.I. Lakkis, M. Elshakankiri, IoT based emergency and operational services in medical care systems, in: 2017 Internet of Things Business Models, Users, and Networks, IEEE, 2017, pp. 1–5.

[97] M. Marjani, F. Nasaruddin, A. Gani, A. Karim, I.A.T. Hashem, A. Siddiqa, I. Yaqoob, Big IoT data analytics: architecture, opportunities, and open research challenges, IEEE Access 5 (2017) 5247–5261.

[98] A. Ukil, S. Bandyoapdhyay, C. Puri, A. Pal, IoT healthcare analytics: the importance of anomaly detection, in: 30th IEEE International Conference on Advanced Information Networking and Applications (AINA), IEEE, Matsue, Japan, 2016, pp. 994–997.

[99] I. Chiuchisan, H.N. Costin, O. Geman, Adopting the internet of things technologies in health care systems, in: International Conference and Exposition on Electrical and Power Engineering (EPE), IEEE, Romania, 2014, pp. 532–535.

[100] Z.K. Zhang, M.C.Y. Cho, C.W. Wang, C.W. Hsu, C.K. Chen, S. Shieh, IoT security: ongoing challenges and research opportunities, in: IEEE 7th International Conference on Service-Oriented Computing and Applications, IEEE, Stockholm, Sweden, 2014, pp. 230–234.

[101] B. Farahani, F. Firouzi, V. Chang, M. Badaroglu, N. Constant, K. Mankodiya, Towards fog-driven IoT eHealth: promises and challenges of IoT in medicine and healthcare, Future Generation Computer Systems 78 (2018) 659–676.

[102] P. Woznowski, D. Kaleshi, G. Oikonomou, I. Craddock, Classification and suitability of sensing technologies for activity recognition, Computer Communications 89 (2016) 34–50.

[103] M. Manas, A. Sinha, S. Sharma, M.R. Mahboob, A novel approach for IoT based wearable health monitoring and messaging system, Journal of Ambient Intelligence and Humanized Computing (2018) 1–12.

CHAPTER 9

A Survey on Machine Learning Techniques for THz Image Analysis

BASABI CHAKRABORTY, PHD • RIKTA SEN • ASHIS KUMAR MANDAL

INTRODUCTION

Terahertz (THz) radiation (often called T-rays) refers to the part of the electromagnetic spectrum lying between infrared and microwave region (100 GHz–10 THz), and this is an area of convergence between the electronics field and the photonics field in the electromagnetic spectrum [1]. As a low energy nonionizing radiation, it has minimal effect on the human body compared to X-rays or gamma rays. Among other characteristics of THz radiation, its high penetration ability through various dielectrics, sensitivity to water content, high reflection by metals, and good tissue differentiation capabilities prompted THz imaging an important modality for many applications in various areas.

THz imaging is now an emerging technology in the area of biological and medical applications, including cancer diagnosis. It can effectively detect the margin of the cancerous cell because THz radiation is very absorptive to water content. THz imaging can be used as an alternative to other diagnostic technologies for imaging the structure of teeth and the identification of dental caries [2]. Another application is wound assessment ranging from the severity of burns to cuts because THz images of the skin can be taken through wound dressings [1].

In the area of security and defense research applications, the possibility of acquiring THz images of concealed objects under clothing has great potential of detecting concealed weapons. THz radiation is readily transmitted through most nonmetallic and nonpolar mediums, thus enabling THz images of finding potentially dangerous materials inside packaging, corrugated cardboard, clothing, shoes, and book bags. Many materials of interest for security applications, including explosives, chemical agents, and biological agents, have characteristic THz image that can be used to identify them [3].

Another important application of THz images is in the area of agriculture and food industry. High water absorption capability of THz radiation enables plant scientist to inspect water content in vegetative tissues [4]. THz technology plays an important role in the food industry, including food inspection, crop inspection, material characterization, etc. Cui et al. reported that THz time-domain spectroscopy (THz-TDS) could be used to detect melamine in milk powders.

As THz imaging systems and techniques are recently being developed, methodologies for their analysis have gradually become important. Although THz radiation has several advantages over X-rays, especially noninvasive and less hazardous to human health, resolution of THz image is lower compared with X-ray images. Sophisticated techniques are needed for their correct analysis. Several techniques based on machine learning tools have been proposed so far. In the following sections, a survey of recently developed various categories of machine learning approaches for object detection and classification in THz images has been described followed by the tabular summarization and conclusion in the final section.

SUPERVISED APPROACHES FOR THZ IMAGE ANALYSIS

Machine learning approaches that have been developed and used so far for analysis, detection, and classification of THz images in different applications can be broadly divided into three groups: supervised approaches, unsupervised approaches, and other approaches that may be a combination of two or more different techniques. In this section, several research works on supervised approaches for THz image analysis have been presented.

Support Vector Machine–Based Approach

Support vector machine (SVM) is a popular and efficient machine learning technique for supervised

Terahertz Biomedical and Healthcare Technologies. https://doi.org/10.1016/B978-0-12-818556-8.00009-4

classification of high-dimensional data into different classes. There are various research works on THz image classification using SVM classifier. In Ref. [5], SVM is used on THz spectral data for differentiating between normal and cancerous tissue. Data are collected from both normal bone tissue cells and osteosarcoma cells using a THz-TDS imaging system. Finite impulse response filter preprocesses the input data, and SVM classifies the normal and cancerous cells within the image. Kernel function, such as radial basis function (RBF), allows SVM to perform separations even in the presence of complex boundaries. They obtained an accuracy of 70.2%, which is substantially better compared to visual screening. Classification system based on SVM in THz (T-ray)-pulsed classification for two datasets, including RNA samples and powder samples, is presented in Ref. [6]. The former dataset is used to classify two classes of objects and the latter is to separate six various types of powdered materials. SVM with Gaussian and polynomial kernels are applied for two-class and multiclass classification, respectively, and high classification accuracy is achieved.

In Ref. [7], SVM is used along with data reduction technique on THz imaging of cancer tissues to separate tumor and normal breast tissue, and 92% accuracy is achieved. Two different approaches are used for dimensionality reduction, popular principal component analysis (PCA) and a heuristic method based on characteristics of the THz pulse in the time and frequency domains. In Ref. [8], an approach in which four wood species are identified using THz-TDS is described. For effective classification, they used PCA for reducing the dimensions of the THz absorption spectrum followed by SVM as a classification model. A new method is proposed in Ref. [9] for the classification of a sand grain. This method combines THz-TDS with chemometrics in which THz spectra of sand samples are analyzed using PCA, partial least squares discriminant analysis (PLS-DA), and SVM-based classification models, with SVM providing the best classification results.

K-nearest Neighbor–Based Algorithms

K-nearest neighbor (KNN) is a simple classification algorithm that does not need any prior assumption. Based on the similarity measure and sample of the training instances for different classes, this algorithm places the new sample into an appropriate class. In Ref. [10], an algorithm is proposed for detecting and classifying breast cancer cells from THz images. THz images are preprocessed using texture features (gray level co-occurrence matrix GLCM) and invariant moment algorithm. Both KNN and artificial neural network (ANN) are used for classification of the normal and the abnormal breast tissues. The results are promising in which ANN performs slightly better than KNN, with accuracy being 98.2% and 96.4%, respectively. Moreover, the processing time was comparatively very fast.

Mahalanobis Distance–Based Approach

Mahalanobis distance (MD) is defined as the distance from a given point to the mean value for a certain class normalized by the variance of the training vectors in that direction. In Ref. [11], the authors explored the identification and classification of the spectroscopic imaging data using MD and compared the results with ANN. Reflective spectroscopic focal-plane imaging of four explosive and biochemical materials at a standoff imaging distance is used as imaging data. The rate of accuracy is observed above 80%, with the accuracy of the MD classifier being slightly higher than that of the neural network. In Ref. [12], authors have used THz pulsed data for biomaterial classification. The biomaterial data are collected from paper, bacterial spores, soda, salt, flour, and Chinese seasoning. This paper also used MD for classification. Before classification, different types of feature extraction methods, such as peak, ARX coefficient, wavelet transform, fast Fourier transform, and Fourier phase, are used. Among these methods, wavelet transform produced the best accuracy of over 99%.

Artificial Neural Network– and Deep Neural networkBased Approach

ANN is a popular approach that is substantially used for THz image classification. With the complex mathematical formulations, ANN maps inputs to outputs. One major advantage of ANN is that, unlike other statistical methods, it does not assume any a priori knowledge. In Ref. [13], ANN is used successfully to separate images of hidden lethal materials and bioagents from images of nonlethal backgrounds. Image dataset, that is, images of an envelope containing a bioagent and a suicide bomber, is generated using simulated multiple frequency (spectral) interferometric imaging. Both multilayer perceptron (MLP) and RBF neural network architectures are used to analyze these THz spectral images. Results suggest that RBF networks are generally more accurate than MLP networks in this classification-type problem. For monitoring and detection of different lethal agents, authors in Ref. [14] proposed a novel screening method where MLP model and Kohonen self-organizing map (KSOM) were studied for identifying the lethal agents in the reconstructed interferometric images. KSOM successfully separated the three classes that are present in the data into three distinct clusters.

Recently, another type of ANN known as a deep neural network, especially convolutional neural network (CNN), has become effective in THz image analysis. For detection of hazardous materials in THz security images, authors in Ref. [15] used the CNN model in the narrow-band domain so that there exists favorable detection and faster recognition process with less false-positive results. In Ref. [16], CNN is used as a model for detecting hidden lethal equipment in both THz images and natural light images. Two-stage deep learning classifiers based on GoogLeNet CNN model have been built here, where the first stage detects in natural light and the second stage detects hidden objects in THz images.

The authors proposed CNN model in Ref. [16], which can identify hazardous possessions in human THz images. Mean filter is used to denoise the THz image due to low signal-to-noise ratio and then faster region-based convolutional neural network (faster R-CNN) was introduced for identification of dangerous goods. The overall recognition rate was better compared with the SVM based approach. In Ref. [17], authors proposed an improved faster R-CNN method based on threshold segmentation for security screening with THz images. This method detects the human body and other objects separately with high speed and high accuracy.

In Ref. [18], a novel Conditional Generative Adversarial Nets (CGANs), named as Mask-CGANs, is proposed to segment weapons using very–poor-quality THz images having a small training dataset.

Extreme Learning MachineBased Approach

Extreme learning machine is a single hidden layer feedforward neural network–based model in which hidden layers are generated irrespective of training data.

In Ref. [19], complex extreme learning machine (CELM) classifier is used on THz pulse transient signals. CELM is designed to address complex value problems for multiclass classification, and in this case, it considers features both from the amplitude and the phase of the recorded spectra. For the experiment, they use RNA samples and powder samples that are binary-class and multiclass datasets, respectively. Compared with the SVM method, CELM exhibits better performance in classifying the samples and generates the results much faster. Authors state that the proposed model has better scalability for very large datasets. In Ref. [20], authors of Ref. [13] also extended their previous research and used CELM classification scheme to solve a multiclass classification problem of THz spectral of six powdered samples. During the training phase of the CELM, they employed the Karush–Kuhn–Tucker theorem to solve the dual optimization problem. The experimental study revealed that during the classification task, CELM is 100 times faster than its SVM counterpart and retains similar classification accuracy.

UNSUPERVISED APPROACHES FOR THZ IMAGE ANALYSIS

Unlike supervised approaches, unsupervised classification approaches do not use the training samples for training of the classifier. In this subsection, THz image classification with unsupervised machine learning approaches is presented.

K-Means Clustering

This is a popular unsupervised classifier for image clustering due to its simplicity and suitability for large datasets. It is a partitional clustering algorithm that continuously categorizes each sample to the nearby cluster until the variation between the cluster mean vectors is small. The iterative procedure starts from an arbitrary assigned initial cluster vector. This approach was first employed in THz image classification by the authors of Ref. [21]. In Ref. [22], authors proposed a novel approach called ranked K-means for segmentation of THz images. The main merit of ranked K-means is that it is less sensitive to the initialization of the cluster centers. They describe the ranked set sampling design and reformulate K-means and tested on several THz images. The performance of ranked K-means exceeds standard K-means, K-means based on SRS sample, and Bradley refinement K-means. For THz image segmentation, Ref. [23] also proposed the integration of simple random sampling and feature weighting method into a K-means algorithm. Feature weighting is used for reducing the feature number so that the clustering accuracy and the computational time can be improved.

In Ref. [24], authors developed a two-stage segmentation strategy for detecting concealed objects from THz images. In the first stage, rough segmentation is accomplished using K-means and region analysis, whereas the active shape model is introduced in the fine segmentation stage. Factor analysis (FA) along with K-means clustering is used for identification and classification of molecules from THz absorption spectrum of the molecules, and better accuracy is obtained than classification based on molecular formulas that are reported in Ref. [25].

Agglomerative Hierarchical Clustering

This is a hierarchical clustering process that does not require an initial parameter like K-means clustering. Although slower than partitional clustering, hierarchical clustering provides more information about clustered groups. Agglomerative clustering starts with each sample as a different cluster, and in each iteration, the closest clusters are united.

In Ref. [26], authors analyzed the THz spectroscopic images that are applied to the diagnosis of the four tumor samples. To extract the cancer information systematically out of the huge amount of multidimensional spectra, initially, PCA has been applied to the observed data. After that, agglomerative hierarchical (AH) clustering and nonhierarchical cluster k-means have been employed. Various AH methods, such as average linkage, centroid linkage, complete linkage, median linkage, and Ward's linkage, are used. Ward's linkage with the square of Pearson's distance shows the best agreement. Another work of AH clustering on THz data identification is proposed by authors in Ref. [27]. To enhance the clustering results, they used preprocessing steps such as windowing in the time domain, filtering out frequencies with a low spectral density, and smoothing in the spectral domain. In order to find the cancer information from the THz spectroscopic images, authors of Ref. [28] also used PCA with AH.

Self-Organizing Map

Unlike MLP, self-organizing map (SOM) does not require training, and it maps higher dimensional data space to lower dimensional subspace, usually form a two-dimensional lattice, and preserves the property of topology. It also works as a powerful tool for identifying THz images. In Ref. [3], authors used SOM to classify THz interferometric images and found it a promising tool for differentiation of C4 explosive metal and semi-transparent barrier materials.

OTHER OR COMBINED APPROACHES

In this section, we basically focus on papers that propose THz image identification using more than one machine learning approaches.

In Ref. [29], a machine learning model is represented for recognition of traumatic brain injury (TBI) from THz images. They proposed a feature extraction method that generates new feature vectors combining the transmittance distribution features in the spatial domain and statistical distribution features in the normalized gray histogram. Three classifiers, including KNN, SVM, and random forest (RF), are applied on TBI datasets with selected features. Among those algorithms, RF exhibits better accuracy and has a lower missed diagnosis rate.

In Ref. [30], authors proposed a classification strategy of formalin-fixed, paraffin-embedded and fresh murine breast tumors from THz images. They used the Bayesian mixture model utilizing a Markov chain Monte Carlo scheme for classifying the tissues, and their experimental outcomes were highly correlated with pathology results in all samples of tissues.

To discriminate genetically modified (GM) and non-GM food, in Ref. [31], the authors analyzed THz spectroscopy images. Eighty-four sugar beet samples were used for experiments, and discriminant analysis (DA) based on PCA discriminates the samples into two classes with the accuracy of 95.8%. In Ref. [32], authors used THz spectroscopic images to locate metal contaminations in sausages. Contaminates are detected using spectral comparison, spectral classification, and one-dimensional scanning spectral analysis. PCA with DA classifier is able to detect metal component in sausages with an accuracy of nearly 100%.

In Ref. [33], hybrid strategies for detecting GM material from THz image samples are presented. The classification model is generated by combining adaptive affine clustering algorithm with SVM. Although appropriate clustering center and the class representative points influence the performance of the model, the proposed approach presents less misjudgment and higher recognition rate compared with other SVM models.

In Ref. [34], THz spectroscopy system is used with different classification models for discrimination of geographical origin of extra virgin olive oils. THz spectroscopy system was examined using least squares support vector machines (LS-SVM), back-propagation neural network (BPNN), RF combined with PCA, and genetic algorithm (GA). The results demonstrated that the maximum accuracy of 96.25% was achieved using the LS-SVM method combined with GA.

To discriminate benign from malignant breast tissue, authors in Ref. [35] collected breast cancer samples from a terahertz pulsed imaging (TPI) handheld probe system, and then image pixels on TPI were classified using two approaches: heuristic parameters in combination with SVM and Gaussian wavelet deconvolution in combination with Bayesian classification individually.

In Ref. [36], a three-step strategy is proposed when dealing with a hidden object in human THz image. Initially, they enhanced THz image using smoothing followed with the gray stretch algorithm. Next, a morphological classification algorithm is used to classify a THz image. Bilateral Contour Tracking

Comparison algorithm is finally used to extract the human body shape.

In Ref. [37], a mechanism to identify GM cotton seeds by combining adaptive dynamic particle swarm optimization SVM (ADPSO-SVM) is proposed for THz spectroscopy. Here, ADPSO is applied to collect information, and SVM is finally used as the classification model. ADPSO-SVM exhibits an accurate, fast, and simple approach to detect transgenic seeds. In their previous study, they used an adaptive decision support vector machine as a classifier for detecting GM cotton seeds [38]. Prior to feeding into the mode, FA is applied to reduce the dimension, and PSO is applied to select feature spectra data. Discrimination of different transgenic cotton seed is also proposed in Ref. [39] by using GA-SVM. PCA is applied to extract relevant features, and GA is applied to select the appropriate feature spectrum. Finally, SVM is used to classify the THz image samples.

To distinguish transgenic rice seeds from nontransgenic rice seeds, authors in Ref. [40] used THz spectroscopy images and classified them based on genotype. They build the classification models using several methods such as PCA, LS-SVM, BPNN, and RF. Similarly in their another study [41], THz spectroscopy images are used for GM organisms of soybean seeds, and above classification models except RF have been used for classification.

In Ref. [42], a tool for detecting wheat grains at different stages of germination using THz image and chemometrics has been developed. THz image of wheat grains was segmented, and features were extracted using PCA; partial least squares regression (PLSR), LS-SVM, and BPNN models are used for classification. Experimental results reveal that the LS-SVM model produced the best discrimination result among the three models, whereas the BPNN model yielded the worst result.

In Ref. [43], a comparative study of four different machine learning algorithm is performed for the classification of images of different THz powder samples obtained using a THz transient spectrometer. They used 2D cross correlation as a feature extraction process prior to the classification task. Multinomial logistic regression (MLR) with ridge estimator classifier, KNN, SVM, and naïve Bayes (NB) are used for classification task. Results confirm that, for most of the datasets, MLR and KNN outperformed SVM and NB.

In Ref. [44], THz images are used for rapid and accurate detection of cervical cancer. Different preprocessing methods such as multiplicative scatter correction, Savitzky–Golay (SG) smoothing and first derivative, principal component orthogonal signal correction (PC-OSC), and emphatic orthogonal signal correction were used for SVM and PLS-DA classification models. SG first derivative and PC-OSC resulted in the best predictive results.

In Ref. [45], affinity propagation clustering algorithm combined with SVM is proposed for identification of THz spectral images of GM cotton samples in which recognition rate of 97.794% is obtained. For discrimination of normal and abnormal tissue samples in colon cancer, THz imaging of the colon tissue is intelligently analyzed by authors in Ref. [46]. Decision tree is used to select the important parameters, and SVM and ANN were used to THz image classification. They observed that linear SVM classifier after using decision tree for reducing features produced the best classification results.

In the paper of Ref. [47], authors proposed an algorithm for segmentation of THz digital holographic images based on the region growth for reducing the boundary blurring problem. In this method, the original image is bilaterally filtered and the morphological erosion operation is carried out to obtain the seeds of region growing followed by GA to optimize threshold for restricting region growth; average structural similarity (MSSIM) is used as an objective function for evaluation of the effectiveness of the proposed algorithm.

Authors in Ref. [48] proposed the component spatial pattern analysis for detecting the illicit drugs hidden in mail envelopes. The spatial distribution of the drugs inside the envelope was extracted from the multispectral images using the absorption spectra. In Ref. [49], four different varieties of Chinese green tea are classified using LS-SVM, NB, and backpropagation artificial neural network (BP-ANN) classifiers. The classification results indicate that the LS-SVM outperforms the NB and BP-ANN significantly for limited training samples.

In Ref. [50], a novel method has been developed for discriminating moldy wheat from THz images. PCA was used for clustering the spectral data, and for classifying the moldy wheat, SVM, a PLSR analysis, and the BP-ANN methods were also used. Among them, PCA-SVM method achieved the highest accuracy for identifying the moldy wheat.

SUMMARY

The various machine learning approaches developed for THz image classification are described in earlier sections. The information regarding different research works is summarized in Table 9.1.

TABLE 9.1
Summary of Some Related Works on THz Image Analysis Using Machine Learning Approach.

Reference	Methods	Application; Remark
Sinyukov et al. [3]	Artificial neural network (ANN) and Kohonen self-organizing maps	Security screening (detection of concealed weapons and explosives)
Berryman et al. [5]	Support vector machines (SVM)	Medical diagnosis (cancer diagnosis)
Yin et al. [6]	SVMs in terahertz (THz) (T-ray)-pulsed classification	DNA sample classification
Fitzgerald et al. [7]	SVM along with data reduction technique	Medical diagnosis (tumor and normal tissue classification)
Wang et al. [8]	Terahertz time-domain spectroscopy (THz-TDS), principal component analysis (PCA), SVM	Wood species identification
Liu et al. [9]	PCA, partial least squares discriminant analysis (PLS-DA), and SVM	Classification of sand grains
Motlak et al. [10]	ANN and k-nearest neighbor (KNN) with pattern recognition	Medical diagnosis (breast cancer classification)
Zhong et al. [11]	Minimum distance classifier and neural network	Explosive and biochemical materials
Te et al. [12]	Statistical pattern classification	Security systems for airports, customs, and post offices
Oliveira et al. [13]	ANN	Security screening (detection of concealed lethal material and bioagents)
Bandyopadhyay et al. [14]	ANN	Security screening (lethal agent identification)
Yang et al. [15]	Convolutional neural network (CNN), faster region-based convolutional neural network (faster R-CNN)	THz security images
Yuan et al. [16]	Two-stage classification system, composed of two deep learning–based classifiers: The CNN and FC (fully connected layer)	Security screening (detection of dangerous equipment)
Zhang et al. [17]	Improved faster R-CNN	Security screening (detection of concealed weapons or other contraband carried on personnel)
Liang et al. [18]	A novel conditional generative Adversarial nets (CGANs), named as Mask-CGANs method to segment weapons	Security screening (detection of concealed weapon)
Yin et al. [19]	Complex extreme learning machine (CELM) classifier	THz sensing technology
Yin et al. [20]	CELM with Karush–Kuhn–Tucker	Multiclass classification problem (THz spectral measurements of six powdered samples)
Berry et al. [21]	Multispectral classification with K-means clustering, unsupervised ISODATA classification	THz pulsed imaging (TPI) in histopathological examination
Ayech ziou [22]	K-means clustering based on ranked set sampling	Agriculture and quality control

(continued)

TABLE 9.1
Summary of Some Related Works on THz Image Analysis Using Machine Learning Approach.—cont'd

Reference	Methods	Application; Remark
Ayech ziou [23]	K-means clustering based on weighted feature learning and random pixel sampling	Agriculture, quality control, life science
Ou et al. [24]	Two-stage segmentation: 1st stage —K-means and region analysis and 2nd stage—ASM	Security screening (detection of concealed objects)
Huang et al. [25]	THz factor analysis along with K-means clustering	Chemistry (molecular classification)
Stephani et al. [27]	Hierarchical agglomerative clustering algorithm	Security and pharmaceutical industry
Nakajima et al. [28]	Agglomerative hierarchical clustering and nonhierarchical clustering K-means with PCA	Medical diagnosis (discriminate cancer tissue from noncancerous tissue) and automatic discrimination of plural components
Shi et al. [29]	KNN, SVM, and random forest (RF) are used for classification	Medical imaging
Bowman et al. [30]	Bayesian mixture model utilizing a Markov chain Monte Carlo scheme	Medical diagnosis
Chen et al. [31]	Discriminant analysis (DA)–based PCA	Food science and genetics (differentiation of genetically modified [GM] and non-GM food)
Wang et al. [32]	Spectral classification with PCA and DA methods and one-dimensional scanning spectral analysis	Food safety and quality control
Liu et al. [33]	Combining adaptive affine clustering algorithm with SVM	Molecular and biomolecular spectroscopy
Liu et al. [34]	Least squares support vector machines (LS-SVM), back-propagation neural network (BPNN), and RF combined with PCA and genetic algorithm (GA)	Food chemistry (differentiation of extra virgin olive oils based on geographical origin)
Grootendorst et al. [35]	TPI systems with SVM and Gaussian wavelet deconvolution in combination with Bayesian classification	Tissue characterization (breast cancer margin detection)
Yue et al. [36]	Gray stretch algorithm, morphological classification algorithm, and Bilateral Contour Tracking Comparison algorithm	Security screening
Liu and Fan [37]	Adaptive dynamic particle swarm optimization SVM algorithm	Food science and genetics
Liu et al. [38]	An novel adaptive decision support vector machine (DSVM)	Food science and genetics (transgenic product differentiation)
Liu et al. [39]	GA-SVM	Food science and genetics (transgenic cotton seeds discrimination)
Liu et al. [40]	PCA, LS-SVM, BPNN, and RF	Food chemistry and genetics (rice seeds classification)
Liu et al.[41]	PCA, LS-SVM, PCA-BPNN	Food science and genetics (transgenic soybean seeds differentiation)
Jiang et al. [42]	PCA used for segmentation and feature extraction; PLSR, LS-SVM, and BPNN used for classification	Food science and agriculture

(continued)

TABLE 9.1
Summary of Some Related Works on THz Image Analysis Using Machine Learning Approach.—cont'd

Reference	Methods	Application; Remark
Siuly et al. [43]	Multinomial logistic regression, KNN, SVM, and naïve Bayes (NB)	Chemistry (powder identification, six different powder samples)
Qi et al. [44]	SVM and PLS-DA	Medical diagnosis (diagnosis of cervical carcinoma)
Liu et al. [45]	ALAP combined with SVM	Food science and genetics (identification of GM cotton samples)
Eadie et al. [46]	Decision tree is used for data reduction; SVM and ANN as classification	Medical diagnosis (colon cancer diagnosis)
Wang et al. [47]	A proposed segmentation algorithm based on the region growth	To solve boundary blurring problem of reconstructed THz digital holographic image
Kawase et al. [48]	Spatial pattern analysis	Border security (detection of illicit drugs)
Xi-Ai et al. [49]	LS-SVM, NB, back-propagation artificial neural network	Agriculture (identification of four different varieties of green tea)
Jiang et al. [50]	SVM, partial least squares regression, and BPNN	Food science and agriculture (moldy wheat classification)

CONCLUSION

This chapter contains a survey of the available machine learning approaches for THz image analysis techniques that are developed in recent days. Due to various favorable characteristics of THz radiation, its use is desirable for imaging system in many application areas. Though THz images have advantages over X-ray images regarding health hazards, their resolution is poor and needs sophisticated techniques for their analysis and interpretation. The area of machine learning is also developing at a fast rate due to availability of increased computational power of computers, and new tools are being developed.

This paper surveys 50 relevant works in the field of detection and classification of objects in THz images by machine learning techniques. The research works are categorized under three main headings: supervised approaches, unsupervised approaches, and other or combined approaches. Under the main categories, research works on different techniques are grouped. The third category contains mainly the works that followed different approaches and combined them. Though every effort has been done so that no important work is left behind, it is extremely difficult to include an exhaustive list as the field is rapidly evolving and newer researches are published day by day. In spite of that we believe that this survey work will be valuable to the new researchers in this emerging filed.

REFERENCES

[1] P. Garbacz, Terahertz imaging - principles, techniques, and limitations, Maintenance problem 1–2016 (2016) 81.

[2] E. Leiss-Holzinger, et al., Imaging of the inner structure of cave bear teeth by novel non-destructive techniques, Palaeontologia Electronica 1–15 (February) (2015).

[3] A. Sinyukov, I. Zorych, Z.H. Michalopoulou, D. Gary, R. Barat, J.F. Federici, Detection of explosives by Terahertz synthetic aperture imaging-focusing and spectral classification, Comptes Rendus Physique 9 (2) (2008) 248–261.

[4] M. Tonouchi, Cutting-edge terahertz technology, Nature Photonics 1 (2) (2007) 97–105.

[5] M.J. Berryman, T. Rainsford, Classification of terahertz data as a tool for the detection of cancer, Biomedical Applications of Micro- and Nanoengineering III 6416 (2006) (2006) 64160X.

[6] X. Yin, B.W.H. Ng, B.M. Fischer, B. Ferguson, D. Abbott, Support vector machine applications in terahertz pulsed signals feature sets, IEEE Sensors Journal 7 (12) (2007) 1597–1607.

[7] A.J. Fitzgerald, Classification of terahertz-pulsed imaging data from excised breast tissue, Journal of Biomedical Optics 17 (1) (2012) 016005.

[8] Y. Wang, S. She, N. Zhou, J. Zhang, H. Yan, W. Li, Wood species identification using terahertz time-domain spectroscopy, BioResources 14 (1) (2019) 1033–1048.

[9] P. Liu, X. Zhang, B. Pan, M. Wei, Z. Zhang, P.B. Harrington, Classification of sand grains by terahertz time-domain spectroscopy and chemometrics, International Journal of Environmental Research 13 (1) (2019) 143–160.

[10] H.J. Motlak, S.I. Hakeem, Detection and classification of breast cancer based-on Terahertz imaging technique using artificial neural network & K-nearest neighbor algorithm, International Journal of Applied Engineering Research 12 (21) (2017) 10661–10668.
[11] H. Zhong, A. Redo-Sanchez, X.-C. Zhang, Identification and classification of chemicals using terahertz reflective spectroscopic focal-plane imaging system, Optics Express 14 (20) (2006) 9130.
[12] C.C. Te, B. Ferguson, D. Abbott, Investigation of biomaterial classification using T-rays, Biomedical Applications of Micro- and Nanoengineering 4937 (2003) 294.
[13] F. Oliveira, et al., Analysis of terahertz spectral images of explosives and bioagents using trained neural networks, Terahertz for Military and Security Applications II 5411 (2004) 45.
[14] A. Bandyopadhyay, et al., Artificial neural network analysis in interferometric thz imaging for detection of lethal agents, International Journal of Infrared and Millimeter Waves 27 (8) (2006) 1145–1158.
[15] X. Yang, et al., CNN with spatio-temporal information for fast suspicious object detection and recognition in THz security images, Signal Processing 160 (2019) 202–214.
[16] J. Yuan, C. Guo, A deep learning method for detection of dangerous equipment,, in: 8th International Conference on Information Science and Technology, ICIST 2018, 2018, pp. 159–164.
[17] J. Zhang, W. Xing, M. Xing, G. Sun, Terahertz image detection with the improved faster region-based convolutional neural network, Sensors 18 (7) (2018).
[18] D. Liang, J. Pan, Y. Yu, H. Zhou, Concealed object segmentation in terahertz imaging via adversarial learning, Optik 185 (2019) 1104–1114.
[19] X.X. Yin, S. Hadjiloucas, Y. Zhang, Complex extreme learning machine applications in terahertz pulsed signals feature sets, Computer Methods and Programs in Biomedicine 117 (2) (2014) 387–403.
[20] X.X. Yin, S. Hadjiloucas, J. He, Y. Zhang, Y. Wang, D. Zhang, Application of complex extreme learning machine to multiclass classification problems with high dimensionality: a THz spectra classification problem, Digital Signal Processing - Journal 40 (1) (2015) 40–52.
[21] E. Berry, et al., Multispectral classification techniques for terahertz pulsed imaging: an example in histopathology, Medical Engineering and Physics 26 (5) (2004) 423–430.
[22] M.W. Ayech, D. Ziou, Segmentation of Terahertz imaging using k-means clustering based on ranked set sampling, Expert Systems with Applications 42 (6) (2015) 2959–2974.
[23] M.W. Ayech, D. Ziou, Terahertz image segmentation using k-means clustering based on weighted feature learning and random pixel sampling, Neurocomputing 175 (PartA) (2015) 243–264.
[24] Z. Ou, H. Geng, X. Zheng, H. Ma, Y. Yu, Segmentation of concealed objects in active terahertz images, in: IST 2018 - IEEE Int. Conf. Imaging Syst. Tech. Proc., 2018, pp. 1–5.
[25] J. Huang, J. Liu, K. Wang, Z. Yang, X. Liu, Classification and identification of molecules through factor analysis method based on terahertz spectroscopy, Spectrochimica Acta Part A: Molecular and Biomolecular Spectroscopy 198 (2018) 198–203.
[26] H. Hoshina, S. Nakajima, M. Yamashita, C. Otani, N. Miyoshi, Terahertz imaging diagnostics of the cancer tissues with chemometrics technique, in: IRMMW-THz 2006 - 31st Int. Conf. Infrared Millim. Waves 14th Int. Conf. Terahertz Electron., 2006, p. 195.
[27] H. Stephani, M. Herrmann, K. Wiesauer, S. Katletz, B. Heise, Enhancing the interpretability of terahertz data through unsupervised classification,, in: XIX IMEKO World Congr. Fundam. Appl. Metrol., No. January, 2009, pp. 2329–2334.
[28] S. Nakajima, et al., Terahertz imaging diagnostics of cancer tissues with a chemometrics technique, Applied Physics Letters 041102 (2007) (2007) 88–91.
[29] J. Shi, et al., Automatic evaluation of traumatic brain injury based on terahertz imaging with machine learning, Optics Express 26 (5) (2018) 6371.
[30] T. Bowman, et al., Pulsed terahertz imaging of breast cancer in freshly excised murine tumors, Journal of Biomedical Optics 23 (02) (2018) 1.
[31] T. Chen, et al., Classification and recognition of genetically modified organisms by chemometrics methods using terahertz spectroscopy, International Journal of Food Science and Technology 50 (12) (2015) 2682–2687.
[32] C. Wang, R. Zhou, Y. Huang, L. Xie, Y. Ying, Terahertz spectroscopic imaging with discriminant analysis for detecting foreign materials among sausages, Food Control 97 (2019) 100–104.
[33] J. Liu, J. Kan, Recognition of genetically modified product based on affinity propagation clustering and terahertz spectroscopy, Spectrochimica Acta Part A: Molecular and Biomolecular Spectroscopy 194 (2018) 14–20.
[34] W. Liu, et al., Discrimination of geographical origin of extra virgin olive oils using terahertz spectroscopy combined with chemometrics, Food Chemistry 251 (2018) 86–92.
[35] M.R. Grootendorst, et al., Use of a handheld terahertz pulsed imaging device to differentiate benign and malignant breast tissue, Biomedical Optics Express 8 (6) (2017) 2932.
[36] G. Yue, Z. Yu, C. Liu, H. Huang, Y. Zhu, Identification and annotation of hidden object in human terahertz image, Information Sciences - Applications 424 (2017) 156–163.
[37] J. Liu, L. Fan, A novel ADPSO-SVM combined with terahertz spectroscopy for recognition of transgenic organisms, Optik 127 (4) (2016) 1957–1961.
[38] J. Liu, Z. Li, F. Hu, T. Chen, A. Zhu, Classification and recognition of transgenic product by terahertz spectroscopy and DSVM, Optik 125 (23) (2014) 6914–6919.
[39] J. Liu, Z. Li, F. Hu, T. Chen, A. Zhu, A THz spectroscopy nondestructive identification method for transgenic cotton seed based on GA-SVM, Optical and Quantum Electronics 47 (2) (2014) 313–322.
[40] W. Liu, C. Liu, X. Hu, J. Yang, L. Zheng, Application of terahertz spectroscopy imaging for discrimination of transgenic rice seeds with chemometrics, Food Chemistry 210 (2016) 415–421.

[41] W. Liu, C. Liu, F. Chen, J. Yang, L. Zheng, Discrimination of transgenic soybean seeds by terahertz spectroscopy, Scientific Reports 6 (October) (2016) 1–7.

[42] Y. Jiang, H. Ge, F. Lian, Y. Zhang, S. Xia, Early detection of germinated wheat grains using terahertz image and chemometrics, Scientific Reports 6 (January) (2016) 1–9.

[43] X. Siuly, S. Yin, Hadjiloucas, Y. Zhang, Classification of THz pulse signals using two-dimensional cross-correlation feature extraction and non-linear classifiers, Computer Methods and Programs in Biomedicine 127 (2016) 64–82.

[44] N. Qi, Z. Zhang, Y. Xiang, Y. Yang, X. Liang, P.D.B. Harrington, Terahertz time-domain spectroscopy combined with support vector machines and partial least squares-discriminant analysis applied for the diagnosis of cervical carcinoma, Anal. Methods 7 (6) (2015) 2333–2338.

[45] J. Liu, Z. Li, F. Hu, T. Chen, Y. Du, H. Xin, "Identification of GMOs by terahertz spectroscopy and ALAP–SVM, Optical and Quantum Electronics 47 (3) (2015) 685–695.

[46] L.H. Eadie, C.B. Reid, A.J. Fitzgerald, V.P. Wallace, Optimizing multi-dimensional terahertz imaging analysis for colon cancer diagnosis, Expert Systems with Applications 40 (6) (2013) 2043–2050.

[47] Y.-T. Wang, Q. Li, A segmentation algorithm on terahertz digital holographic image, in: Proc.SPIE, vol. 11170, 2019.

[48] K. Kawase, Y. Ogawa, Y. Watanabe, H. Inoue, Non-destructive terahertz imaging of illicit drugs using spectral fingerprints, Optics Express 11 (20) (2003) 2549.

[49] C. Xi-Ai, Z. Guang-Xin, H. Ping-Jie, H. Di-Bo, K. Xu-Sheng, Z. Ze-Kui, Classification of the green tea varieties based on support vector machines using terahertz spectroscopy, in: Conference Record - IEEE Instrumentation and Measurement Technology Conference, vol. 1, 2011, pp. 905–909, no. 1.

[50] Y. Jiang, H. Ge, F. Lian, Y. Zhang, S. Xia, Discrimination of moldy wheat using terahertz imaging combined with multivariate classification, RSC Advances 5 (114) (2015) 93979–93986.

CHAPTER 10

Amalgamation of Machine Learning and Artificial Intelligence for Breast Cancer Detection

BRIGHT KESWANI, PHD • LOKESH VIJAY, MBBS • POONAM KESWANI, PHD • PRITY VIJAY, PHD • AMBARISH G. MOHAPATRA, PHD

INTRODUCTION

Cells are the building blocks of our body. These cells merge to form different organs and tissues performing numerous functions. Each of these cells repairs and divides themselves in a scrupulous system. In some situation, these cells start growing in strange style forming lumps identified as tumor. The overgrowth of cells in the region of the breast duct forms breast tumor. The breast tumor can be classified as benign or malignant. Benign tumors are not cancers and can be detached easily without any risk. But malignant tumor can spread around breast duct and lobules causing breast cancer. Breast cancer is curable if symptoms are pragmatic in an early stage but late stages of it are dangerous. Among all types of cancer occurring in women, breast cancer is the most common one. Approximately one out of every eight women in United States is suffering from breast cancer. Statistics proves almost 25% of the female having cancer is diagnosed with the breast cancer [1]. Although medical tools such as mammograms, ultrasounds, and others are available, they sometime fail to impart truthful result in the early stage of disease. This creates risk for physician in predicting cancerous tumors appropriately. Therefore, a demand for new strategies for detection of breast cancer is needed. Enormous amount of patient big data motivates researchers to apply different machine learning (ML) approach and build predictive models for prediction of breast cancer [2].

Breast Cancer Epidemiology

Breast cancer is the most common malignancy around the world in women. 1,671,149 new cases of breast cancer were detected and 521,907 mortality were reported due to breast cancer in 2012 [3]. In India also breast cancer has been reported as the most common cancer in women with incidence of 25.8 per 100,000 women and death rate approaching as high as 12.7 per 100,000 women [4]. Overall, it has been attributed as second most common cause of cancer-related deaths. Changes in lifestyle are increasing in the risk for breast cancer. Till the era of 1999, life expectancy increased due to better healthcare facilities. As hormone replacement therapy proved to be an established factor in breast cancer and thus its use was decreased, it led to a decrease in the breast cancer cases from year 1999–2006 by almost 2% annually [5].

Risk Factors

Age has been ascribed as most important risk factor. Increasing life expectancy has been attributed to increase in incidence of breast cancer. Female sex is no doubt an important risk factor with only less than 1% cases occurring in male. Some other factors include overall increased estrogen exposure in the female increases the risk, in terms of early menarche and delayed menopause, no pregnancy or late pregnancy, low parity, lack of breast feeding, and use of hormone replacement therapy. Other lifestyle-related factors include obesity, alcohol intake, and smoking. Family history of breast cancer is another risk factor, and substantial amount of breast cancer patients have positive family history. Personal history of breast cancer is also a risk factor for cancer in the contralateral breast. History of chest wall radiotherapy at younger age is a potential risk factor for development of breast cancer at later age [6,7].

Terahertz Biomedical and Healthcare Technologies. https://doi.org/10.1016/B978-0-12-818556-8.00010-0

Genes Associated With Breast Cancer

Various mutations in the genes have been attributed as a risk factor for breast cancer development and hence termed as hereditary breast cancer. The most important are BRCA1 followed by BRCA2, together constituting major cases of hereditary breast cancer. Breast cancer-associated gene1 (BRCA1) is located on chromosome 17q21 and BRCA2 on 13q12. Other gene mutations responsible with very less incidence (1% or <1%) are p53, STK11/LKB1, PTEN, MSH2/MLH1, and ATM [5,8].

Historical Risk Factors

Histological findings on biopsy may characterize and appear as additional risk factor weather an individual carries a risk of developing breast cancer in future. The relative risk of various histological findings and development into breast cancer are [5]

Historical Findings	Relative Risk
Nonproliferative disease	1
Proliferative disease without atypia	1.3–1.9
Proliferative disease with atypia	3.7–4.2
Proliferative disease with atypia with strong family history	4–9
Lobular carcinoma in situ	>7

Risk Assessing Models and Tools

Various models were constructed for breast cancer risk assessment. Some of those models are discussed below [5,8].

Gail model

Gail models include age, age at menarche and at first birth, number of breast biopsy specimens, history of atypical hyperplasia, and total first-degree relatives with breast cancer. It assesses the aggregate/total risk of breast cancer according to decade of life.

Claus model

Claus model gives individual assessment of breast cancer risk according to decade of life according to the presence of first- and second-degree relatives with breast cancer and their age at presentation/diagnosis.

Brcapro model

BRCAPRO model as name suggests overcomes the drawback of both Gail model and Claus model, i.e., it takes into consideration molecular factors like mutation in BRCA1 and BRCA2 genes which has been an established risk factor. It works on Mendelian principle which looks for chances whether a person is possessing mutation in genes responsible for breast or ovarian cancer.

Tyrer-Cuzick model

Tyrer-Cuzick model involves both family history and personal risk factors. By incorporating family history details, this model derives chances whether an individual carries mutation in genes that may lead to breast cancer. This information is then added to other risk factors, namely age at menarche, first live birth and menopause, number of pregnancy, history of atypical hyperplasia or LCIS, height, and body mass index.

Molecular Marker and Assay

Various molecular markers are there which have proven role in deciding the response to treatment and prognosis. Markers which have been studied extensively are steroid hormone receptors—(a) estrogen receptor (ER), (b) progesterone receptor (PR), and human epidermal growth receptor (HER), *p53*. ER assessment is done nowadays in almost all cases of breast cancer to direct hormonal therapy. HER-2 protein is produced from erb-B2 gene and increased amount is found in 20% patients of breast cancer. Trastuzumab therapy may be given to patient positive for HER-2. Prognosis may be determined by presence and absence of receptors. For example, ER, PR, and HER-2 negative cancer, which are also known as triple negative cancer, have poor prognosis as these tumors are almost resistant to chemotherapy [5,8]. In a similar way to ER, PR, and HER-2, multiple gene products may be used for determining the prognosis and response to therapy. Following are the various tests that have come across.

21-Gene Test

21-gene test gives a recurrence score for ER-positive breast cancer, thus guiding whether to give chemotherapy along with hormonal therapy or not.

Mamma print assay

Mamma Print assay assess 70 genes and provides details whether disease is low-risk or high-risk disease.

Screening in Breast Cancer

Women aged 40 to 49 with average risk are prescribed with mammograms every year. Women aged 50 to 74 with average risk are also prescribed for mammograms every year. Women higher than average risk are recommended for magnetic resonance imaging (MRI) and mammogram every year from age of 40 years [9].

Pathological Classification of Breast Cancer

Breast cancer can be classified pathologically into three parts as shown below [5].

Noninvasive epithelial cancers

1. Lobular carcinoma in situ
2. Ductal carcinoma in situ or intraductal carcinoma
   a. Papillary
   b. Cribriform
   c. Solid
   d. Comedo

Invasive epithelial cancers

1. Invasive lobular carcinoma
2. Invasive ductal carcinoma—most common
   a. Invasive ductal carcinoma, not otherwise specified
   b. Tubular carcinoma
   c. Mucinous or colloid carcinoma
   d. Medullary carcinoma
   e. Invasive cribriform carcinoma
   f. Invasive papillary carcinoma
   g. Adenoid cystic carcinoma
   h. Metaplastic carcinoma

Mixed connective and epithelial tumors

1. Phyllodes tumor
2. Carcinosarcoma
3. Angiosarcoma
4. Adenocarcinoma

A Clinical Approach: Patient Suspected As Breast Cancer/Breast Lump and Management

Clinical evaluation

Most of the patients with complaint of breast lump are considered as a suspected case of carcinoma and should be approached in a similar way to rule out the disease while evaluating other risk factors, like age, family history, etc. Other complaints may be asymmetrical breasts, nipple discharge or recent nipple retraction, swelling in axilla, and ulceration over breast. After assessing patient history, proper examination with inspection and palpation on bilateral breast and bilateral axillary region (to rule out axillary lymph node enlargement) is recommended. Systemic and general examination is prescribed to rule out any signs suggestive of metastasis; however, metastatic workup is mandatory with the help of radiological and blood investigations in advanced cases as only clinical examination never rules out metastases [5,8,10].

Clinical investigations

Clinical investigation of a patient suspected to breast cancer is categorized into several divisions which are given below.

Imaging. Several popular imaging techniques which are currently in trend to the detection of breast cancer are given below.

Mammography. Mammography is one of the oldest investigations for diagnosis as well as screening of the breast carcinoma. Mammography techniques have evolved over the time. Conventionally for screening purposes, two views are taken: mediolateral oblique and Craniocaudal view. For diagnostic purposes, these views can be adjusted along with 90° lateral views or with spot compression views. Conventional mammography delivers 0.1 cGy of radiation. Features suggestive of breast carcinoma are solid mass with or without stellate features, asymmetrical thickening of breast parenchyma, and clustered microcalcification.

Ductography. In ductography, radiopaque contrast is injected in one of the major ducts and then mammography is performed. It is done when patient with bloody nipple discharge is reported.

Ultrasonography. Ultrasonography is an important imaging technique particularly in young women with heavy breast. It is useful in distinguishing benign from malignant disease of breast. Axillary lymph node can be diagnosed—malignant or benign based on certain sonographic findings. Ultrasound-guided biopsy or cytology can be taken in previous inconclusive specimen. It has no radiological exposure but drawback is that it is operator dependent.

Magnetic resonance imaging. MRI is not used commonly; however, it is nowadays recommended in high-risk cases, i.e., strong family history and with known susceptible mutated genes.

Breast imaging reporting and data system. Breast imaging reporting and data system investigation consists of several stages depending upon the patient problem. Incomplete assessment needs additional imaging evaluation or prior mammograms for comparison. Benign finding usually recommend annual screening. Probably benign finding (<2% malignant) than initial short-interval follow-up was suggested. If suspicious abnormality (2%–95% malignant) is reported, then biopsy is recommended. Appropriate action should be taken in case of highly suggestive malignancy (>95% malignant). Known biopsy is mandatory in case of proven malignancy.

Biopsy. Breast biopsy can be fine needle aspiration cytology, core needle biopsy, or vacuum-assisted core biopsy. In FNAC 22 gauze needle is used; however, only feature it can determine is presence/absence of malignant cells. In core needle biopsy, 14 gauze needles are used. It determines whether the malignancy is invasive or not. Also it determines the status of receptors. Vacuum-assisted biopsy devices use 8 to 10 gauze needle and is commonly done under image guidance. All these techniques need image guidance like such as mammography, ultrasound, or MRI.

Metastatic work up. According to the stage of the cancer, metastatic workup can be done such as complete blood count, liver function tests, and alkaline phosphatase level, chest radiogram, bone scan, abdominal computed tomographic scan, or MRI.

Terahertz technique. Terahertz imaging is an alternative approach for the detection and diagnosis of breast cancer. It is a type of electromagnetic radiation technique which has been successfully adapted for providing highly specific images of tumors, which help in cancer detection. Traditional imaging technique of breast cancer sometimes fails to produce clear picture of breast tissue on the margins of a tumor. Due to unavailability of clear picture of margin between healthy tissue and tumor, surgeons cannot judge appropriately about the removal of entire tumor during the surgery. Due to which chances of secondary surgery maximizes near about 20%–40%. Terahertz imaging reduces the chances of second surgeries, cancer reoccurrence, and metastasis through fast and precised tumor margin assessment. Terahertz spectroscopy gives high quality tissues images. It emits very few waves than radiography thus enabling deeper imaging into an object. The radiation is nonionizing and therefore produces least harmful effects on human body. Its absorption property is large due to which water and metals highly reflect terahertz radiation. Combinational power of pattern reorganization and terahertz can provide a potential solution for rapid and noninvasive detection and diagnosis of disease. Terahertz technology is capable enough of producing precise image and therefore can be used as efficient diagnostic tool, but extracting important information from these images is very difficult. Therefore, there is a need of multivariate statistical tools of pattern recognition that are used in analysis and classification of these images [11].

Staging breast cancer

TNM Staging.

T (PRIMARY TUMOR)	
TX	Primary tumor cannot be assessed
T0	No evidence of primary tumor
Tis	Carcinoma in situ (DCIS, LCIS, Paget's disease of nipple alone)
T1	Tumor<2 cm
T2	Tumor>2 cm and <5 cm
T3	Tumor>5 cm
T4	Tumor of any size with extension to either chest wall or skin
T4a	Extension to chest wall (excluding pectoralis major)
T4b	Ulceration, satellite nodules, or edema of skin
T4c	Both T4a and T4b
T4d	Inflammatory carcinoma
N (REGIONAL LYMPH NODES)—CLINICAL	
NX	Regional lymph nodes cannot be assessed
N0	No regional lymph nodes
N1	Metastasis to ipsilateral axillary lymph nodes level I and II—are mobile
N2a	Metastasis to ipsilateral axillary lymph nodes level I and II—are fixed, matted
N2b	Metastasis to ipsilateral internal mammary lymph nodes in absence of axillary lymph nodes
N3a	Metastasis in ipsilateral infraclavicular lymph nodes
N3b	Metastasis to ipsilateral internal mammary lymph nodes and axillary lymph nodes
N3c	Metastasis in ipsilateral supraclavicular lymph nodes
N (REGIONAL LYMPH NODES)—PATHOLOGICAL	
pNX	Regional lymph nodes cannot be assesse
pN0	No regional lymph nodes metastases assessed histologically
pN1	Micrometastases; or metastases in 1–3 axillary lymph nodes; and/or in internal mammary nodes with metastases detected by sentinel lymph node biopsy but not clinically detected
pN2	Metastases in 4–9 axillary lymph nodes; or in clinically apparent internal mammary lymph nodes in the absence of axillary lymph node metastases
pN3	Metastases in 10 or more axillary lymph nodes; or in infraclavicular (level III axillary) lymph nodes; or in clinically detected ipsilateral internal mammary

	lymph nodes in the presence of one or more positive level I and II axillary lymph nodes; or in more than three axillary lymph nodes and in internal mammary lymph nodes with micrometastases or macrometastases detected by sentinel lymph node biopsy but not clinically detected; or in ipsilateral supraclavicular lymph nodes
M (DISTANT METASTASES)	
M0	No clinical or radiographic evidence of distant metastases
M1	Distant detectable metastases as determined by classic clinical and radiographic means and/or histologically proven larger than 0.2 mm
Stage 0	TisN0M0
Stage IA	T1 N0 M0
Stage IB	T0 N1mi M0
	T1 N1mi M0
Stage IIA	T0 N1 M0
	T1 N1 M0
	T2 N0 M0
Stage IIB	T2 N1 M0
	T3 N0 M0
Stage IIIA	T0 N2 M0
	T1N2 M0
	T2 N2 M0
	T3 N1 M0
	T3 N2 M0
Stage IIIB	T4 N0 M0
	T4 N1 M0
	T4 N2 M0
Stage IIIC	Any T N3 M0
Stage IV	Any T Any N M1

Treatment in Breast Cancer

Treatment modality differs in each case and depends on stage of the disease, patient's factors, and receptor status. Therefore, individualization of treatment in breast cancer forms a very essential part taking into consideration each and every factor. Treatment modalities of breast cancer are given below.

Surgery

In early days, consideration was that by extensive locoregional resection mortality can be brought down; however, through experience and advancement in screening and other treatment modalities, surgical techniques have been traveled from extensive dissection of Halsted radical mastectomy to breast conserving surgery (BCS) and oncoplastic techniques. Various factors determine mastectomy or BCS but mortality rates remain same in both.

Chemotherapy

Chemotherapy can be given in neoadjuvant or adjuvant form. Most frequently used regimens are CAF (cyclophosphamide, adriamycin, 5-FU) or CMF regimen.

Radiotherapy

In an era of BCS, its use has increased. Any contraindication to radiotherapy means that BCS is to be avoided. Radiotherapy is also used in postmastectomy cases of locally advanced breast cancer.

Hormonal therapy

Tamoxifen is used in ER-positive female in reproductive age group. In postmenopausal women, aromatase inhibitors like anastrozole are used to prevent extraovarian source of estrogen.

NEED OF INCORPORATING MACHINE LEARNING AND ARTIFICIAL INTELLIGENCE

Breast cancer is considered as the maximum number of cancer worldwide. In 2012, more than 522,000 women have been estimated as a victim of breast cancer and rises to 20% in next 5 years. Only key to reduce mortality rate is early detection of a disease. One of the efficient techniques for detection of breast cancer is mammography screening. It has been reported that there is a reduction of 20% mortality rates by mammography screening program. Abnormalities in mammography can be an indication of breast cancer which required further investigation. Breast imaging such as ultrasound imagery is common for the further investigation. Breast biopsy is the step which is carried out after the confirmation of the disease which involves microscopic investigation of cells' features in order to conclude cells as normal or cancerous. But disadvantage of surgical biopsy is that it can cause anxiety and stress in patient which brings lots of risk. During this process, breast tissues also distort, causing problem for radiologist to observe the results of mammography. Due to several risks factors of biopsies, detection of breast cancer needs be done carefully and therefore breast cancer technique should move to an alternate direction. Mammography is broadly divided into screening and diagnostic mammography. Screening mammogram is a simple and suggested to all women above age 40 and considered as a first step of investigation. Any abnormality in the screening mammograms can help in early detection of breast cancer, which further helps doctor to operate correct area. Second type of mammogram is diagnostic mammography; a complex X-ray examination process of a breast suggested after the symptoms of the breast cancer has been discovered during the screening mammography. It is a time-consuming process because precise size along with location of an abnormal region and its surrounding tissues has to be investigated. This process is more expensive and time consuming when compared with screening because several images of each breast with different orientation of the breast parenchyma have to be taken. Therefore, machine-aided tools and techniques are required to avoid complicated process of clinical investigations for breast cancer detection.

Rising trend had been recognized in the demands and usage of ML in the last few years for diagnosis and prognosis of breast cancer. Conventional method using statistics for data extraction and interpretation had been modified by automatic generic methods set through ML. ML provides a smart solution in terms of fast and efficient tools and data-driven models for processing real-time breast cancer data with accurate results. Robustness of ML techniques can help physicians as an efficient alternative tool for many manual works. Breast cancer if detected earlier can save life where ML classification algorithms are playing important role for classification of malignant and benign tumors of breast cancer patient. Precise prediction can help physician in prescribing further treatment. Many classification ML techniques such as artificial neural network (ANN), K-nearest neighbor (KNN), decision tree (DT), support vector machine (SVM), etc., have been widely used for the detection of BC. ML algorithms are very helpful while making decisions of positive and negative test of several diseases. Therefore, classifiers are playing important role everywhere from CAD systems to digital mammograms. ML technique makes use of feature vector in classifying mammogram images into benign or malignant tumors.

Machine Learning and Artificial Intelligence

ML and artificial intelligence is the branch of computer science having the ability to self-train a system in an efficient way, so that system learns automatically from a data and also improves with the experiences without being programmed explicitly. It consists of sets of algorithms that offer a possibility to a software application to predict the precise outcome. The fundamental goal of ML is to construct a model, receiving an input and using statistics formula for the prediction of an output when new data are arrived in the system. ML looks into the data examples to search patterns and construct decision rules for building a predictive model which can be used to predict future data. These predictive models are capable enough of self-learning with experience without any human interruption and take a decision based on certain circumstances [12]. ML can broadly categorize into supervised and unsupervised learning containing wide sets of algorithms in each category.

Types of Machine Learning Algorithms

Supervised ML algorithms are useful for a dataset which contains target class. Supervised models are functional to unseen data with the usage of past examples of the target class [13]. It acquires advantages of evaluating outcome prediction through comparison with that of original output, calculates the error, and modifies it accordingly. On the other hand, unsupervised ML algorithms are in use when the dataset is not having labels. It is basically applied to extract a hidden pattern from the dataset in an absence of target variable. The common process for ML model is shown in Fig. 10.1.

Depending on the noisiness of the system and how the system responds, the training sets vary to achieve success. In general, a system may have more than a 100 example training sets. But, the solution solely depends on the context of the problem and behavior of the dataset. However, training a model as per requirement is a very tedious job to do and subject to matter of expert.

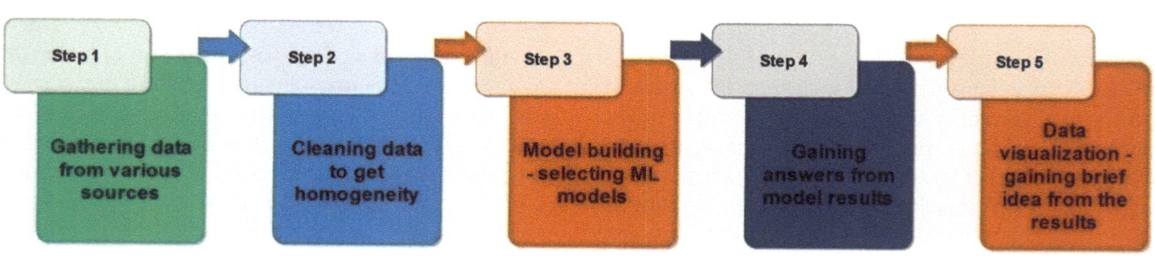

FIG. 10.1 Machine learning process.

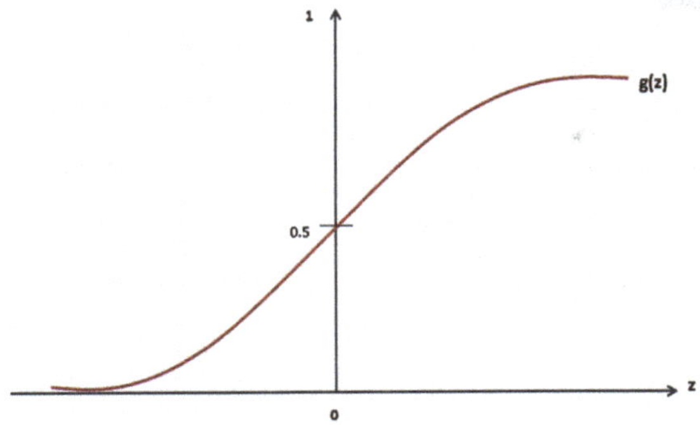

FIG. 10.2 S-shaped sigmoid curve.

Several Machine Learning Algorithms

ML algorithms learn and improve automatically from past experience. Several ML classification algorithms for breast cancer diagnosis have been used (SVM, KNN, DT, Neural Net) on dataset and their performances have been compared while constructing a predictive model for automatic prediction of unseen data. Performance evaluation of which has been done through various matrices and measures.

Logistic regression

Logistic regression (LG) [14] is simple and widely used classifier that classifies the target through returning its probabilities either as 0 or 1. It can be used for email spam detection, cancer detection, credit card fraud detection, and many such classification problems. LG is almost similar to linear regression, except linear regression predicts continuous number but LG expects true and false. LG computes the correlation between the features variable and dependent variable based on probabilities output concluded logistic function. These probabilities must be transformed into either 0 or 1 by a sigmoid or S-shaped curve. It is also known as logistic function and a curve is constructed using natural logarithm of the odds of the target value rather than probability. The logistic function can be written as

$$g(Z) = \frac{1}{1 + e^{-x}} \tag{10.1}$$

Hypothesis representation of LG can be defined as

$$h\theta(x) = g(\theta^T n) \tag{10.2}$$

Above function can be combined to form an equation

$$h\theta(x) = \frac{1}{1 + e^{-\theta Tx}} \tag{10.3}$$

In Fig. 10.2, g(Z) calculates class output depending on input features. Value for sigmoid function ranges from 0 to 1, it predicts 0 when an input (Z) is $-\infty$ and 1 when an input (Z) is ∞. The threshold value is kept at 0.5. It can be clearly observed in Eqs. (10.4) and (10.5), when x is an input, it passes to the sigmoid function and output is greater than 0.5, then class is equal to 1 ($y = 1$) or output is less than 0.5, then class is equal to 0 ($y = 0$).

$$\text{if } h\theta(x) \geq 0.5 \text{ then } y = 1 \tag{10.4}$$

$$\text{if } h\theta(x) < 0.5 \text{ then } y = 0 \tag{10.5}$$

Optimization is needed to obtain the best fit line by using the right parameters for building models. Optimization algorithms are used to maximize the likelihood for accurate classification and known as maximum likelihood estimator. Gradient descent or gradient ascent, etc., are some of the different optimization algorithms that can be used to maximize the likelihood in the case of LG.

Support vector machine

SVM is a supervised ML algorithm used individually in classifications as well as a regression problem. SVM classifies target feature through constructing optimum hyperplane. Value of each feature is plotted in n-dimensional space as a particular coordinate value. Then separation hyperplane is calculated based on the coordinates which actually differentiate two classes precisely [15] (Fig. 10.3).

Support vectors are the feature that separates two classes and helps in calculating hyperplane. Many hyperplane can be constructed for target classification but best among them should contain the widest margin. Among all, best hyperplane is chosen get the most out of the distance between the support vectors of either class, which is known as margin. In real and complex

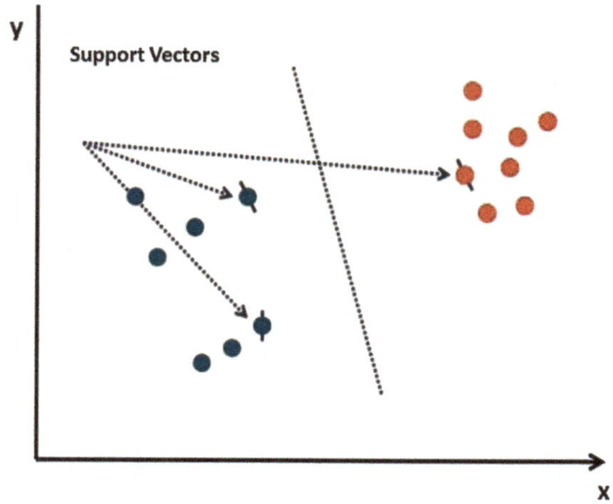

FIG. 10.3 Support vectors.

dataset, most of the time linear hyperplane is hard to construct; in such cases, SVM uses a technique called kernel. A kernel can easily convert low-dimensional input space into high-dimensionality space (Fig. 10.4).

Decision boundary is a term referred to separation line or hyperplane, and it helps to separate two classes. Decision boundary is calculated only for one time throughout the training process. Therefore, SVM can classify a large amount of data. SVM classification is done first by calculating support vectors of the different class that are maximally separated by each other. Optimization is done by minimizing ||w|| and maximizing b, where b is a bias and ||w|| is the magnitude of a vector. Eq. (10.6) is a formula for constructing properly separable hyperplane.

$$Yi(X^i \cdot W + b) \geq 1 \qquad (10.6)$$
$$\text{Class (known feature} + \text{b}) = 1$$

K-nearest neighbor

KNN [16] is simplest and versatile classifier useful for both classification and regression problem. KNN takes plenty of computational space memory for all the training data. KNN classifier detects the unknown feature by calculating it with a nearest known feature in a dataset and predicts the output based on (K) number of features situated near to it (Fig. 10.5).

In this study, the value of K is fixed to 5. It means KNN will try to find the distance of the unknown feature with five nearest neighbors. Distance is calculated between each of the row of training data and test data and then sorted in an ascending order. Among them, predicted class belongs to the frequent number of features depending on k. Euclidean distance is a famous metrics which is used to calculate the distance between the unknown feature with that of K number of the nearest data sample. Euclidean squared, Chebyshev, and city

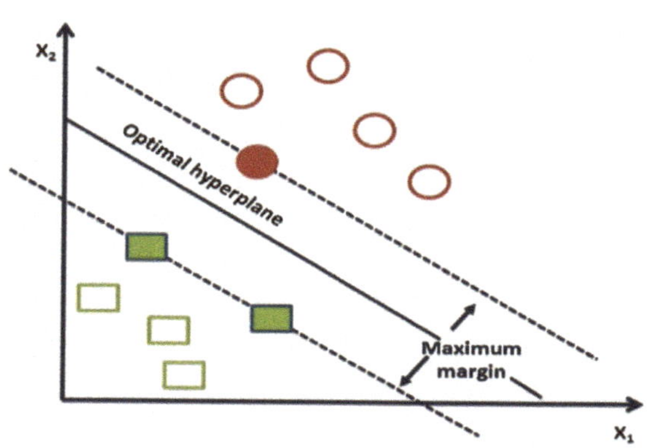

FIG. 10.4 Hyperplane constructed through support vector.

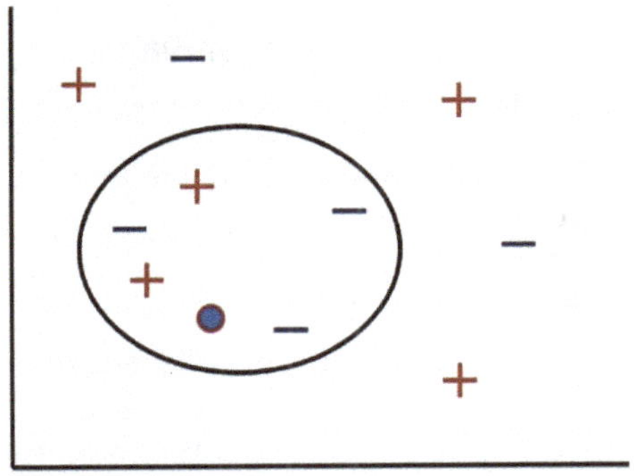

FIG. 10.5 K-nearest neighbor with k = 5 neighbors.

block are other such matrices. Euclidean distance can be formulated as Eq. (10.7):

$$\text{Distance}(P, Y) = \sqrt{\sum_{i=1}^{n} (P_i - Y_i)^2} \tag{10.7}$$

Decision tree

A DT can be used for solving classification as well as a regression problem [17]. DT predicts the result, learning through decision-making rules constructed from the training data. DT uses a tree-like structure to accomplish the problem and flash the result. A DT is easily understandable when compared with other ML algorithm. A DT forms tree-like structure where class labels are represented as a leaf node and attribute is represented as the internal node. In order to generate the tree-like structure from the training set, the best attribute is picked as the root of a tree. Then the training set splits into a different subset. The process of searching root and its subset is repeated at each branch of the tree to find leaf nodes in all the branches of the DT.

Graphical representation of a DT is easy to understand. A DT is less affected by outliers and missing values. Trees constructed by learning the decision rule consist of a root node, decision node, terminal node, branch, parent node, and child node. Splitting is a key process of separating nodes into one or more subnodes. DT uses various algorithms such as the Gini index and information gain for a splitting process. Here, in an experiment, we use a DT with the Gini index to build the model.

Gini index

Gini index is a type of metric used to measure how randomly selected attribute as root node can identify incorrectly. It can be calculated from below mentioned formula and attribute with lower Gini index is preferable to be selected as the root node. Gini index is calculated by adding the weighted sum of squared possibilities of attributes and then subtracting it from 1. This study uses the Gini index for calculating the root node for a DT.

$$\text{Gini Index} = 1 - \sum_{x=1}^{n} P_x^2 \tag{10.8}$$

Information gain

Information gain is used to estimate the information contained by each attribute. Entropy is defined to measure the randomness of a random variable. In order to calculate information gain, it is required to measure entropy of each attribute. Entropy is a process to measure impurity. Information gain is calculated in two steps. In first step, entropy of the target class is calculated:

$$\text{Entropy} = \sum_{x}^{class} -Plog_2\,P_x \tag{10.9}$$

In Eq. (10.9), P_x is the probability of class x and entropy is calculated based on the proportion of target values. In the second step, information gain is calculated with the help of entropy. Information gain helps in making the decision about the best split in a training dataset and best variable to split a node. Counting of entropy of parent and child nodes is needed for calculation of information gain due to split. A variable with the highest information is selected for the split.

Naïve bayes

Naïve Bayes (NB) classifier as the name suggests is based on Bayes theorem. NB presumes dataset features are not related to each other, even if they are correlated. It requires a very small portion of a dataset to detect parameters necessary to predict the output. It is a fast classifier. NB predicts the output based on probability which is calculated by every feature individually. It is an easy going model for a large dataset.

Neural network

Neural network (NN) is most powerful ML algorithm, which is nowadays applied in most of data mining tools. Its working fundamental is just like human brain system. It is a set of numerous interconnected neurons for processing of data into meaningful information. The NN is capable of training a big amount of data very easily and efficiently. NN guarantees to extract meaningful information from a highly complex dataset and forms pattern and trends for analysis which is not possible for general human being [18].

NN is utilized nowadays for mining data, especially for decision support application. Human being learns from experience and computers are good in following instructions. NN takes best of both the systems, i.e., it constructs a model that behaves just like human brain neurons in a computer system. NN acquired attractiveness because of its precision during classification and its technique to distinguish complex pattern without difficulty.

NN is sometime referred as ANN models that are extremely efficient and accurate when compared with other ML models. NN fabricates the output by mapping multiple input nodes into numerous output nodes. NN learns from a set of examples provided to it as an input. Single layer architecture of the NN is capable of solving the linear separable problem. But the exceedingly complex problem becomes a challenge for ANN. Therefore, in order to conquer this obscurity, multilayered perceptron (MLP) was developed in 1950. MLP provides the user a flexibility to add a number of the hidden layer between the input and output layer to solve the respective problem competently.

Feedforward is the essential architectural procedure of an NN, intending propagation of the inputs from the input layer to the complete hidden layer present in between the architecture until it reaches the output layer. Back propagation NN method calculates the error by propagating again from the output layer to hidden layer and then to the input layer. The process is repeated for a number of times until error is reduced. A number of neurons are connected together to form feedforward NN architecture. The NN architecture consists of a number of the layers where the first layer is an input layer and the last layer is the output layer in between a hidden layer of any number. Below NN is present feed forward NN architecture of three layers.

The error is computed through back propagation method with the help of gradient descent. During back propagation, in order to minimize the error, weight is regularly updated through gradient descent in each epoch. Gradient descent minimizes loss occurred in training by comparing actual value with that of predicted output. As shown in Fig. 1.4, each layer connected to the other layer is represented through a weight coefficient. Input feature present in the dataset is received by the input layer. Hidden layer calculates weight sum of all the given input and redirect it to the activation function.

$$Neural\ Net_x = \sum_{i=0}^{n} A_i w_{ji} + W_o \tag{10.10}$$

In Eq. (10.10), i is an input layer unit, j is a hidden layer unit, and w_{ji} is a weight at hidden layer j. Feed forward back propagation architecture can also be applied to MLP. NN multilayer architecture has been used during this research because of its high performance when compared with other ML classification algorithms and its efficiency during processing of huge volume of data.

Performance Evaluation Matrices and Measures

Once an experiment has been conducted, performance evaluation is the most important task to be performed, for checking accuracies of different learning algorithms, used to construct the model. In this experiment, different types of matrices and measures to ensure the accurateness of an algorithm for prediction are confusion matrix, accuracy, classification error, sensitivity, specificity, precision, F1-score, ROC curve, and AUC. All of these matrices and measures are explained below.

Confusion matrix

Confusion matrix [19] is a table-like structure containing one value in each row and a column for the recitation of classifier performance in an experiment. If the dependent variable is consisting of two responses, confusion matrix construct - 2*2 size of the matrix for the comparison of the predicted value, with the test set value. Then the output of the evaluation is placed in respective boxes (TP, FP, TN, and FN) of the confusion matrix. In this study, format of confusion matrix used is as follows (Table 10.1)

Each of the boxes in a confusion matrix has a special meaning which clearly explains the number of times model is correct and the number of times model is incorrect during prediction. True negative (TN) is the total count of correct prediction of negative class. False positive (FP) is a total count of the wrong prediction of positive class. False negative (FN) is a total count of the wrong prediction of negative class. It is also known as type error II. True positive (TP) is a total count of correct prediction of the positive class. Apart from a confusion matrix, there are numbers of performance measures, derived from confusion used here.

TABLE 10.1
Confusion Matrix for Binary Classification.

-Ve / +Ve (Predicted) / - Ve / +Ve (Actual)		Negatives	Positives
		Predicted (0)	Predicted (1)
Negatives	Actual (0)	True Negative (TN)	False Positive (FP)
Positives	Actual (1)	False Negative (FN)	True Positive (TP)

Classification accuracy

Classification accuracy [19] is a measure of the total number of correct prediction over a total number of predictions as shown in Eq. (10.11), detected by a classification model (Table 10.2).

Classification error

Classification error of misclassification [19] is a measure of a total number of incorrect predictions as shown in Eq. (10.12), detected by a classification model over a total number of predictions. It is also known as the misclassification rate (Table 10.3).

Sensitivity

Sensitivity (SN) is an important measure derived from the confusion matrix [19] through the division of a total number of correct positive predictions over the total number of positive as shown in Eq. (10.13). True positive rate (TPR) or recall (REC) is a synonym for sensitivity. It responses the total number of times model prediction is correct for positive class (Table 10.4).

Specificity

Specificity (SP) is an important measure derived from a confusion matrix [19] through the division of a total number of correct negative predictions over a total number of negatives as shown in Eq. (10.14). True negative rate is a synonym for specificity. It responses a total number of times model prediction is correct for negative class (Table 10.5).

Precision

Precision (PR) is an important measure derived from the confusion matrix [19] through the division of a total number of correct positive prediction over the total number of positive predictions as shown in Eq. (10.15). It is also known as positive prediction value (Table 10.6).

F1-score

F1-score is a weighted average of recall and precision as shown in Eq. 3.15 [19].

$$\text{F1} - \text{Score} = \frac{2 \ * \text{Precision} * \text{Recall}}{\text{Precison} \ + \ \text{Recall}} \tag{10.16}$$

Receiver operatic characteristic curve

Receiver operatic characteristic curve or ROC curve [68] is used for visualization of performance of classifier at all possible thresholds. It is two-dimensional curves with TPR or sensitivity on Y-Axis and false positive rate (FPR) or 1-sensitivity on X-axis.

TABLE 10.2
Classification Accuracy.

Test Data	Predictive Negative	Predicted Positive
Actual negative	TN	**FP**
Actual positive	**FN**	TP

$$\text{Classification Accuracy} = \frac{TN + TP}{TP \ + \ TN \ + \ FP \ + \ FN} \tag{10.11}$$

TABLE 10.3
Classification Error.

Test Data	Predictive Negative	Predicted Positive
Actual negative	**TN**	FP
Actual positive	FN	**TP**

$$\text{Classification Error} = \frac{FP + FN}{TP + TN + FP + FN} \tag{10.12}$$

TABLE 10.4
Sensitivity or Recall Rate.

Test Data	Predictive Negative	Predicted Positive
Actual negative	TN	FP
Active positive	FN	**TP**

$$\text{Sensitivity} = \frac{TP}{TP + FN} \tag{10.13}$$

TABLE 10.5
Specificity.

Test Data	Predictive Negative	Predicted Positive
Actual negative	**TN**	FP
Active positive	FN	TP

$$\text{Specificity} = \frac{TN}{TN + FP} \tag{10.14}$$

TABLE 10.6
Precision.

Test Data	Predictive Negative	Predicted Positive
Actual negative	TN	FP
Actual positive	FN	**TP**

$$\text{Precision} = \frac{TP}{TP + FP} \tag{10.15}$$

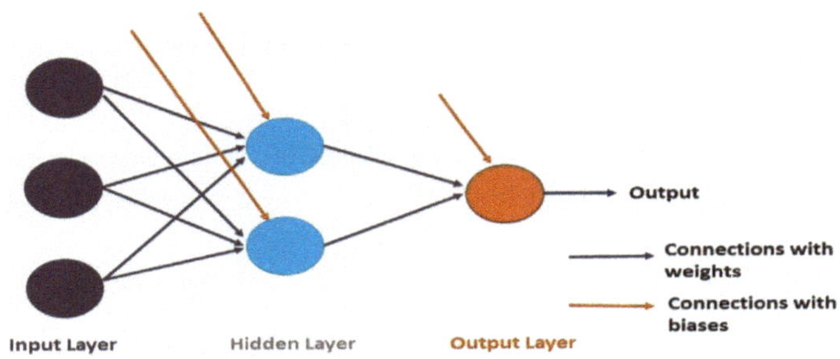

FIG. 10.6 Three-layer neural network architecture.

$$\textbf{Neural Net}_x = \sum_{i=0}^{n} A_i w_{ji} + W_O \tag{10.10}$$

Area under curve

Area under curve or AUC or area under the ROC curve is a measure of the complete region beneath the ROC curve [19].

Machine Learning-Aided Breast Cancer Detection

We are using the dataset obtained from the University of Wisconsin Hospitals, Madison, from Dr. William H. Wolberg. Our aim is to classify target attribute of the dataset consisting two types of tumor (benign or malignant). As discussed earlier, benign is nondangerous tumor, while malignant can cause cancer and hence should be predictable for further investigation. The Wisconsin Breast Cancer Database is consisting of 699 records and 11 attributes. As presented in Fig. 10.6, 458 cases of benign and 241 cases of malignant have been presented [20].

Computed features from fine needle aspirate digitized image of a breast mass is taken. A feature depicts individuality of the present cell nuclei of current image. The mean and standard error of largest values (worst) of these features were computed for each image resulting in 30 features (Figs. 10.7 and 10.8).

Dataset statistics

Features containing in a dataset are a core characteristic to predict a class through ML. Figure below is a histogram showing radius mean of malignant and benign tumor where most frequent malignant mean is 20 (Table 10.7 and Figs. 10.9 and 10.10).

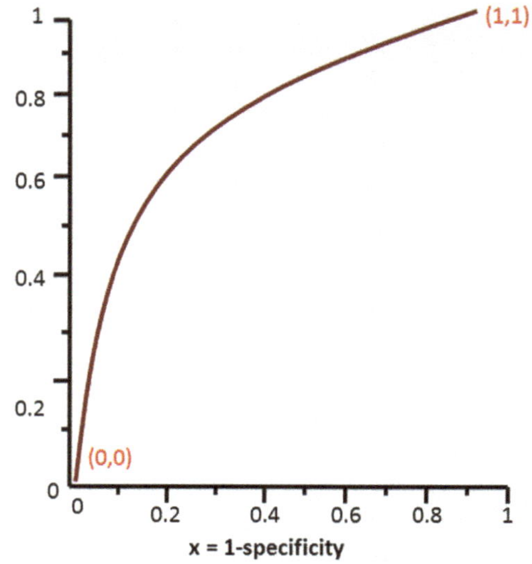

FIG. 10.7 ROC curve showing sensitivity (TPR) and 1-specificity (FPR) at different classification cut-off (threshold).

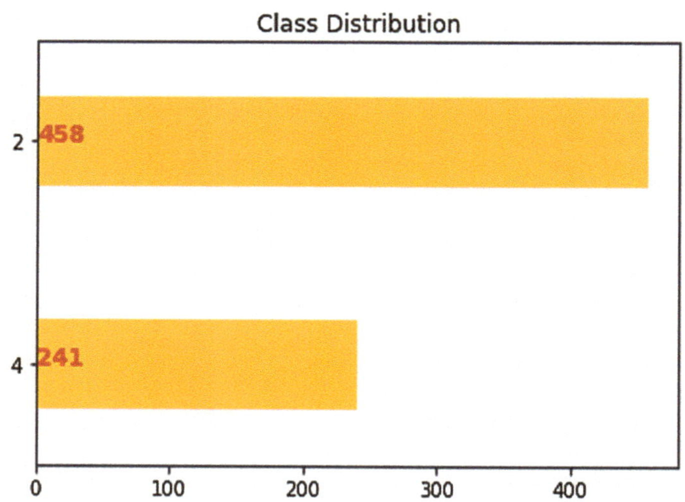

FIG. 10.8 Breast cancer dataset class distribution.

TABLE 10.7
ML Classifier Result of Breast Cancer Dataset.

Matrices & measures	Logistic Regression	SVM	KNN	NB	DT	NN
Accuracy	93%	93%	95%	92%	93%	98%
Precision	96%	94%	98%	92%	88%	96%
Recall	91%	86%	89%	84%	93%	96%
F1 – Score	56%	90%	93%	88%	90%	96%
Misclassification	.64%	.64%	.04%	.04%	.64%	.03%
Confusion Matrices: Actual Negative (TN, FP)	108, 7	112, 3	114, 1	111, 4	108, 7	113, 2
Confusion Matrices: Actual Positive (FN, TP)	4, 52	8, 48	6, 50	9, 47	4, 52	5, 51

Total test Sample	Predictive Negative	Predictive Positive
Actual Negative	TN	FP
Actual Positive	FN	TP

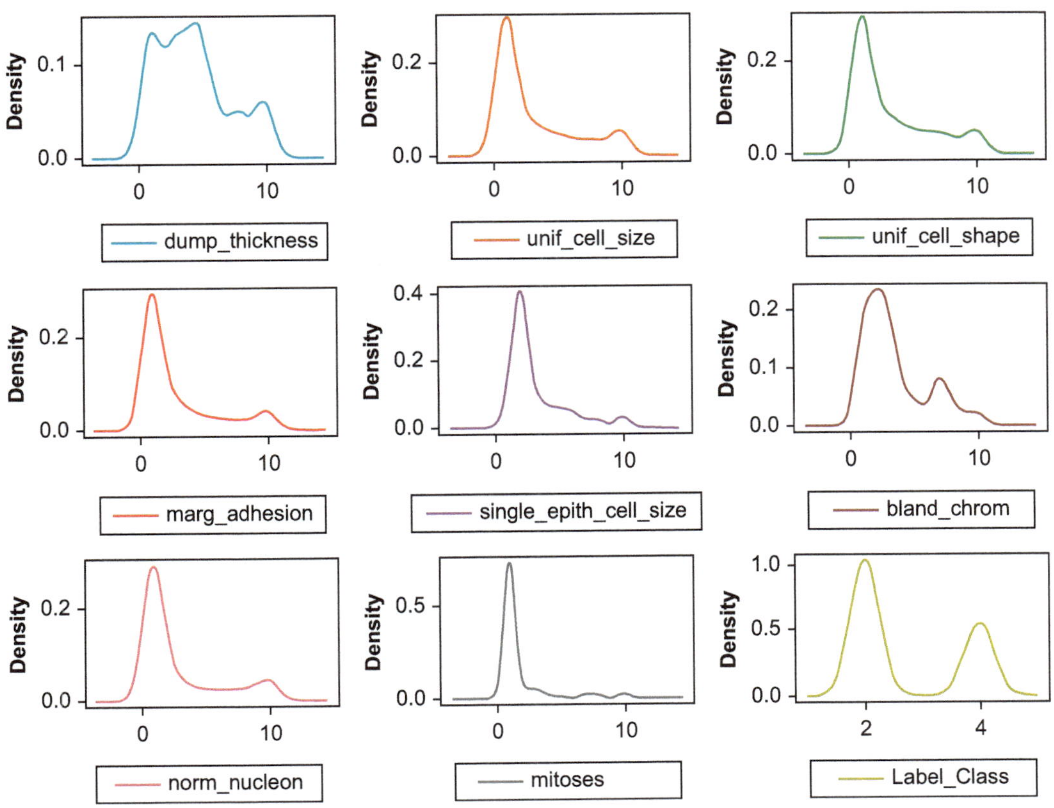

FIG. 10.9 Density graph attribute of breast cancer dataset.

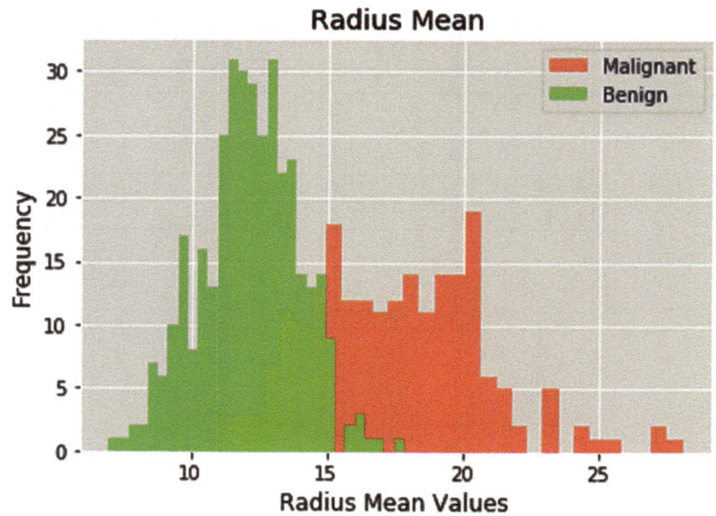

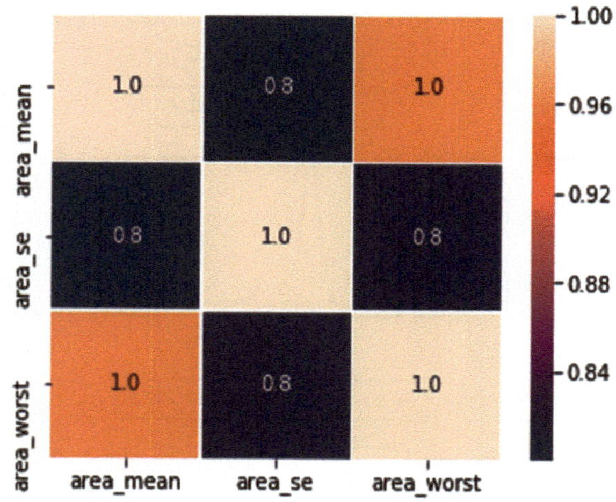

FIG. 10.10 Correlation Map (area_mean, area_se, area_worst).

CONCLUSION

Various concepts, risk factors, models, and available tools related to breast cancer are discussed in this chapter. Primary challenges and available treatment of breast cancer and possible breast cancer investigation are discussed. In addition to this, amalgamation of AI and ML with respect to breast cancer diagnosis and prognosis are discussed which definitely help in reduction of painful surgeries for precise confirmation of disease. Various ML algorithms such as LG, SVM, KNN, NB, DT, and NN are applied on breast cancer dataset for constructing breast cancer detecting system. Model constructed through NN is observed as best model for breast cancer detection with very less FP and FN. It can help medical domain in early diagnosis and prognosis of breast cancer.

REFERENCES

[1] V. Chaurasia, et al., Prediction of benign and malignant breast cancer using data mining techniques, Journal of Algorithms and Computational Technology 12 (2) (2018) 119–126.

[2] P. Vijay, B. Keshwani, Emergence of big data with hadoop: a review, IOSR Journal of Engineering 6 (3) (March 2016) 50–54.

[3] M. Ghoncheh, et al., Incidence and mortality and epidemiology of breast cancer in the world, Asian Pacific Journal of Cancer Prevention 17 (S3) (2016).

[4] S. Malvia, et al., Epidemiology of breast cancer in Indian women, Asia-Pacific Journal of Clinical Oncology 13 (4) (August 2017) 289–295.

[5] M. Courtney, et al., Textbook of Surgery, Diseases of the Breast, Elsevier, June 2016.

[6] Y.-S. Sune, et al., Risk factors and preventions of breast cancer, Internatoional Journal of Biological Sciences 13 (11) (November 2017) 1387–1397.

[7] S. Eva Singletary, Rating the risk factors for breast cancer, Annals of Surgery 237 (4) (April 2003) 474–482.

[8] K.K. Hunt, et al., Schwartz Textbook of Surgery, McGraw-Hill, May 2017.

[9] K.C. Oeffinger, et al., American Cancer Society, Breast cancer screening for women at average risk: 2015 guideline update from the American Cancer Society, Journal of the American Medical Association 314 (15) (2015) 1599–1614.

[10] N.S. Williams, P.R. O'connell, A.W. McCaskie, Bailey & Love's Short Practice of Surgery, March 2010.

[11] H.J. Motlak, S.I. Hakeem, Detection and classification of breast cancer based-on terahertz imaging technique using artificial neural network & K-nearest neighbor algorithm, International Journal of Applied Engineering Research 12 (21) (2017).

[12] A. Conner-Simons, Using Artificial Intelligence to Improve Early Breast Cancer Detection, CSAIL, 2017.

[13] M. Awad, R. Khanna, Efficient Learning Machines, vol. 2, Springer, April 2015, 1.

[14] D. Barbic, et al., Logistic regression analysis of financial literacy implications for retirement planning in Croatia, CRORR Journal 7 (December 2016).

[15] P. Vijay, B. Keswani, Support vector machine (SVM) kernels based approach for detection of breast cancer, CASS 2 (2) (November 2018).

[16] X. Yu, X. yu, The research on an adaptive k-nearest Neighbors classifier, IEEE International Conference on Cognitive Informatics 5 (8) (July 2006).

[17] B.S. Mounika Yadav, S.B. Velagaleti, Challenges in handling imbalanced big data: a survey, International Journal of Current Engineering and Scientific Research 5 (3) (2018).

[18] A.J. Mehta, et al., A multi-layer artificial neural network architecture design for load forecasting in power systems, World Academy of Science, Engineering and Technology International Journal of Electrical and Computer Engineering 5 (2) (July 2011).

[19] Hossin, Sulaiman, A review on evaluation metrics for data classification evaluations, International Journal of Data Mining and Knowledge Management Process 5 (March 2015).

[20] Breast Cancer Wisconsin (Original) Data Set. https://archive.ics.uci.edu/ml/datasets/Breast+Cancer+Wisconsin+%28Original%29.

CHAPTER 11

Terahertz Molecular Imaging and Its Clinical Applications

PRAVEEN KUMAR POOLA, PHD • YOGEENTH KUMARESAN, PHD •
ILYA KRASNIKOV, PHD • ALEKSEI SETEIKIN, PHD

INTRODUCTION

Terahertz (THz) waves lies in the electromagnetic spectrum in the range from 0.1 to 10 THz. This frequency range has a corresponding wavelength range from 3 mm to 30 μm, wavenumber range from 3.3 to 333 cm^{-1}, energy range from 0.41 to 41 meV, and a temperature range from 1 to 100 K respectively. THz spectrum lies in between the microwave spectrum and infrared spectrum as shown in Fig. 11.1. The THz spectrum was unexplored and unutilized as of now, so the name became popular as "Terahertz gap." The main obstacle in using this THz band is its lack of THz wave generation and detection. To bridge this gap and use this spectrum efficiently, during 1980–90s, various groups have worked on the generation and detection of ultrafast lasers to make it possible to work with the THz waves [1–9]. Optical rectification was used for the generation of THz [10], and electro-optic effect was developed for the detection of THz signal [11]. These developments have provided with the larger bandwidths compared with the earlier THz developmental techniques. Using these new developments combined with the photoconductive switching principle has allowed to perform live imaging [12]. Mickan et al. [12] have performed THz imaging on leaf to study the THz radiation with varying water content from the leaf base to its apex, margin, veins, and midribs. The experimental results from Hu and Nuss et al. [13] have revealed the spectroscopic information of the sample using the absorption (Ab) and refraction of THz waves. Later, THz waves also experimentally demonstrated on water containing specimens to correlate the Ab and refraction coefficients to physically meaningful parameters. This THz wave feature of relating THz wave properties to physical parameters is absent in other spectral regions has opened the new door to study the plethora of applications. The main industries which benefitted by using this THz waves are food, biology, metrology, and forensic to identify the whole range of molecules present in the sample [14,15].

THz spectroscopy uses low-energy and nonionizing radiation, which makes the THz energy interaction with the living matter different from that of ionizing radiation techniques such as X-rays, and gamma rays, which uses high energy. Moreover, many biological studies have revealed strong spectral fingerprints in THz spectrum [16–22]. The above advantages make the THz technology to sit in a front seat as a diagnostic tool to identify these biomolecules in various intrabiomedical branches.

The increase in number of publications from Fig. 11.2 shows the THz radiation potential as a clinical tool to identify various cancer stages in a label-free and noninvasive manner by identifying intrinsic THz spectroscopic biomarkers [23,24]. Recent experiments have suggested that in the absence of thermal effects, THz radiation can provoke the changes in tissues and cells at molecular level [25–28]. To analyze the thermal effects with respect to THz radiation, a number of numerical simulation were performed and reported in the literature [29–32].

To reveal the biological effects due to THz waves, in vitro cell cultures were the good start because of the consistency and reproducibility of experiments [25,26,33–35]. In order to evidently discriminate the THz effects on cells from other thermal and spurious effects, maintaining the cells in their living physiological conditions is important. The living condition parameters such as temperature, pH, and CO_2 should be constantly maintained throughout the THz exposure time period [35].

THz can provide submillimeter imaging resolution in axial direction and up to a few hundred microns of spatial resolution [36,37]. THz imaging suffers less from scattering effects in tissue when compared with

Terahertz Biomedical and Healthcare Technologies. https://doi.org/10.1016/B978-0-12-818556-8.00011-2

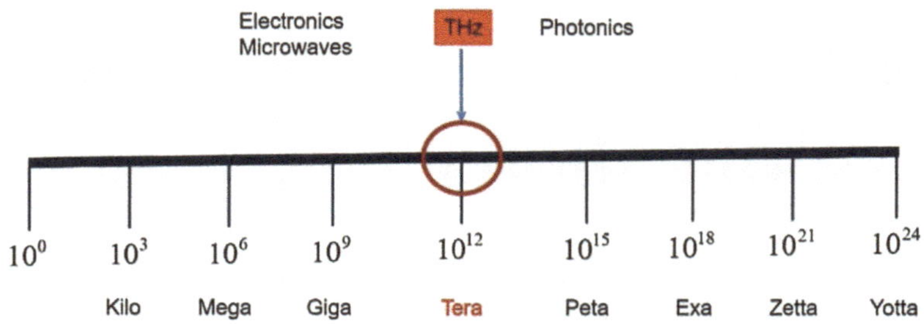

FIG. 11.1 Electromagnetic spectrum.

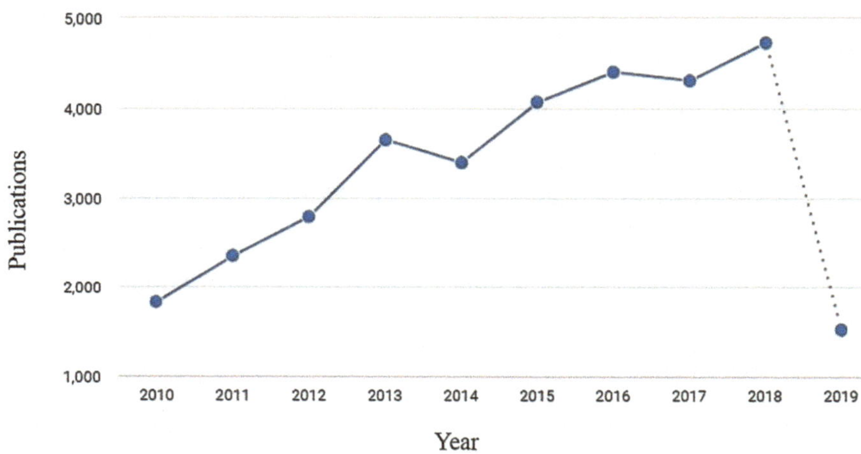

FIG. 11.2 The progress in terahertz imaging research measured as number of publications per year.

visible light imaging. THz imaging was first demonstrated on human skin to differentiate the benign and malignancy [38]. After this, many researchers have started investigating THz imaging on breast tissues, oral tissues, skin burns to assess tumor margin identification, and brain tissues [24,29,39–45]. This progress is evident from Fig. 11.2 as the number of publications increases from year to year. Using the keyword "Terahertz Imaging," we have generated Fig. 11.2 using "https://app.dimensions.ai./ In this chapter, we cover the THz applications on various biomedical fields and explore THz potential in clinical applications as an intraoperative tool.

THz imaging uses different methods to generate the contrast to identify the molecular changes occurring at the microscopic level. In soft tissues, THz imaging achieves better contrast than many other imaging techniques. Tissue fixation using formalin is a routine method for the tissue to preserve, but this process will reduce the achievable contrast while imaging [46,47]. Some of the other contrast mechanisms are explained below.

DARK-FIELD TECHNIQUE

Dark-field image will be formed with no illumination around the sample and only the scattered light from the sample alone is responsible for image formation. This simple technique produces useful image contrast to differentiate between the stained and unstained biological tissues [48].

PHASE CONTRAST IMAGING TECHNIQUE

Phase contrast image is formed due to the difference in phase between the sample and reference arm. So basically the phase contrast image is formed with the help of interferometer concept. The phase difference between the sample arm and reference arm will change due to the difference in refractive index (RI) between the specimen and its surrounding area [49].

ADDING CONTRAST AGENTS

The other way to enhance the contrast is by using contrast agents such as gold nanorods (GNRs). When IR light is illuminated on to the tissue with GNRs injected into it, it results into a generation of strong THz radiation because of the temperature rise around the GNR due to the generation of plasma polarities around the GNRs. This target-specific GNR Ab effect is more prominent in the case of cancer cells. This phenomenon of GNRs has successfully explored in oncology [50–52].

TERAHERTZ CLINICAL APPLICATIONS

The Ab and refraction of THz waves are explored in soft tissues for disease diagnostics in the skin, breast oral and colon, etc. The investigations from the number of biological samples have signified a greater RI and Ab coefficient values for tumor tissues when compared with healthy tissues. These studies make the THz imaging as a golden standard to discriminate normal tissue from the diseased tissue. THz imaging has been explored immensely in various fields ranging from food, metrology, forensic sciences, medicine, and biology. In this chapter, we focused exclusively on the healthcare and biomedical applications using THz waves.

THZ IMAGING OF SKIN

The THz amplitude E_{max} reveals the surface features, whereas the same amplitude normalized by the $|E_{min}|$ provides depth information. Woodward et al. [45] have performed THz imaging experiments to discriminate healthy tissues from the in vitro basal cell carcinoma (BCC). Woodward et al. have clearly distinguished the *in vitro* skin regions with inflammation, disease, and normal using THz image. The depth information of the skin tissue was also clearly shown using the THz time-domain image.

Wallace et al. [53–55] have reconfirmed that using the terahertz pulsed imaging (TPI), it is possible to delineate the tumor margins from the normal regions prior to surgery. This THz technology in a portable form was used to conduct this study in a clinical setting. This portable system results on a primary BCC, bland-looking lesion, and nodular BCC (diseased). Wallace et al. have shown the excised tissue THz image at t = 3.12 ps and t = 2.8 ps signifying the size of the tumor directly after excision at depth. In an another study, Wallace et al. have shown the differentiation of inflammatory crust and normal tissue from the surface image (E_{min}) formed at t = 2.8 ps. They has also reported a tumor depth of ~0.25 mm indicating the extent of tumor below the surface. All the THz image results from this study are well correlated with the histology results. For further experimental details and figures, refer to Ref. [45,53–55].

Pickewell et al. [56] have applied THz imaging on human skin epidermis from the mean volar forearm. The results of RI and Ab coefficient are shown in Fig. 11.3.

Fig. 11.4 shows the mean spectral data of RI and Ab coefficient with 95% confidence interval from 10 patients having BCC and normal skin. BCC tissue shows a higher RI than the normal tissue and is more pronounced between the 0.25 and 0.75 THz range. This observation

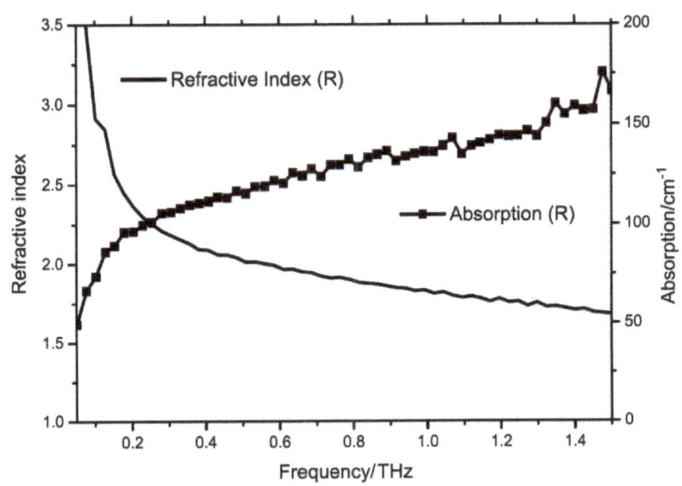

FIG. 11.3 Complex refractive index and absorption coefficient of an epidermis calculated from a volar forearm using the terahertz pulsed imaging reflection measurements. (All images were reproduced with permission from E. Pickwell, B.E. Cole, A.J. Fitzgerald, M. Pepper, V.P. Wallace, In vivo study of human skin using pulsed terahertz radiation, Physics in Medicine and Biology 49(9) (2004) 1595.)

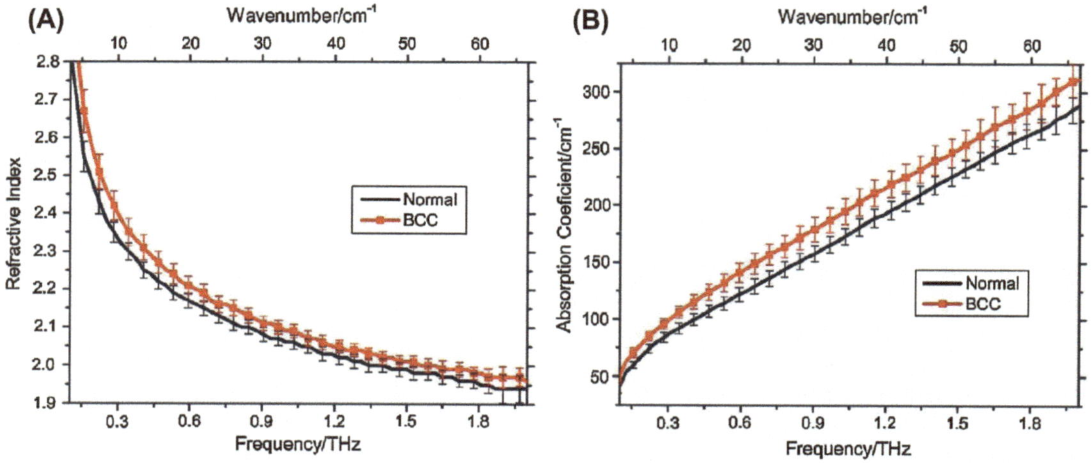

FIG. 11.4 **(A)** The measured refractive index. **(B)** The measured absorption coefficient on a basal cell carcinoma (BCC) and normal tissue. (All images were reproduced with permission from E. Pickwell, A.J. Fitzgerald, B.E. Cole, P.F.Taday, R.J. Pye, T. Ha, V.P. Wallace, Simulating the response of terahertz radiation to basal cell carcinoma using ex vivo spectroscopy measurements, Journal of Biomedical Optics 10(6) (2005) 064021.)

can act as a good biomarker for cancer detection. Fig. 11.4A shows the RI coefficient, whereas Fig. 11.4B shows the Ab coefficient α, which is consistently higher for BCC than for normal tissue at 0.5 THz. The difference increases by 25 cm^{-1} at two THz [57].

Similarly, Pickwell et al. [58] have applied the THz imaging to calculate the RI and Ab coefficient on a water, ex vivo human skin, and adipose tissue. It is evident from Refs. [58] that skin and water have similar RI values, while the Ab coefficient indicates similar trend for water, skin, and adipose tissue. The inference from this study is that THz radiation would propagate deeper into the adipose tissue than in the skin.

This study is more focused on THz imaging of tissues at 22 and -33^0. Hiromichi et al. [59] have used the TPI system to measure the frozen porcine biological tissue properties. Fig. 11.5 A–E shows the time-domain waveforms on no sample, adipose tissue, striated muscle, and interface at 22 and −33°C. Fig. 11.5 F–I shows the measured RI on different tissue samples mentioned above. Fig. 11.5J shows a 2-D plot of the measured Ab at 1.0 THz representing tiny spots on the adipose tissue in a striated muscle. While Fig. 11. 5K image maps the THz time-domain maximum peak positions showing the difference of adipose tissue, striated muscle, and interface.

Parrott et al. [60] have studied the effect of THz signal at five positions namely forehand, cheek, chin, forearm, and palm. From Fig. 11.6, it is evident that at first three positions, the THz signal has shown similar response with a small variation in the initial peak signal followed by a large trough. But in contrast, a more pronounced peak is observed in the THz signal for the dorsal forearm and palm [60].

In another application, THz imaging was explored to measure human scars. Fan et al. [61] have explored the THz imaging to calculate the in vivo human skin scars for improving scar treatment and management as shown in Fig. 11.7. In this work, authors have shown that the RI plays a prominent role even after months of postinjury in comparison to the Ab coefficient. The results are nicely summarized and visualized in Figs. 11.7 and 11.8 showing the images and coefficients of RI and Ab values of the human scars postinjury.

THZ IMAGING OF ORAL LESION SCREENING

The need for accurate 3D reconstruction of teeth tissue structure is essential for resolving the clinical problems. At present, there is an urgent need for a nondestructive technique to perform fast disease screening method. In order to test the THz imaging in this direction, Crawley et al. [62] have made an attempt to measure the thickness of dental enamel and also to quantify the enamel erosion problems. The study was conducted on a pilot human incisor. Teeth structures up to depth are shown accurately to within 10 mm in Fig. 11.9. Using THz radiation, tooth sample was imaged. The palatal and labial surfaces are images for this study. In the THz image, the enamel–dentine interface looks light on dark, whereas the enamel–air interface looks dark on light. The thickness of the enamel was calculated to be

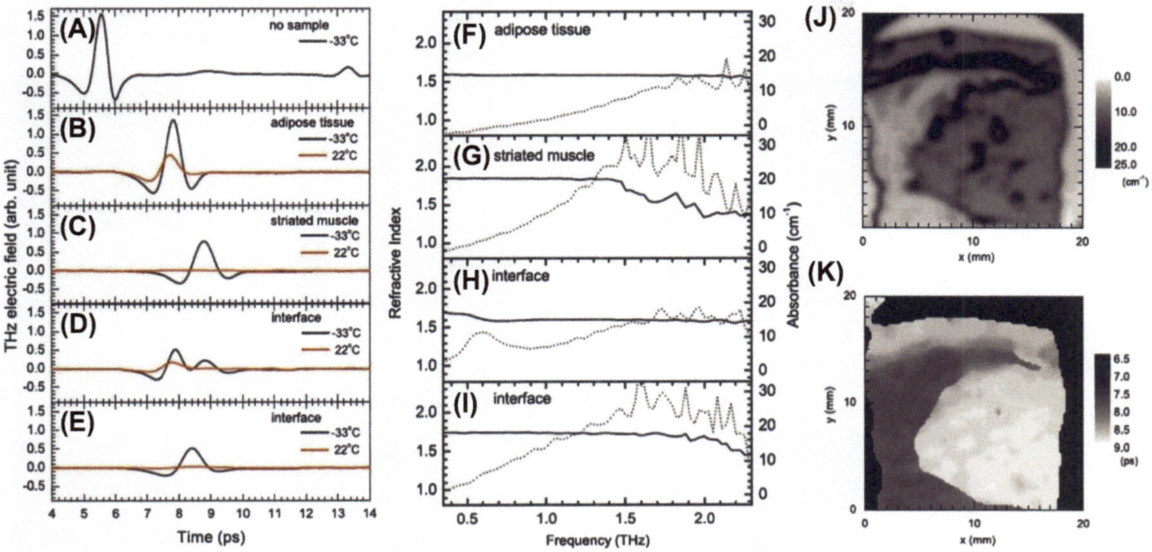

FIG. 11.5 **(A–E)** Terahertz (THz) signal representing the traced positions at 22^0 and -33^0. **(F–I)** Refractive index (RI) and absorption (Ab) coefficients measured on a porcine tissue at −33°C. **(J, K)** Ab corresponding images at 1.0 THz. (All images were reproduced with permission from H. Hoshina, A. Hayashi, N. Miyoshi, F. Miyamaru, C. Otani, Terahertz pulsed imaging of frozen biological tissues, Applied Physics Letters 94 (12) (2009) 123901.)

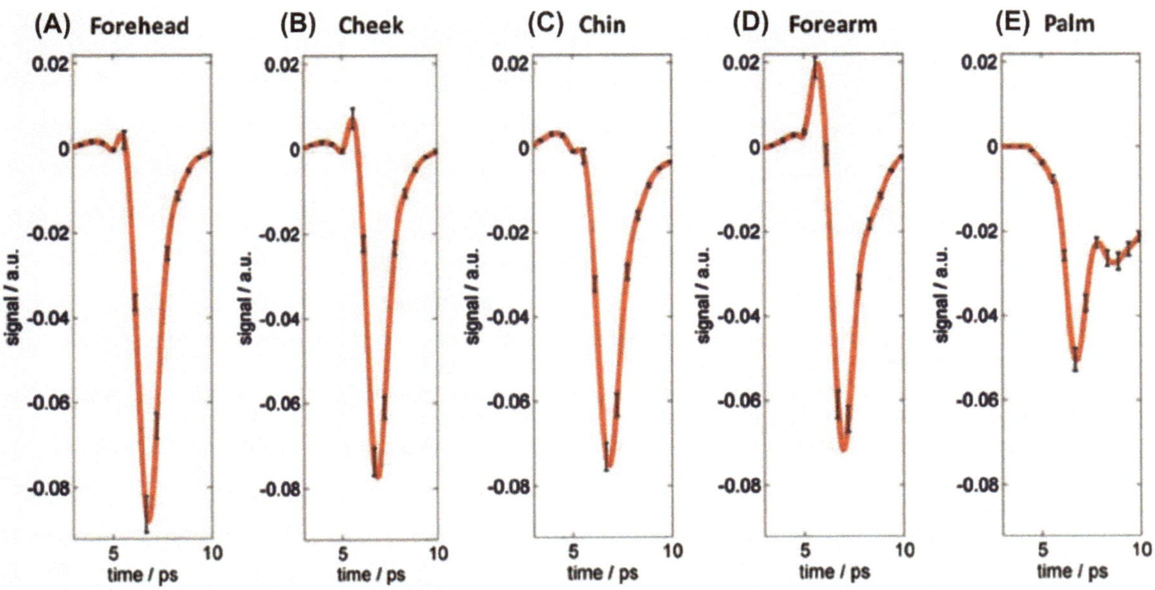

FIG. 11.6 Terahertz signal measured at **(A)** forehand, **(B)** cheek, **(C)** chin, **(D)** forearm, and **(E)** palm, respectively. (All images were reproduced with permission from E.P. Parrott, S.MY Sy, T. Blu, V.P. Wallace, E. Pickwell-MacPherson, Terahertz pulsed imaging in vivo: measurements and processing methods. Journal of Biomedical Optics 16(10) (2011) 106010.)

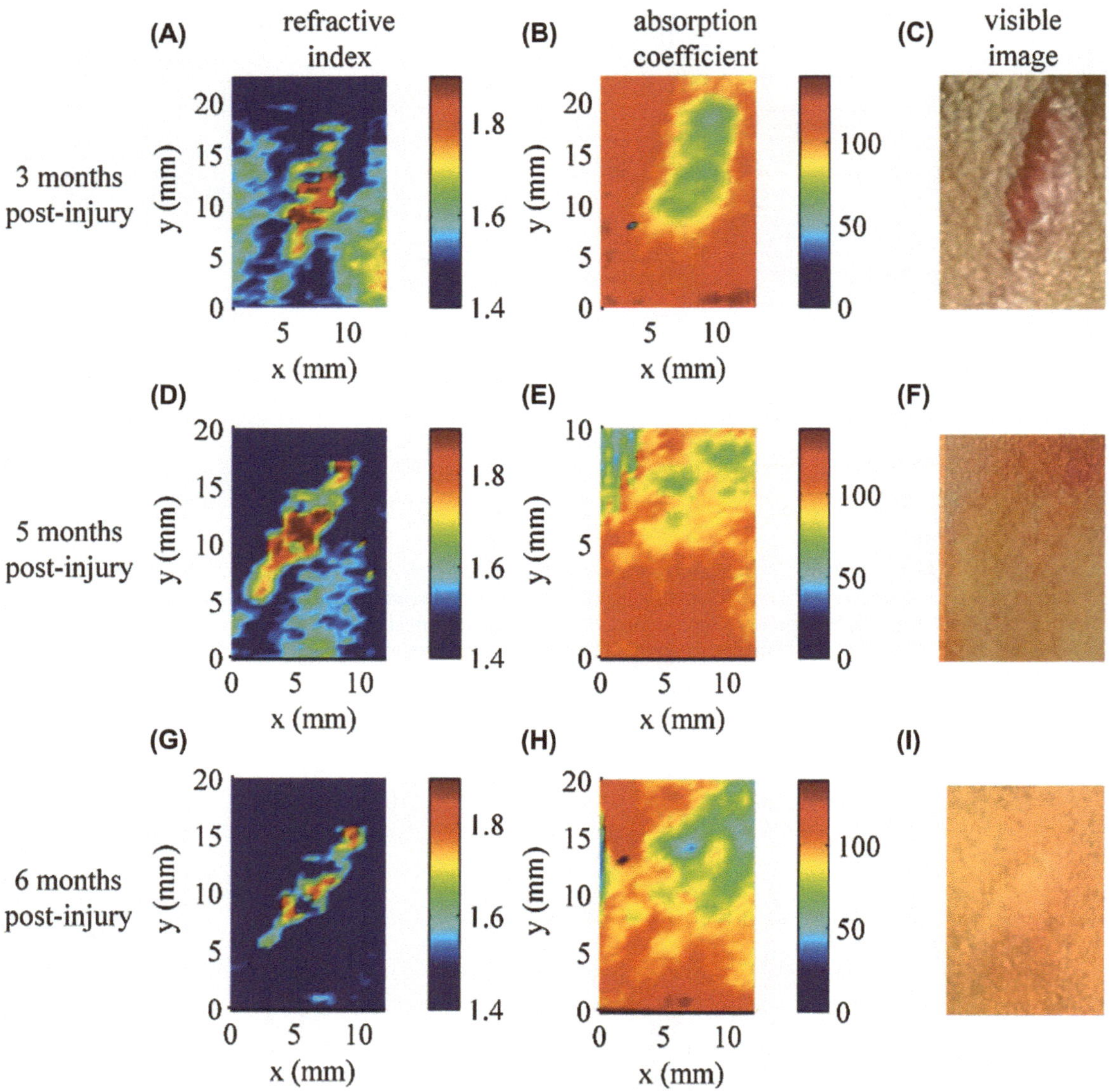

FIG. 11.7 Terahertz images of refractive index and absorption coefficient measurements at different time periods. **(A, B, C)** Measurements are acquired after 3 months postinjury. **(D, E, F)** Measurements are acquired after 5 months postinjury. **(G, H, I)** Measurements are acquired after 6 months postinjury. (All images were reproduced with permission from S. Fan, B.S.Y. Ung, E.P.J. Parrott, V.P. Wallace, E. Pickwell-MacPherson, In vivo terahertz reflection imaging of human scars during and after the healing process, Journal of biophotonics 10(9) (2017) 1143–1151.)

between 0.4 and 0.9 mm. This study was conducted systematically on a set of 12 dental samples.

The in vitro healthy tooth images with several continuous ranges of frequencies at 0.21 THz, 0.43 THz, 0.6 THz, 1.28 THz, and 1.49 THz are shown in Fig. 11.10. Each of the images has 56 × 56 pixels with a pixel size of 180 μm. We can observe from Fig. 11.10 that with the increase in THz frequency, the spatial resolution also increases which in turn clearly differentiates the dentine and enamel area. Using these demonstration abnormalities in the sample can be located very easily [29].

Nazarov et al. [63] have used THz imaging to measure the Ab and RI coefficient at various enamel and dentin areas marked with circles on the optical images as shown in Fig. 11.11. This study has used a frequency range of 0.1–3 THz. The sample thickness varies among

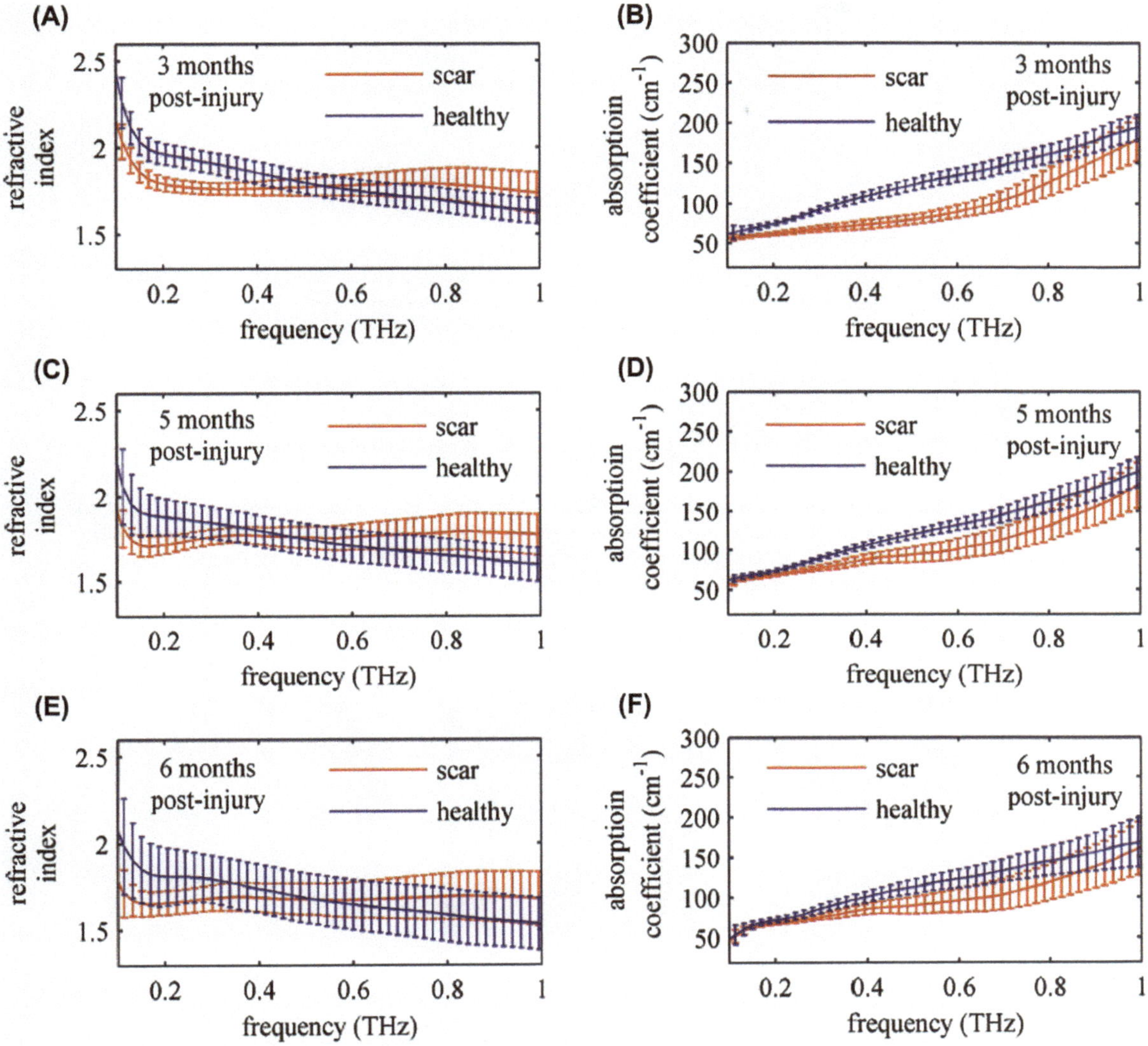

FIG. 11.8 The measured postinjury optical properties like refractive index (RI) and absorption (Ab) coefficients on a healthy and scar skin. **(A)** and **(B)** show the RI and Ab coefficients measured after 3 months postinjury; **(C)** and **(D)** show the RI and Ab coefficients measured after 5 months postinjury; **(E)** and **(F)** show the RI and Ab coefficients measured after 6 months postinjury. (All images were reproduced with permission from S. Fan, B.S.Y. Ung, E.P.J. Parrott, V.P. Wallace, E. Pickwell-MacPherson, In vivo terahertz reflection imaging of human scars during and after the healing process, Journal of biophotonics 10(9) (2017) 1143–1151.)

230–470 μm. We can observe from Fig. 11.11 that different tooth areas have similar Ab spectra, whereas refraction spectra show a big difference for various areas on the tooth in comparison with Ab spectra.

Sim et al. [43,44] have explored the THz imaging for the analysis of oral cancer at −20°C and 20°C temperatures. The study was performed between 0.2 and 1.2 THz frequency range. The experimental results demonstrated in this work could easily distinguish the healthy tissue (mucosa) from the oral lesion. From Fig. 11.12, we can see that THz imaging results where the first column (A) shows the optical images of six oral samples, second column (B) shows the THz images at frozen temperature, third column (C) shows the THz images at room temperature, and the fourth (D) is the histology images of the six tissues for

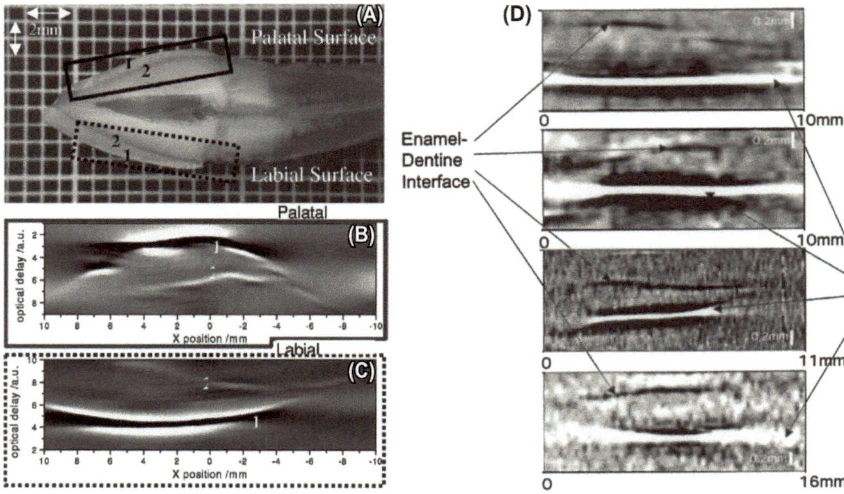

FIG. 11.9 **(A)** Optical image of a human incisor. **(B, C)** Terahertz images of the corresponding palatal and labial surfaces. **(D)** Enamel–air interface and enamel–dentine interface. (All images were reproduced with permission from D.A. Crawley, C. Longbottom, V.P. Wallace, B.E. Cole, D.D. Arnone, M. Pepper, Three-dimensional terahertz pulse imaging of dental tissue, Journal of Biomedical Optics 8, (2) (2003) 303–308.)

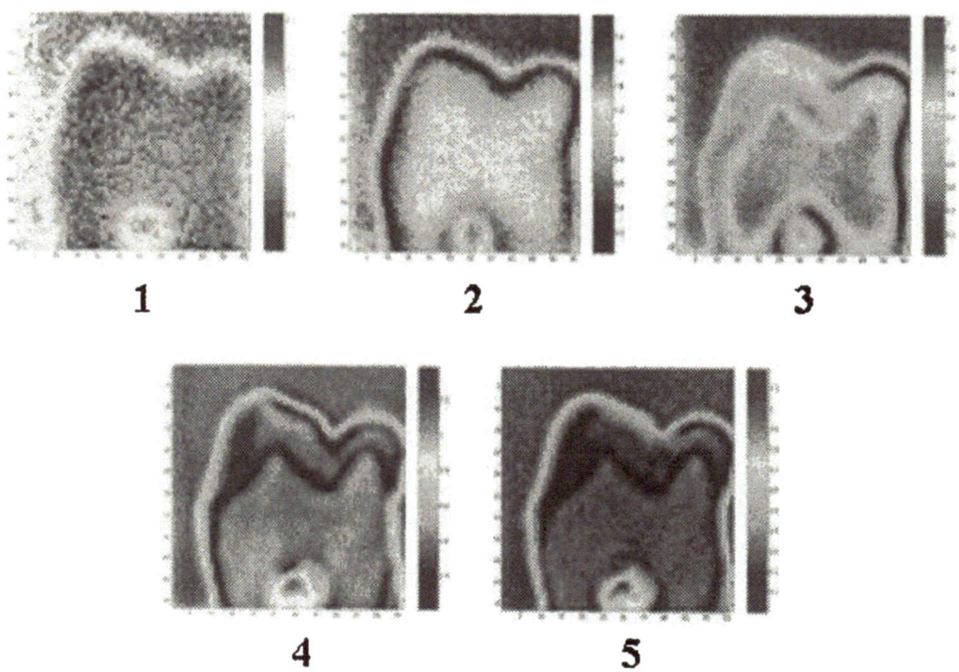

FIG. 11.10 THz images at **(1)** 0.21 THz, **(2)** 0.43 THz, **(3)** 0.6 THz, **(4)** 1.28 THz, and **(5)** 1.49 THz continuous frequency range. (All images were reproduced with permission from A.J. Fitzgerald, E. Berry, N.N. Zinovev et al., An introduction to medical imaging with coherent terahertz frequency radiation, Physics in Medicine and Biology 47 (2002) R67.)

comparison. The cancer lesions are marked with blue in Fig. 11.12D. Fig. 11.13 has shown the THz Ab and RI spectra of normal mucosa and oral cancer at 20^0 and -20^0 temperature with a 95% confidence interval. The average values of Ab and RI coefficient have shown a smaller value in oral cancer tissue than in normal mucosa at 20^0 temperatures. This analysis serves as a marker for identifying the cancer tissue.

Kistenev et al. [64] have performed THz spectroscopy on saliva sample to diagnose the oral lichen planus with subgroups of erosive and reticular form as shown in Fig. 11.14. The absorption of the THz radiation was plotted in terms of $\log(I_c/I_b)$ on the frequency, where I_c and I_b are the intensities passing through cuvette "b" and "c." The results demonstrated have shown a 100% differential classification accuracy between the oral lichen subgroups and control group.

THZ IMAGING OF BREAST CANCER TISSUES

THz radiation was used to investigate the breast cancer tissues due to its noninvasive nature of this imaging modality. For this purpose, Ashworth et al. [41] have used a portable THz spectrometer and a mouse model. In the frequency range 0.15–2.0 THz, the THz system distinguish the healthy breast tissue from the cancerous breast tissue. The tumor with its surrounding adipose tissue is visible in the E_{max} image and is well correlated with the E_{max}/E_{min} image, where only the tumor is visible.

Simultaneously, complex RI and Ab coefficient values are used for classification of adipose, fibrous breast, and breast cancer tissues. Tissues with tumor have shown a higher RI and Ab coefficient than the other tissues.

THz surface imaging on ex vivo breast carcinoma tissue was measured by calculating the E_{max}. THz image could easily discriminate the adipose, fibrosis, and tumor areas. The exact correlation between the THz image and histology image shown in Wallace et al. [53,55] have clearly shows the potential of THz imaging as a future histology method in breast cancer analysis [53,55].

Fitzgerald et al. [65] have used excised human breast specimen to investigate the TPI to find the margins between the tumor and healthy tissue. This study has revealed that under controlled conditions, TPI can differentiate in situ ductal carcinoma from the invasive carcinoma with lobular features. From the THz images shown in Ref. [65], we will know the exact size and shape of the tumor regions.

Chui-Min Chiu et al. [66] have used THz fiber-scanning near-field imaging system to identify the breast tumor from the normal tissue. The developed system uses a 0.3 THz frequency and has a compact size can easily fit into the pathology lab in place of optical microscope due to its better contrast.

Using the same system, different breast cancer case studies were performed to study the potential of THz system potential in evaluating the tumor tissue with different states or grades. Overall Hua Chen et al. [66a] have shown the capability of THz imaging system on 20 different cancer grades.

THZ IMAGING OF BRAIN TISSUES

THz time-domain spectroscopy (TDS) investigations on the mouse model were performed by Shi et al. [67], to distinguish the Alzheimer disease (AD) tumor brain tissue from the normal tissue. In this comparative study, Ab coefficient has revealed more information than the RI, in particular, the number of tryptophan molecules closely associated with the AD brain tissue was strongly shown at 1.44, 1.8, and 2.114 THz frequencies as shown in Fig. 11.15A and B. The results demonstrated in this study will be useful for the early diagnosis of AD. In addition, the absorption spectrum of normal tissue and AD tissue has suggested that tryptophan in AD brain tissue is less bonded to other molecules than in normal brain tissue. Fig. 11.15A and C measurements were performed on tissues with thickness 150 μm, whereas Fig. 11.15B and D measurements are on tissue with thickness 250 μm.

Meng et al. [68] have investigated paraffin-embedded brain glioma (PEBG) using THz-TDS system. The experimental parameters such as Ab, RI coefficients, and dielectric constants on PEBG show higher Ab, RI coefficient, and dielectric constants than the normal brain tissue. As it was observed from Fig. 11.16A and B that relative rates of various experimental parameters like Ab, RI coefficient, dielectric constant (both real and imaginary), and datum line have shown a better contrast for frequencies below 1.0 THz. Whereas between 1.7 and 2.0 THz range only RI and real part of the dielectric constant shows better contrast.

THz pulsed spectroscopy investigation on ex vivo human brain gliomas was performed by Gavdush et al. [69] to study the THz response of edema. The results demonstrated in these experiments have suggested that edema and tumor have similar THz responses. The experimental parameters investigated are Ab coefficient (Fig. 11.17B and E, H, K), RI (Fig. 11.17A and D, G, J), and H&E-stained histology

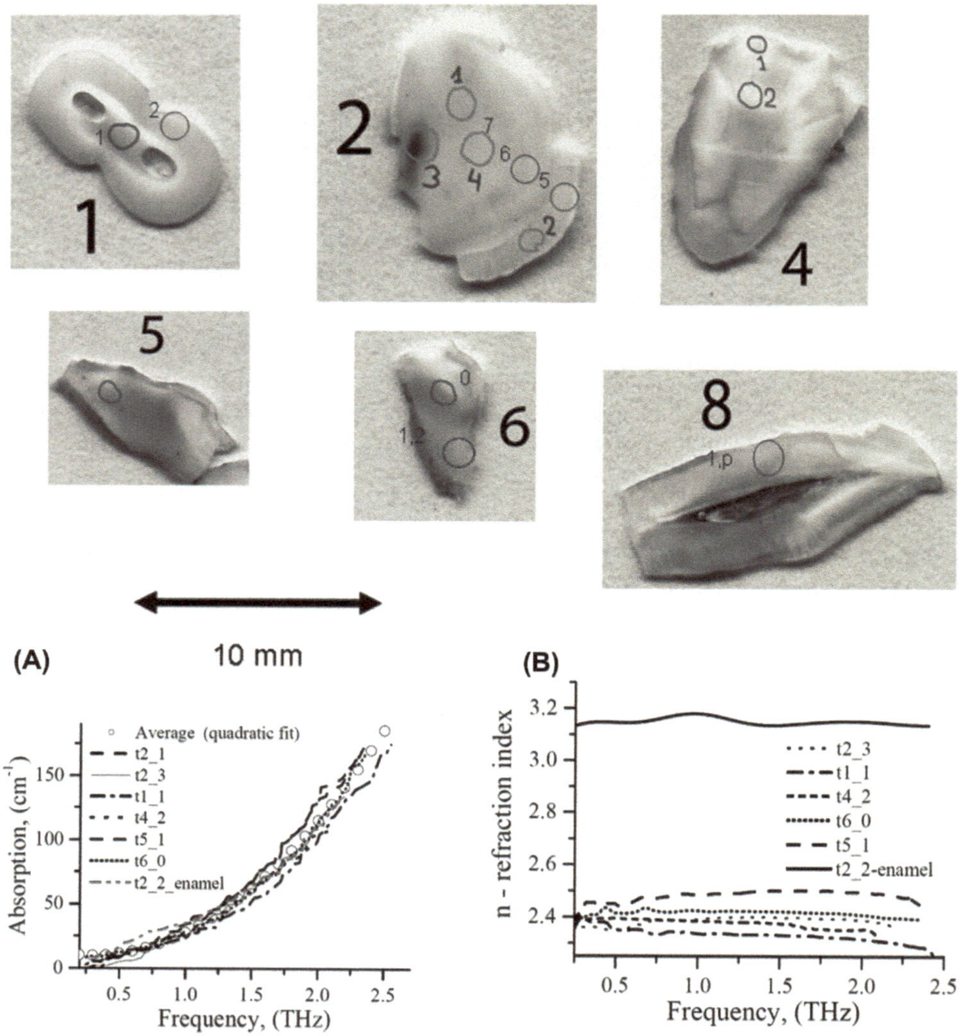

FIG. 11.11 Teeth specimen areas marked by circles are scanned by terahertz (THz) radiation. **(A, B)** Measured absorption and refraction index spectra of different teeth specimen at different tooth areas. (All images were reproduced with permission from M. M. Nazarov, A. P. Shkurinov, V. V. Tuchin. Tooth study by terahertz time-domain spectroscopy, in: Saratov Fall Meeting 2007: Optical Technologies in Biophysics and Medicine IX, vol. 6791, International Society for Optics and Photonics, 2008. p. 679109.)

images (Fig. 11.17C and F, I, L), which are measured on ex vivo human brain containing graded gliomas regions with intact and edematous tissues. The error bars represent a 2.0σ confidential interval of measurements, assuming fluctuation of optical properties within each tissue sample and each tissue class. To unalter the THz response, human glioma tissues are embedded in gelatin.

THz spectroscopy investigation on fresh rat brain tissue was performed by yamaguchi et al. [70] to distinguish the tumor tissue from the normal tissue. Fig. 11.18A shows the optical image of brain tissue consists of the tumor inside marked red in color. Fig. 11. 18B shows the H&E image, whereas Fig. 11.18C and D shows the normal and tumor tissue images. The recorded RI and Ab coefficient are shown in

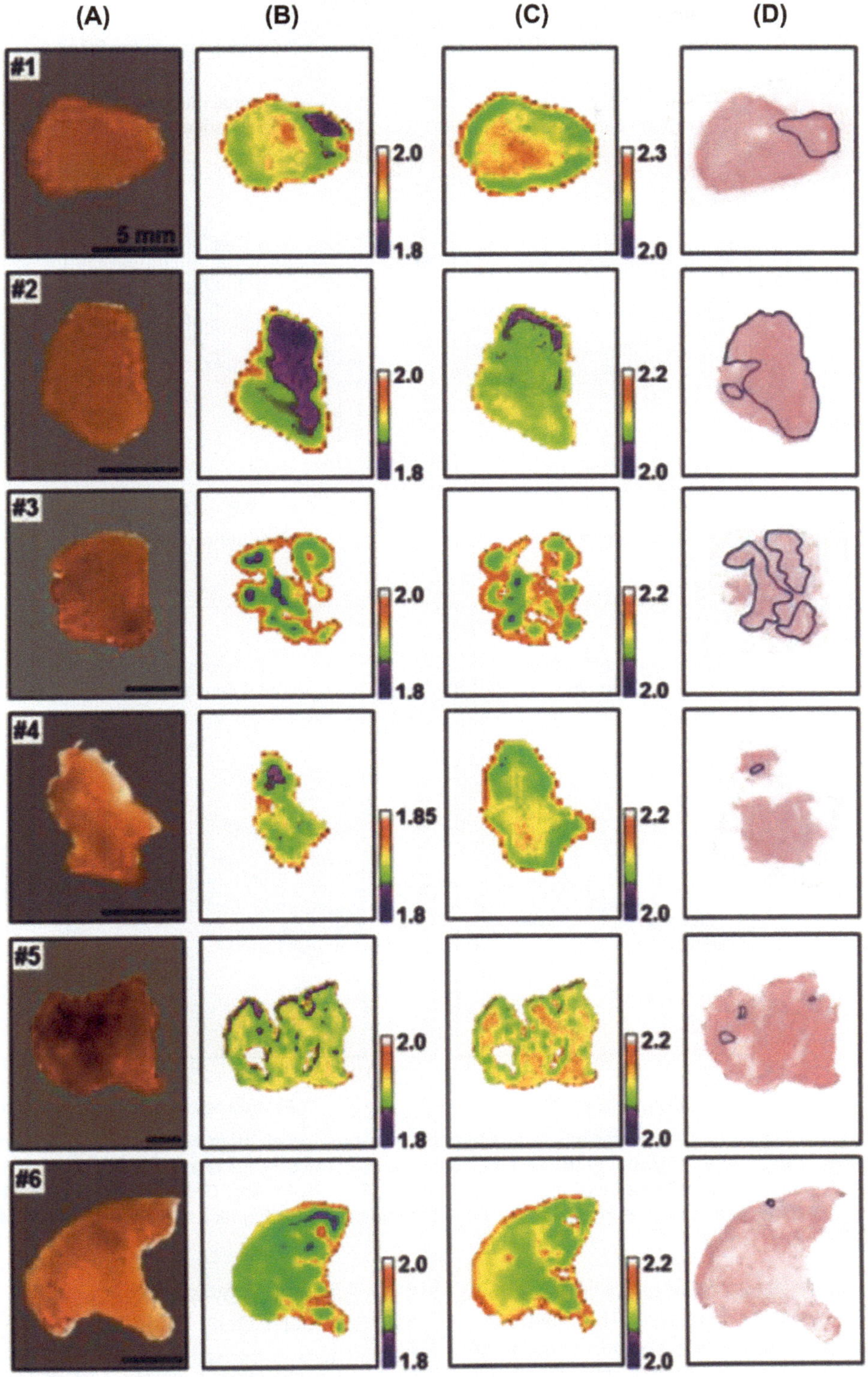

FIG. 11.12 Analysis of six oral lesions, **(A)** optical images of tissue lesions, **(B)** Terahertz (THz) images measured at frozen temperature, **(C)** THz images measured at room temperature, and **(D)** histopathological images. (All images were reproduced with permission from Y.C. Sim, J.Y. Park, K.-M. Ahn, C. Park, J.-H. Son, Terahertz imaging of excised oral cancer at frozen temperature, Biomedical Optics Express 4 (8) (2013b) 1413–1421.)

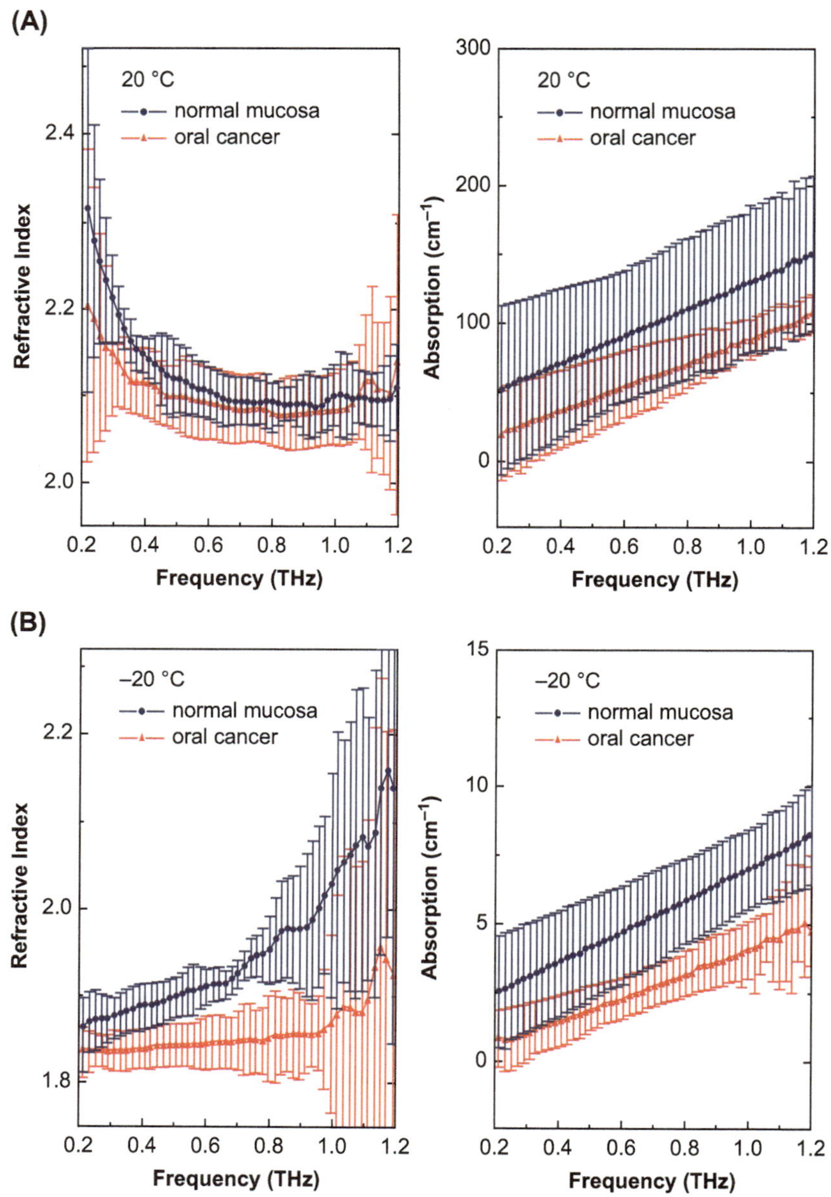

FIG. 11.13 The RI and Ab coefficient parameters are measured on six normal mucosa and oral cancer specimens at **(A)** a 20°C temperature **(B)** a −20°C temperature in the 0.2–1.2 THz frequency range. (All images were reproduced with permission from Y.C. Sim, J.Y. Park, K.-M. Ahn, C. Park, J.-H. Son, Terahertz imaging of excised oral cancer at frozen temperature, Biomedical Optics Express 4 (8) (2013b) 1413–1421.)

Fig. 11.18E and F suggest that tumor regions have higher RI than normal tissue regions. The experiments were repeated on 10 fresh tissue samples without any preprocessing. The data consistency on 10 samples shows the potential of THz imaging as a future in vivo diagnostic tool in brain tumor imaging.

THZ IMAGING OF VARIOUS MISCELLANEOUS TISSUES

Several tissues excised from rat model were investigated using the THz spectroscopy using reflection geometry. Huang et al. [71] have examined tissues include liver, kidney, heart muscle, leg muscle,

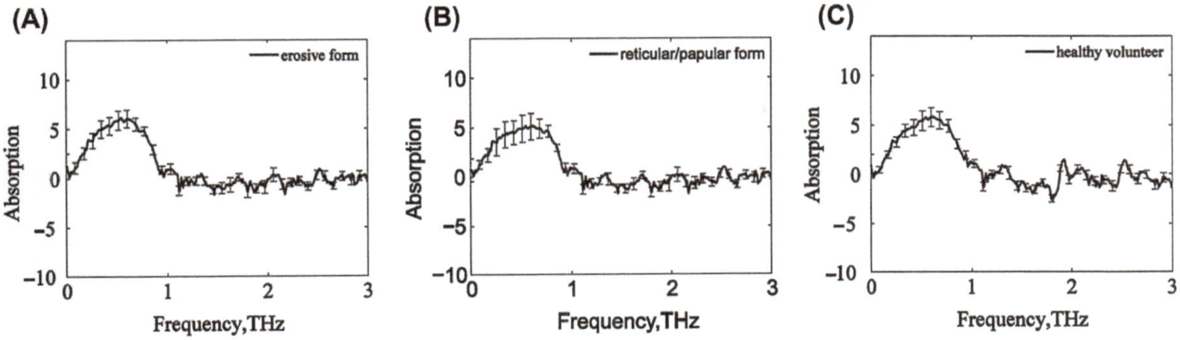

FIG. 11.14 Absorption of terahertz (THz) radiation on **(A)** patients with erosive oral lichen planus (OLP), **(B)** reticular/papular OLP, and **(C)** the control group (healthy). (All images were reproduced with permission from Y.V. Kistenev, A.V. Borisov, M.A. Titarenko, O.D. Baydik, A.V. Shapovalov, Diagnosis of oral lichen planus from analysis of saliva samples using terahertz time-domain spectroscopy and chemometrics, Journal of Biomedical Optics 23 (4) (2018) 045001.)

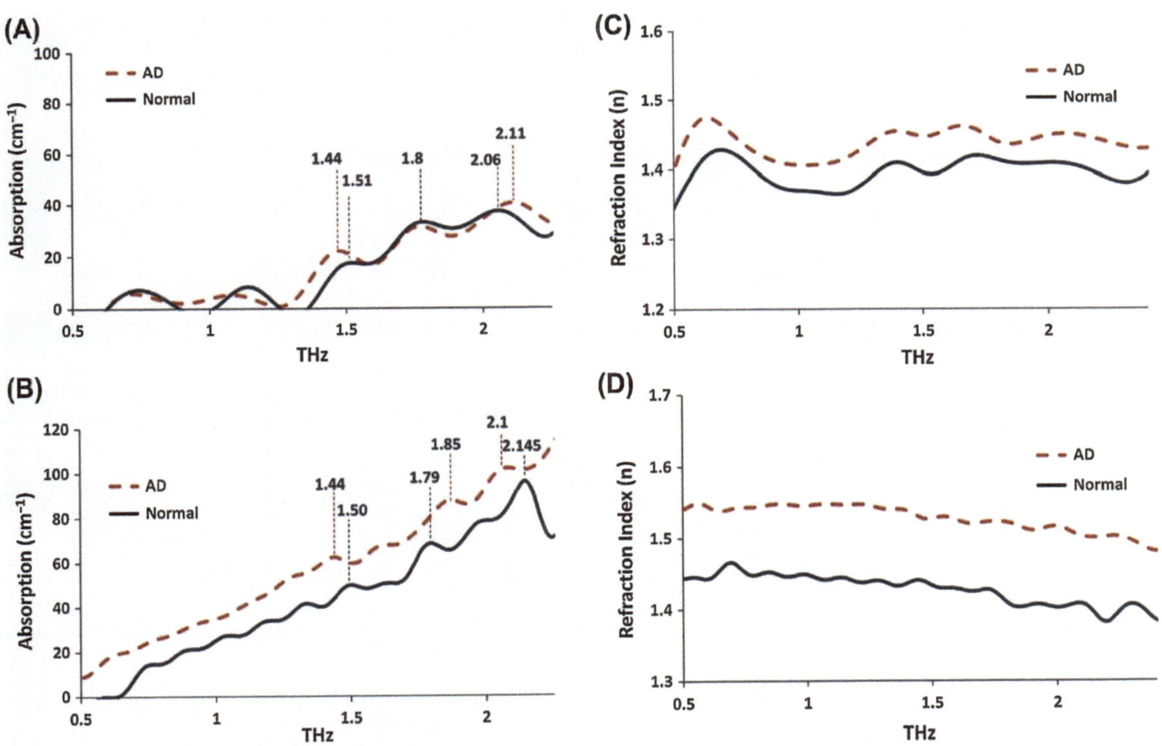

FIG. 11.15 Absorption (Ab) and refractive index (RI) spectra of terahertz (THz) radiation on Alzheimer disease (AD) and normal brain tissue. **(A)** Ab coefficient measured on tissue thickness of 150 μm. **(B)** Ab coefficient measured on tissue thickness of 250 μm. **(C)** RI of THz waves transmitted through AD and normal tissues (thickness of tissue was 150 μm). **(D)** RI of THz waves transmitted through AD and normal tissues (thickness of tissue was 250 μm). (All images were reproduced with permission from L. Shi, P. Shumyatsky, A. Rodríguez-Contreras, R.R. Alfano, Terahertz spectroscopy of brain tissue from a mouse model of Alzheimer's disease, Journal of Biomedical Optics 21 (1) (2016) 015014.)

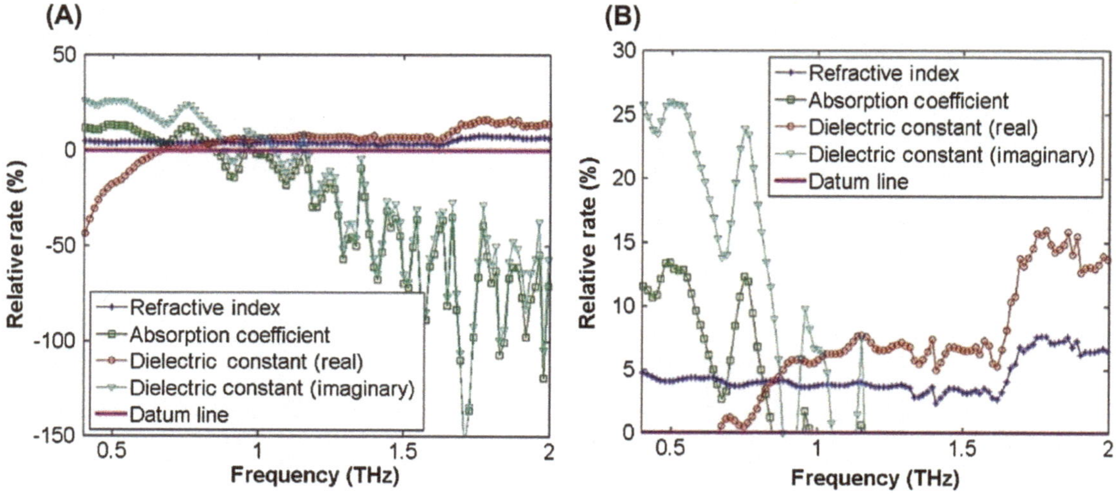

FIG. 11.16 Relative rates of the refractive index, absorption coefficient, and dielectric constant. **(A)** The full cycle of the curves. **(B)** Only the positive cycle of the curves. (All images were reproduced with permission from K. Meng, T.-nan Chen, T. Chen, L.-guo Zhu, Q. Liu, Z. Li, F. Li et al., Terahertz pulsed spectroscopy of paraffin-embedded brain glioma, Journal of Biomedical Optics 19 (7) (2014) 077001.)

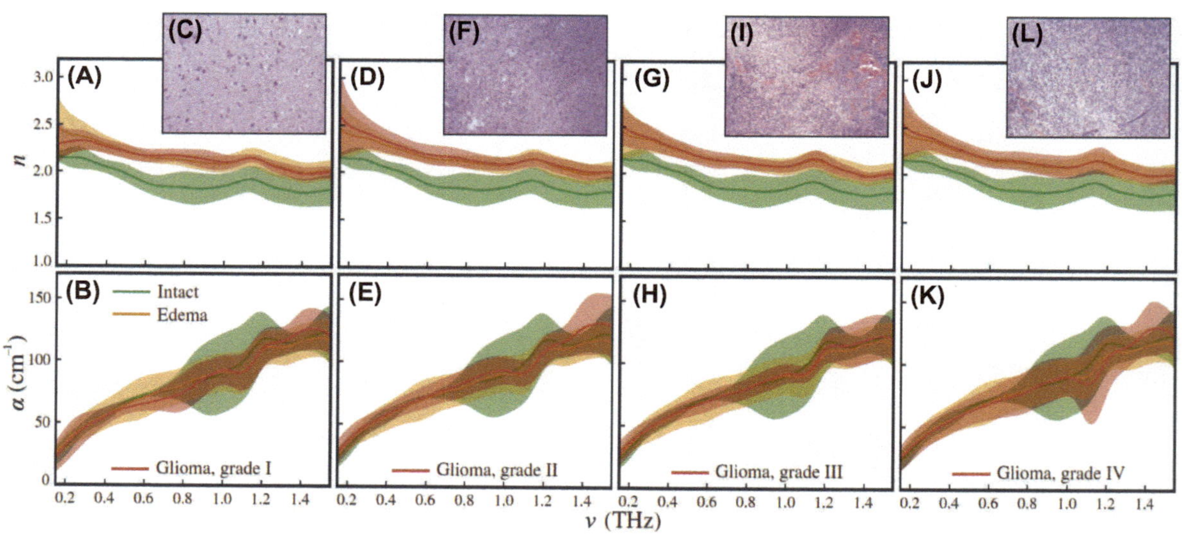

FIG. 11.17 Refractive index (n), amplitude absorption coefficient (α), and the histology of gelatin-embedded human brain gliomas of various ex vivo graded samples. **(A–C)** Belongs to the measured n, α, and histology on grade I glioma; **(D–F)** belongs to the measured n, α, and histology on grade II glioma; **(G–I)** belongs to the measured n, α, and histology on grade III glioma; **(J–L)** belongs to the measured n, α, and histology on grade IV glioma. The THz optical properties n and α of gliomas are compared with equal data for the intact and edematous tissues, averages within the entire set of brain tissue specimens. (All images were reproduced with permission from A.A. Gavdush, N.V. Chernomyrdin, K.M. Malakhov, S.-I.T. Beshplav, I.N. Dolganova, A.V. Kosyrkova, P.V. Nikitin et al. Terahertz spectroscopy of gelatin-embedded human brain gliomas of different grades: a road toward intraoperative THz diagnosis, Journal of Biomedical Optics 24 (2) (2019) 027001.)

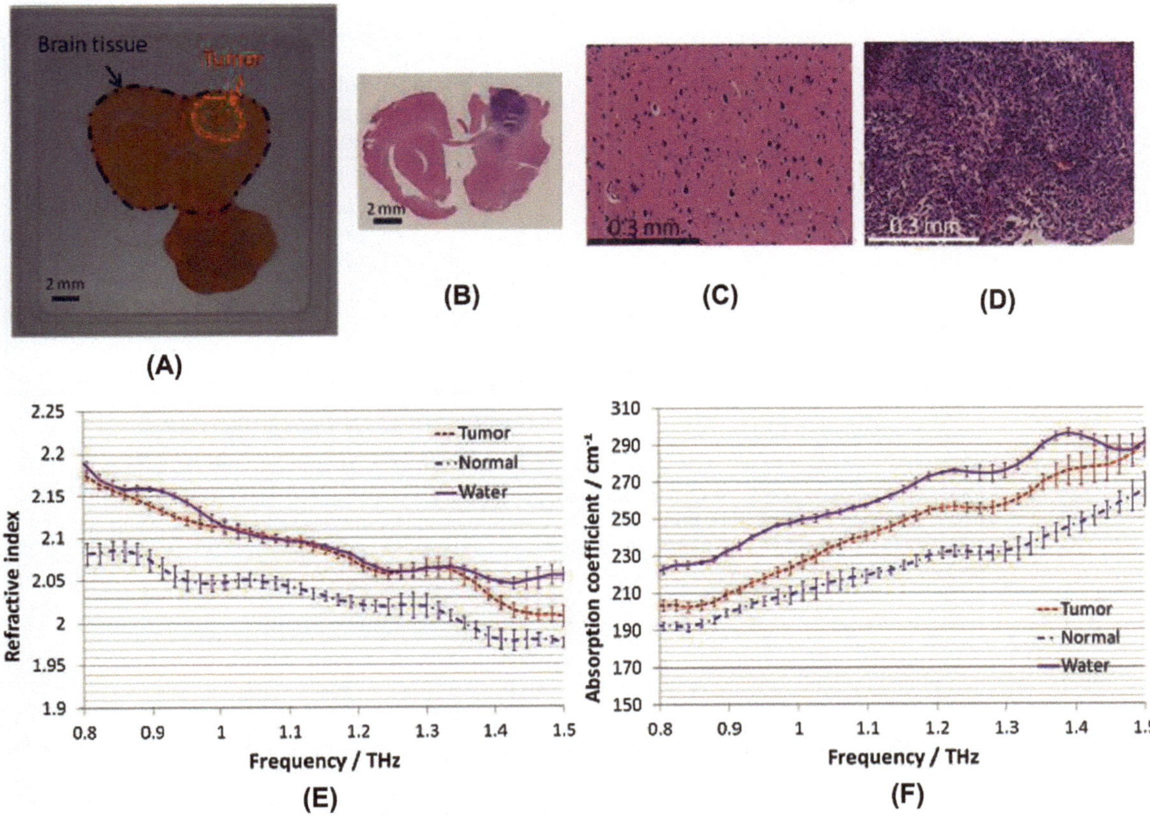

FIG. 11.18 **(A)** Optical image of a rat brain tissue sample. **(B)** Histology of whole brain tissue, **(C)** normal region, and **(D)** tumor region of an H&E stained image. **(E)** Measured RI and **(F)** measured Ab coefficient on a tumor, normal, and water regions of the rat brain tissue sample from the frequency range 0.8–1.5 THz. (All images were reproduced with permission from S. Yamaguchi, Y. Fukushi, O. Kubota, T. Itsuji, S. Yamamoto, T. Ouchi, Terahertz spectroscopy and detection of brain tumor in rat fresh-tissue samples, in: Optical Interactions with Tissue and Cells XXVI, vol. 9321. International Society for Optics and Photonics, 2015. p. 93210O.)

pancreas, and abdominal fat tissue and found that Ab coefficient measured from the several tissues clearly distinguishes each of the tissue types with 95% confidence interval.

THz reflection imaging and spectroscopy was investigated by Ji et al. [72] on gastrointestinal tract tissues including large intestine (LI), glandular stomach (GS), and fore stomach (FS) excised from a rat model. From Fig. 11. 19A and B, it was observed that RI of LI and GS are 0.18–0.21 times greater than that of FS at 0.5 THz. Similarly, Ab coefficient of LI and GS are 22 cm^{-1} greater than that of FS at 0.5 THz. The RI and Ab coefficients of LI and GS are greater than those of FS due to a difference in water content.

The THz signal is sensitive to the changes in the cartilage within a knee joint. This signal was analyzed by wai chi kan et al. [73] on rabbit femoral condyle samples. The results from this study suggest that THz imaging has a potential to measure up to 0.5 mm cartilage thickness and it was shown in Fig. 11.20. Thus, in future, THz imaging could improve the study of early-stage osteoarthritis and reduce the number of animals sacrificed by allowing the repeated measurements on the same animal.

FUTURE DIRECTIONS

Being the safest imaging modality, THz technology will find an infinite number of applications in medicine and therapeutics and can surely benefit from the harmless penetrating of THz waves to make it visualize the internal information about the physical objects. The increasing theoretical and experimental data suggest that THz waves may impact the biological systems

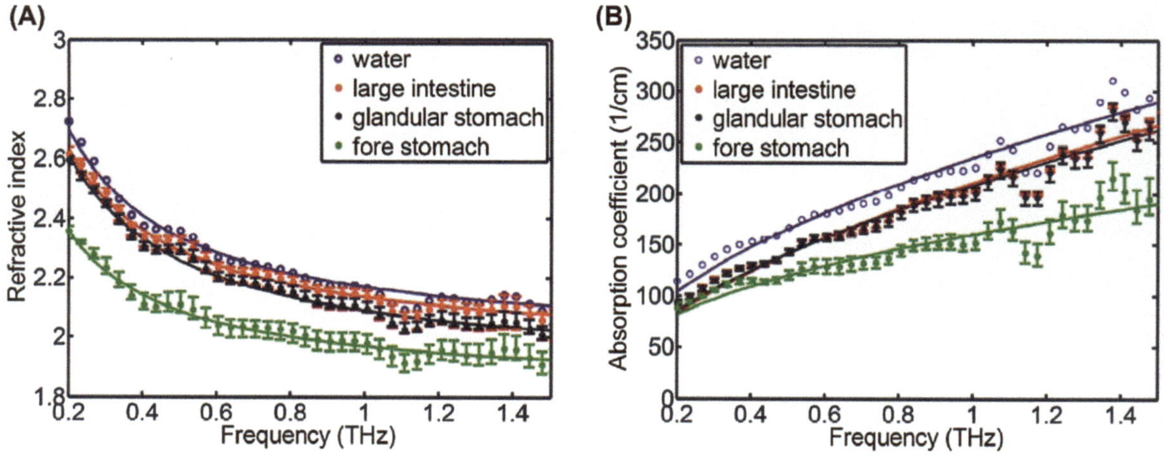

FIG. 11.19 **(A)** The measured RI of water and three gastrointestinal (GI) tract samples. **(B)** The measured absorption coefficients of water and three GI tract samples. (All images were reproduced with permission from Y.B. Ji, S.-H. Kim, K. Jeong, Y. Choi, J.-H. Son, D.W. Park, S.K. Noh et al., Terahertz spectroscopic imaging and properties of gastrointestinal tract in a rat model, Biomedical Optics Express 5 (12) (2014) 4162–4170.)

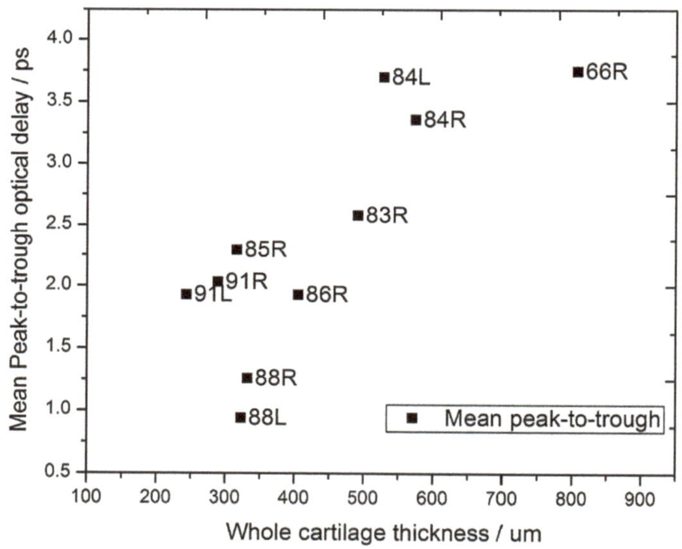

FIG. 11.20 The graph of the mean peak-to-trough THz optical delay against the mean total cartilage thickness from histology. (All images were reproduced with permission from W.-C. Kan, W.-S. Lee, W.-H. Cheung, V.P. Wallace, E. Pickwell-MacPherson. Terahertz pulsed imaging of knee cartilage, Biomedical Optics Express 1 (3) (2010) 967–974.)

and their functions. In order to create a safety THz standard for the technology and its future medical applications, the effect of THz radiation on human tissue needs to be carefully examined. These safety standards will become the benchmark for future THz technology clinical applications. The miniaturization of the THz systems for portability and ease of use also needs to be addressed because the current THz systems are bulky and complex. The need for low power THz source is also one of the future requirements, which is useful for a portable system. The next frontier in medical diagnostics is the noninvasive *in vivo* molecular imaging using THz waves. THz imaging can be used as an intraoperative tool to avoid unnecessary surgical resection of healthy tissue during the surgical operations. This intra-operative tool can, in turn, reduce the need for repeated invasive operative interventions. The challenge to address the penetration depth of THz waves at higher frequencies due to the water absorption should also be addressed.

REFERENCES

[1] P. Smith, D. Auston, A. Johnson, W. Augustyniak, Picosecond photoconductivity in radiation-damaged silicon on-sapphire films, Applied Physics Letters 38 (1981) 47–50.
[2] G. Mourou, C. Stancampiano, A. Antonetti, A. Orszag, Picosecond microwave pulses generated with a sub picosecond laser-driven semiconductor switch, Applied Physics Letters 39 (1981a) 295.
[3] G. Mourou, C.V. Stancampiano, D. Blumenthal, Picosecond microwave pulse generation, Applied Physics Letters 38 (1981b) 470–472.
[4] J.A. Valdmanis, G. Mourou, C.W. Gabel, Picosecond electro-optic sampling system, Applied Physics Letters 41 (1982) 211.
[5] D.H. Auston, K.P. Cheung, J.A. Valdmanis, D.A. Kleinman, Cherenkov radiation from femtosecond optical pulses in electro-optic media, Physical Review Letters 53 (1984) 1555.
[6] M. Ketchen, D. Grischkowsky, T. Chen, et al., Generation of subpicosecond electrical pulses on coplanar transmission lines, Applied Physics Letters 48 (1986) 751–753.
[7] J. Valdmanis, R. Fork, Design considerations for a femtosecond pulse laser balancing self phase modulation, group velocity dispersion, saturable absorption, and saturable gain, IEEE Journal of Quantum Electronics 22 (1986) 112–118.
[8] D.E. Spence, P.N. Kean, W. Sibbett, 60-fsec pulse generation from a self-mode-locked Ti:sapphire laser, Optics Letters 16 (1991) 42–44.
[9] J.-H. Son, J.V. Rudd, J. Whitaker, Noise characterization of a self-mode-locked Ti:sapphire laser, Optics Letters 17 (1992) 733–735.
[10] X.C. Zhang, X. Ma, Y. Jin, et al., Terahertz optical rectification from a nonlinear organic crystal, Applied Physics Letters 61 (1992) 3080–3082.
[11] Q. Wu, X.C. Zhang, Free-space electro-optic sampling of terahertz beams, Applied Physics Letters 67 (1995) 3523–3525.
[12] S. Mickan, D. Abbott, J. Munch, X.-C. Zhang, T. Van Doorn, Analysis of system trade-offs for terahertz imaging, Microelectronics Journal 31 (2000) 503–514.
[13] B. Hu, M. Nuss, Imaging with terahertz waves, Optics Letters 20 (1995) 1716–1718.
[14] Y.S. Lee, Principles of Terahertz Science and Technology, Springer, New York, 2009.
[15] X.C. Zhang, J. Xu, Introduction to THz Wave Photonics, Springer, New York, 2009.
[16] Y. Feng, E.W. Prohofsky, Vibrational fluctuations of hydrogen bonds in a DNA double helix with nonuniform base pairs, Biophysical Journal 57 (1990) 547–553.
[17] A. Markelz, S. Whitmire, J. Hillebrecht, R. Birge, THz time domain spectroscopy of biomolecular conformational modes, Physics in Medicine and Biology 47 (2002) 3797–3805.
[18] B.M. Fischer, M. Walther, P.U. Jepsen, Far-infrared vibrational modes of DNA components studied by terahertz time-domain spectroscopy, Physics in Medicine and Biology 47 (2002) 3807.
[19] S.M. Chitanvis, Can low-power electromagnetic radiation disrupt hydrogen bonds in dsDNA? Journal of Polymer Science Part B: Polymer Physics 44 (2006) 2740–2747.
[20] S.J. Kim, B. Born, M. Havenith, M. Gruebele, Real-time detection of protein-water dynamics upon protein folding by terahertz absorption spectroscopy, Angewandte Chemie International Edition 47 (2008) 6486–6489.
[21] O.P. Cherkasova, V.I. Fedorov, E.F. Nemova, A.S. Pogodin, Influence of terahertz laser radiation on the spectral characteristics and functional properties of albumin, Optics and Spectroscopy 107 (2009) 534–537.
[22] R.J. Falconer, A.G. Markelz, Terahertz spectroscopic analysis of peptides and proteins, Journal of Infrared, Millimeter and Terahertz Waves 33 (2012) 973–988.
[23] C.S. Joseph, A.N. Yaroslavsky, M. Al-Arashi, et al., Terahertz spectroscopy of intrinsic biomarkers for non-melanoma skin cancer, in: Presented at Proceedings of SPIE, 2009, 72150I-I-10.
[24] C. Yu, S. Fan, Y. Sun, E. Pickwell-MacPherson, The potential of terahertz imaging for cancer diagnosis: a review of investigations to date, Quantitative Imaging in Medicine and Surgery 2 (2012) 33–45.
[25] B.S. Alexandrov, K.Ø. Rasmussen, A.R. Bishop, et al., Non-thermal effects of terahertz radiation on gene expression in mouse stem cells, Biomedical Optics Express 2 (2011) 2679.
[26] B.S. Alexandrov, M.L. Phipps, L.B. Alexandrov, et al., Specificity and heterogeneity of terahertz radiation effect on gene expression in mouse mesenchymal stem cells, Scientific Reports 3 (2013) 1184.
[27] K.-T. Kim, J.H. Park, S.J. Jo, et al., High-power femtosecond-terahertz pulse induces a wound response in mouse skin, Scientific Reports 3 (2013) 2296.
[28] L.V. Titova, A.K. Ayesheshim, A. Golubov, et al., Intense picosecond THz pulses alter gene expression in human skin tissue in vivo, in: Presented at Proceedings of SPIE 8585: 85850Q-Q-10, San Francisco, CA, 2013.
[29] A.J. Fitzgerald, E. Berry, N.N. Zinovev, et al., An introduction to medical imaging with coherent terahertz frequency radiation, Physics in Medicine and Biology 47 (2002) R67.
[30] E. Berry, G.C. Walker, A.J. Fitzgerald, et al., Do in vivo terahertz imaging systems comply with safety guidelines? Journal of Laser Applications 15 (2003) 192.
[31] T.T.L. Kristensen, W. Withayachumnankul, P.U. Jepsen, D. Abbott, Modeling terahertz heating effects on water, Optics Express 18 (2010) 4727e4739.
[32] G. Wilmink, J. Grundt, Invited review article: current state of research on biological effects of terahertz radiation, Journal of Infrared, Millimeter and Terahertz Waves 32 (2011) 1074e1122.

[33] R.H. Clothier, N. Bourne, Effects of THz exposure on human primary keratinocyte differentiation and viability, Journal of Biological Physics 29 (2003) 179–185.

[34] J. Bock, Y. Fukuyo, S. Kang, et al., Mammalian stem cells reprogramming in response to terahertz radiation, PloS One 5 (2010) e15806.

[35] R. Williams, A. Schofield, G. Holder, et al., The influence of high intensity terahertz radiation on mammalian cell adhesion, proliferation and differentiation, Physics in Medicine and Biology 58 (2013) 373–391.

[36] P.H. Siegel, Terahertz technology in biology and medicine, IEEE Transactions on Microwave Theory and Techniques 52 (2004) 2438–2447.

[37] X.-C. Zhang, Terahertz wave imaging: horizons and hurdles, Physics in Medicine and Biology 47 (2002) 3667–3677.

[38] R.M. Woodward, B.E. Cole, V.P. Wallace, et al., Terahertz pulse imaging in reflection geometry of human skin cancer and skin tissue, Physics in Medicine and Biology 47 (2002) 3853.

[39] R.M. Woodward, V.P. Wallace, R.J. Pye, et al., Terahertz pulse imaging of ex vivo basal cell carcinoma, Journal of Investigative Dermatology 120 (2003a) 72–78.

[40] P.C. Ashworth, P. O'Kelly, A.D. Purushotham, et al., An intra-operative THz probe for use during the surgical removal of breast tumors, in: Presented at 33rd International Conference on Infrared, Millimeter and Terahertz Waves, Pasadena, CA, 2008, pp. 1–3.

[41] P.C. Ashworth, E. Pickwell-MacPherson, E. Provenzano, et al., Terahertz pulsed spectroscopy of freshly excised human breast cancer, Optics Express 17 (2009) 12444–12454.

[42] M.H. Arbab, T.C. Dickey, D.P. Winebrenner, et al., Terahertz reflectometry of burn wounds in a rat model, Biomedical Optics Express 2 (2011) 2339.

[43] Y.C. Sim, K.-M. Ahn, J.Y. Park, C. Park, J.-H. Son, Temperature-dependent terahertz imaging of excised oral malignant melanoma, IEEE Journal of Biomedical and Health Informatics 17 (2013a) 779–784.

[44] Y.C. Sim, J.Y. Park, K.-M. Ahn, C. Park, J.-H. Son, Terahertz imaging of excised oral cancer at frozen temperature, Biomedical Optics Express 4 (8) (2013b) 1413–1421.

[45] R.M. Woodward, V.P. Wallace, D.D. Arnone, E.H. Linfield, M. Pepper, Terahertz pulsed imaging of skin cancer in the time and frequency domain, Journal of Biological Physics 29 (2e3) (2003b) 257–259.

[46] P.C. Ashworth, E. Pickwell-MacPherson, S.E. Pinder, et al., Terahertz spectroscopy of breast tumors, in: Infrared and Millimeter Waves, 2007 and the 15th International Conference on Terahertz Electronics, 2007. IRMMWTHz. Joint 32nd International Conference on IEEE, 2007, pp. 603–605.

[47] Y. Sun, B.M. Fischer, E. Pickwell-MacPherson, Effects of formalin fixing on the terahertz properties of biological tissues, Journal of Biomedical Optics 14 (2009) 064017.

[48] T. Löffler, T. Bauer, K.J. Siebert, et al., Terahertz dark-field imaging of biomedical tissue, Optics Express 9 (2001) 616–621.

[49] K. Edward, T.W. Mayes, B. Hocken, F. Farahi, Trimodal imaging system capable of quantitative phase imaging without 2p ambiguities, Optics Letters 33 (2008) 216–218.

[50] X. Huang, I.H. El-Sayed, W. Qian, M.A. El-Sayed, Cancer cell imaging and photothermal therapy in the near infrared region by using gold nanorods, Journal of the American Chemical Society 128 (2006) 2115–2120.

[51] J.W. Lee, J.M. Yang, H.J. Ko, et al., Multifunctional magnetic gold nanocomposites: human epithelial cancer detection via magnetic resonance imaging and localized synchronous therapy, Advanced Functional Materials 18 (2008) 258–264.

[52] S.J. Oh, J. Kang, I. Maeng, et al., Nanoparticle-enabled terahertz imaging for cancer diagnosis, Optics Express 17 (2009) 3469–3475.

[53] V.P. Wallace, A.J. Fitzgerald, E. Pickwell, et al., Terahertz pulsed spectroscopy of human basal cell carcinoma, Applied Spectroscopy 60 (2006a) 1127–1133.

[54] V.P. Wallace, A.J. Fitzgerald, S. Shankar, et al., Terahertz pulsed imaging of basal cell carcinoma ex vivo and in vivo, British Journal of Dermatology 151 (2004) 424–432.

[55] V.P. Wallace, E. MacPherson, A.J. Fitzgerald, T. Lo, E. Provenzano, S. Pinder, A. Purushotham, Terahertz pulsed imaging and spectroscopy of breast tumors, in: Optical Methods in the Life Sciences, Vol. 6386, International Society for Optics and Photonics, 2006, p. 638610.

[56] E. Pickwell, B.E. Cole, A.J. Fitzgerald, M. Pepper, V.P. Wallace, In vivo study of human skin using pulsed terahertz radiation, Physics in Medicine and Biology 49 (9) (2004) 1595.

[57] E. Pickwell, A.J. Fitzgerald, B.E. Cole, P.F. Taday, R.J. Pye, T. Ha, et al., Simulating the response of terahertz radiation to basal cell carcinoma using ex vivo spectroscopy measurements, Journal of Biomedical Optics 10 (6) (2005) 064021.

[58] E. Pickwell, V.P. Wallace, Biomedical applications of terahertz technology, Journal of Physics D: Applied Physics 39 (17) (2006) R301.

[59] H. Hoshina, A. Hayashi, N. Miyoshi, F. Miyamaru, C. Otani, Terahertz pulsed imaging of frozen biological tissues, Applied Physics Letters 94 (12) (2009) 123901.

[60] E.P. Parrott, S.M.Y. Sy, T. Blu, V.P. Wallace, E. Pickwell-MacPherson, Terahertz pulsed imaging in vivo: measurements and processing methods, Journal of Biomedical Optics 16 (10) (2011) 106010.

[61] S. Fan, B.S.Y. Ung, E.P.J. Parrott, V.P. Wallace, E. Pickwell-MacPherson, In vivo terahertz reflection imaging of human scars during and after the healing process, Journal of Biophotonics 10 (9) (2017) 1143–1151.

[62] D.A. Crawley, C. Longbottom, V.P. Wallace, B.E. Cole, D.D. Arnone, M. Pepper, Three-dimensional terahertz pulse imaging of dental tissue, Journal of Biomedical Optics 8 (2) (2003) 303–308.

[63] M.M. Nazarov, A.P. Shkurinov, V.V. Tuchin, Tooth study by terahertz time-domain spectroscopy, in: Saratov Fall Meeting 2007: Optical Technologies in Biophysics and Medicine IX, Vol. 6791, International Society for Optics and Photonics, 2008, p. 679109.

[64] Y.V. Kistenev, A.V. Borisov, M.A. Titarenko, O.D. Baydik, A.V. Shapovalov, Diagnosis of oral lichen planus from analysis of saliva samples using terahertz time-domain spectroscopy and chemometrics, Journal of Biomedical Optics 23 (4) (2018) 045001.

[65] A.J. Fitzgerald, V.P. Wallace, M. Jimenez-Linan, L. Bobrow, R.J. Pye, A.D. Purushotham, D.D. Arnone, Terahertz pulsed imaging of human breast tumors, Radiology 239 (2) (2006) 533–540.

[66] C.-M. Chiu, H.-W. Chen, Y.-R. Huang, Y.-J. Hwang, W.-J. Lee, H.-Y. Huang, C.-K. Sun, All-terahertz fiber scanning near-field microscopy, Optics Letters 34 (7) (2009) 1084–1086;
[a] H. Chen, W. Lee, H. Huang, C. Chiu, Y. Tsai, T. Tseng, J. Lu, W. Lai, C. Sun, Performance of THz fiber-scanning near-field microscopy to diagnose breast tumors, Optics Express 19 (2011) 19523–19531.

[67] L. Shi, P. Shumyatsky, A. Rodríguez-Contreras, R.R. Alfano, Terahertz spectroscopy of brain tissue from a mouse model of Alzheimer's disease, Journal of Biomedical Optics 21 (1) (2016) 015014.

[68] K. Meng, T. nan Chen, T. Chen, L. guo Zhu, Q. Liu, Z. Li, F. Li, et al., Terahertz pulsed spectroscopy of paraffin embedded brain glioma, Journal of Biomedical Optics 19 (7) (2014) 077001.

[69] A.A. Gavdush, N.V. Chernomyrdin, K.M. Malakhov, S.-I.T. Beshplav, I.N. Dolganova, A.V. Kosyrkova, P.V. Nikitin, et al., Terahertz spectroscopy of gelatin embedded human brain gliomas of different grades: a road toward intraoperative THz diagnosis, Journal of Biomedical Optics 24 (2) (2019) 027001.

[70] S. Yamaguchi, Y. Fukushi, O. Kubota, T. Itsuji, S. Yamamoto, T. Ouchi, Terahertz spectroscopy and detection of brain tumor in rat fresh-tissue samples, in: Optical Interactions with Tissue and Cells XXVI, Vol. 9321, International Society for Optics and Photonics, 2015, p. 93210O.

[71] S.Y. Huang, Y.X.J. Wang, D.K.W. Yeung, A.T. Ahuja, Y.T. Zhang, E. Pickwell-MacPherson, Tissue characterization using terahertz pulsed imaging in reflection geometry, Physics in Medicine and Biology 54 (1) (2008) 149.

[72] Y.B. Ji, S.-H. Kim, K. Jeong, Y. Choi, J.-H. Son, D.W. Park, S.K. Noh, et al., Terahertz spectroscopic imaging and properties of gastrointestinal tract in a rat model, Biomedical Optics Express 5 (12) (2014) 4162–4170.

[73] W.-C. Kan, W.-S. Lee, W.-H. Cheung, V.P. Wallace, E. Pickwell-MacPherson, Terahertz pulsed imaging of knee cartilage, Biomedical Optics Express 1 (3) (2010) 967–974.

CHAPTER 12

Waveguides for Terahertz Endoscopy

PRAVEEN KUMAR POOLA, PHD • ILYA KRASNIKOV, PHD • ALEKSEI SETEIKIN, PHD

INTRODUCTION

Terahertz (THz) wavelengths covering from micrometers (μm) to millimeters (mm) is emerging as a robust platform for clinical studies [1]. THz spectrum offers a significant technological potential in the fields such as biology [2–5], spectroscopy [6–8], and sensing [9–12]. Though THz technology is fascinating to examine the surfaces of an organ or tissue, it is difficult to examine the interior organs without a surgery. At present, the current diagnostic imaging techniques available for the detection of local and distant cancer tissues are positron emission tomography [13], magnetic resonance imaging [14], and computed tomography [15]. All these imaging modalities have a number of limitations including the high cost, poor resolution, and limitation in the detection of inactive tumors [16,17]. In this scenario, the invention of THz endoscope has played a crucial role in the diagnosis of internal organs such as colon or gastrointestinal [18–20]. These THz endoscopes have revolutionized the way of medical practitioners for faster and cheaper diagnosis. Particularly, THz endoscopy unwraps the numerous internal cancers [21–25]. The THz endoscope unit consists of a flexible tube to move inside the body and a delivery system, but is hard to realize in reality because most of the THz waveguides are rigid and will contain significant propagation loss [26]. In order to over come these problems, researchers have developed attachable miniaturized transmitter and receiver endoscope modules [18].

CHARACTERIZING THE WAVEGUIDES

The characterization of waveguide follows two methods. In the first approach, sample and reference pulses are measured accordingly. Then the THz radiation loss and dispersion can be calculated using these two measurements as reported in Gallot et al. [27], Mendis and Grischkowsky et al. [28], McGowan et al. [29], and Mendis and Grischkowsky et al. [30]. In other method, THz pulses are propagated through a waveguides of two dissimilar sizes to calculate the THz dispersion and losses [31].

Grischkowsky et al. [32] have provided the governing equation of input and output fields with the assumption of single mode propagation in free space, however, in case of waveguide, the electromagnetic (EM) equation governing the waveguide is given by

$$E_{out}(\omega) = E_{ref}(\omega) T_1 T_2 C^2 \exp(-\alpha_{eff} L/2) \exp(-j\beta_{eff} L) \quad \textbf{(12.1)}$$

where $E_{out}(\omega)$ and $E_{ref}(\omega)$ are complex electric fields at angular frequencies ω. T_1 and T_2 are total transmission coefficients at the entrance and exit faces, respectively, C is the coupling coefficient, α_{eff} is the effective material loss, L is the length of the sample, and β_{eff} is propagation constant.

TERAHERTZ WAVEGUIDES

Waveguides are categorized into metallic and dielectric groups. In this chapter, both of these waveguides are discussed in details.

METAL CIRCULAR WAVEGUIDES

McGowan et al. [29] have demonstrated the first THz metal submillimeter–diameter circular tube. Freely transmitting THz radiation was properly coupled into metal tube using two hyperhemispherical silicon lenses. Because of strong group velocity dispersion (GVD), the amplitude of the THz pulse was stretched about 70 ps from its initial value 0.5 ps.

Since the THz radiation is not dissipative in metallic components, metallic structures are able to guide the THz waves. A number of authors have proposed a different types of waveguides to propagate the THz spectrum in metallic waveguides. Gallot et al. [27], Mendis and Grischkowsky [28], and Mcgowan et al. [29] have proposed a hollow metallic circular/rectangular waveguides, whereas McGowan et al. [28], Mendis and Grischkowsky [30], and Mendis and Mittleman [33,34] have proposed a parallel-plate waveguides (PPWGs) [35], Jeon et al. have proposed coaxial waveguides, Jeon et al. [36], Wachter et al. [37], and wang

Terahertz Biomedical and Healthcare Technologies. https://doi.org/10.1016/B978-0-12-818556-8.00012-4

et al. [38] have proposed a metal wire waveguide, Bingham et al. [39] have proposed parallel-plate photonic waveguides, Jeon et al. [40] have proposed a metal sheet waveguide, and at last Wachter et al. [41] have proposed a metallic slot waveguides. All these configurations have significantly reduced the propagation dissipation losses.

Gallot et al. [27] have theoretically calculated the field absorption, phase and group velocities for circular waveguide. The absorption coefficient of every mode is viably unbounded underneath the cutoff frequency and gradually moves toward a constant value with the increase in frequency.

METAL WIRE WAVEGUIDES

Goubau et al. [42], Sommerfeld et al. [43], and Wentworth et al. [44] have used millimeter waves to study the absorption and dispersion properties of single metal wires. The high conductivity of metal wires makes the EM waves to transmit along the exterior of the wires. Only the TEM mode can sustain and propagate along the metal wires, whereas due to the very high absorption coefficients the remaining EM modes vanish immediately. Recently, Jeon et al. [36] have used silicon-on-sapphire (SOS) chips for the THz pulse generation and detection. Along with the Jeon et al. [36], Mendis and Mittleman [34] have also studied the THz pulse absorption and dispersion properties. The schematic diagram of this configuration was shown in Fig. 12.1.

Using different wire lengths, THz pulse spectra and its absorption coefficient are measured and are shown in Fig. 12. 2A–C, respectively. The THz pulses look identical because of minute differences in the amplitude absorption signal and low GVD in the transmitted THz pulses. However, the problem of EM loss with flexibility persists in the single metal wire. Single metal has a small skin depth (high conductivity), due to which when a metal wire is twisted, as a result, most of the THz waves will be radiated into the air at this bending point. This drawback has limited the applicability of single metal wire as a waveguide for a THz endoscope.

PARALLEL-PLATE WAVEGUIDES

Low propagation loss, flexibility, no cutoff frequency, and low GVD are the ideal parameters for THz endoscope waveguide. Metal wires and tubes failed to meet these requirements. PPWG is prepared out of two thin metal strips that satisfy the aforementioned parameters. As mentioned previously, TEM mode has low loss and low GVD, and also it maintains TEM mode irrespective of the curved shape. The curve depths are shown to the corresponding transmitted THz pulses in Fig. 12.3.

Mendis and Grischkowsky et al. [28,30] have used the two cylindrical silicon lenses to create a THz wave focused at the air gap of the PPWG. The demonstrated THz pulse in the TEM mode shows a good SNR. The waveguide dimension used for this endoscopic application is 10 mm, but PPWG has a large dimension than this, because of this difference in dimension PPWG has failed to find THz endoscopic applications.

Two totally unique metallic structures are appraised in this section. (1) Metallic waveguides with circular cross sections: the propagating mode (TE and additional metal modes) is firmly bound to the structure (metallic walls) resulting in high losses because of finite physical

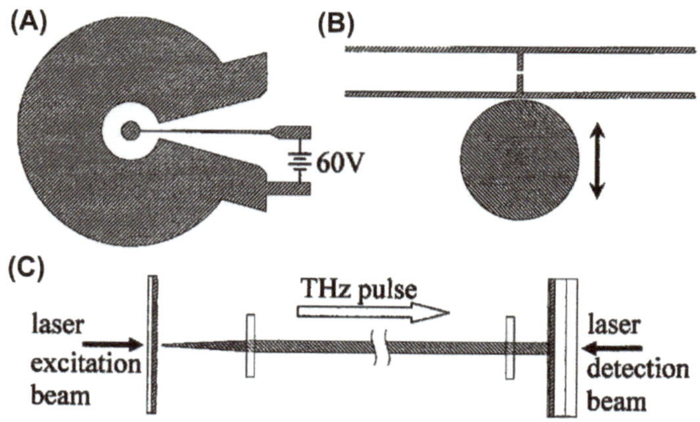

FIG. 12.1 Schematic diagram of a metal wire waveguide system. **(A)** Schematic diagram of the transmitter chip. **(B)** The receiver antenna and the output face of the copper wire. **(C)** Cross section of the transmitter chip, the copper wire, and the detection chip. (All images were reproduced with permission from T.I. Jeon, J. Zhang, D. Grischkowsky, THz Sommerfeld wave propagation on a single metal wire, Applied Physics Letters, 86 (16) (2005) 161904.)

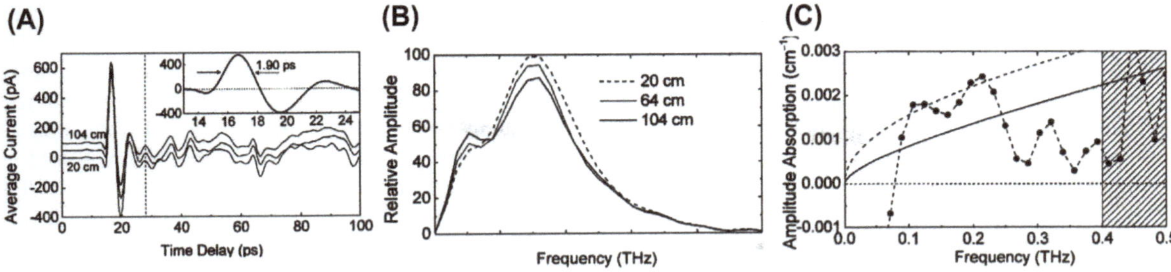

FIG. 12.2 **(A)** Transmitted terahertz (THz) pulses for 20, 64, and 104 cm long copper wires. **(B)** The spectrum of the pulses is truncated at the dashed line shown in (A). **(C)** Amplitude absorption coefficients. (All images were reproduced with permission from T.I. Jeon, J. Zhang, D. Grischkowsky, THz Sommerfeld wave propagation on a single metal wire, Applied Physics Letters 86(16) (2005) 161904.)

phenomenon of the metals in THz frequencies. The propagating mode inside these metallic waveguides experiences high scattering near the cutoff frequency of the mode. (2) PPWGs: TEM mode stays limited in between the plates in single direction with a lower attenuation coefficient compared with circular and rectangular metallic waveguides. Moreover, to bring down the loss, these waveguides supply scattering-free propagation. The repression winds up in higher loss for the metal slot conductor in contrast to metal wire, demonstrating there is an exchange off between sturdy mode restriction and low attenuation in metallic waveguides. As we will in general see inside the following section, there is a closely resembling exchange off for dielectric waveguides.

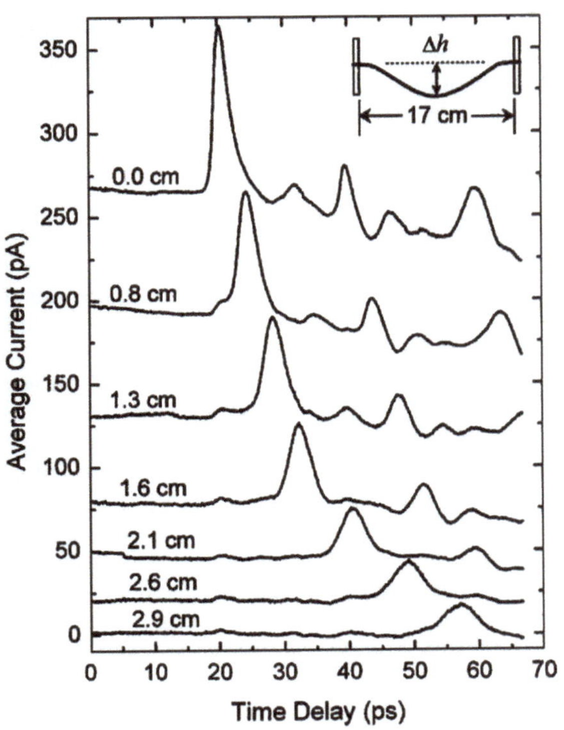

FIG. 12.3 Transmitted terahertz pulses for the indicated curve depths Dh. (All images were reproduced with permission from T.I.Jeon, J.Zhang, D.GrischkowskyTHz Sommerfeld wave propagation on a single metal wire, Applied Physics Letters 86(16) (2005). 161904.)

DIELECTRIC WAVEGUIDES

Another significant class of nonplanar waveguides proposed for the THz range is dielectric waveguides. These waveguides are otherwise called fibers on the off chance that they are bendable and have circular cross sections and are consistently utilized at higher frequencies.

Predominantly, the dielectric waveguides proposed are characterized into three classes: (1) hollow-core, (2) solid-core, and (3) porous-core waveguides. The creation of either antiresonances or photonic bandgaps makes the immediate cladding structure to guide the THz radiation through hollow-core waveguides. Then again, solid-core and porous-core waveguides work on the total internal reflection which fulfills the condition, for example, refractive index (RI) of the core is more than the cladding RI. On the off chance that this condition is turned around, i.e., RI of the core is not exactly the cladding RI, at that point the THz radiation core value relies upon the development of the photonic bandgap [45]. Under the porous-core bandgap waveguide, Nielsen et al. [46] have theoretically reported the formation of honeycomb bandgap.

The dielectric waveguides creation process has supported from the advanced manufacture strategy of optical waveguides, especially IR waveguides and microstructured optical fibers. In the instance of hollow-core and solid-core microstructured waveguides, the waveguide preforms without anyone else's input are proper for THz direction.

Here, first we evaluate the hollow-core waveguides, then solid-core waveguides and finally porous-core waveguides, respectively. The one normal controlling system in all these dielectric waveguide categories is that core RI is more prominent than the cladding RI leading to total internal reflection.

HOLLOW-CORE WAVEGUIDES

As reported by Benabid et al. [47] and Rowland et al. [48], the controlling mechanisms in all the dielectric hollow-core waveguides are fueled by either the establishment of photonic bandgaps or with instant cladding structure because of antiresonances. Knight et al. [49,50], Temelkuran et al. [51], and Katagiri et al. [52] have proposed a class of waveguides in which the cladding structures resonantly echo the mode back into the core, and the transmission band will be decided by the cladding thickness. In the previous mechanism, the cladding does not bolster modes for specific modes for certain ranges of frequency, so the guided modes remain in the core. Microstructured bandgap fibers and Bragg fibers are instances of this sort of waveguides.

The relationship between the antiresonance and bandgap decides the THz radiation guiding mechanism confining to the particular band in the core [53,54]. Couny et al. [55], Argyros and Pla et al. [56], Couny et al. [57], and Argyros et al. [58] have proposed Kagomé-lattice hollow-core microstructured fibers of this class of waveguides for the endoscopy applications.

Hollow-core waveguides have a low absorption in the THz range as THz frequency is predominately focused in the air core. But as already mentioned, the dimension of the hollow waveguides limits its applicability in the THz endoscopy. Generally, for a broad THz spectrum, the transmission is restricted to particular frequency bands in this class of waveguides. They are classified as (1). single/hybrid-clad waveguides, (2) microstructured bandgap waveguides, and (3) Kagomé microstructured waveguides. The principle of bandgap and Kagomé is used as waveguiding mechanism for the second and third cases, respectively.

HOLLOW-CORE SINGLE/HYBRID-CLAD WAVEGUIDES

To expand the transmission coefficient of hollow-core waveguides, Hidaka et al. [59] have proposed a hollow-core THz waveguide prepared with ferroelectric polyvinylidene fluoride (PVDF), a flexible polymer. For the frequencies higher than 0.3 THz, PVDF has a negative dielectric constant, which leads to the similar imaginary RI of metals. Because of this, PVDF behaves like metal for both the TM and TE polarization modes from 1 to 2 THz, which was reported by Hidaka et al. [60,61]. So the PVDF will reflect radiation like a metal. For the frequency range 1−2 THz, PVDF shows higher reflectivity of TM polarization than the Cu metal. In this scenario, the aim of increasing the transmission coefficient has increased to three times higher for an 8 mm bore diameter PVDF pipe ($\alpha = 1.5\ m^{-1}$) when compared with that of an analogous Ni−Cu pipe ($\alpha = 5\ m^{-1}$).

HOLLOW-CORE MICROSTRUCTURED BANDGAP WAVEGUIDES

If there should arise an occurrence of hollow-core microstructured bandgap waveguides, hollow core is encompassed by a micrometer scale air gaps in the cladding. When a THz radiation propagates through a cladding 2D photonic crystal band formation confines the propagated light to limit within the bandgap of cladding. But this type of waveguides having the finite number of air holes and scattering loss at the air−dielectric interface suffer from higher losses [62,63]. However, the loss can be compensated either by integrating the adequate concentric rings of air gaps around the core or by expanding the proportion of cladding air gap width to gap to gap positioning pitch. But the advantage of compensating the loss makes the fabrication process complex. On the other hand, scattering losses can be suppressed by tuning the fiber fabrication parameters.

KAGOMÉ HOLLOW-CORE MICROSTRUCTURED WAVEGUIDES

The materialization of Von-Neumann Wigner quasi-bound states within a continuum allows the waveguide to propagate THz spectrum in Kagomé hollow-core microstructured waveguides [47,55,56,64,65]. Because of the antiresonance impact of the Kagomé lattice, the wave guided modes restricted to hollow core and are stopped from proficiently coupling to the cladding. When compared with the Bragg waveguide, Kagomé-lattice waveguide offers three times wider transmission band [66]. But the losses due to absorption are eight times higher in Kagomé-lattice waveguide in comparison to the Bragg waveguides.

The low absorption and dispersion losses make the hollow-core waveguides suitable for sensing applications. But these advantages are confined to a specific band of THz spectrum, so the offered low loss and dispersion are for the designed narrow window and are not suitable for the broad THz range. Another significant downside of hollow-core waveguides is the bigger measurement size of the waveguide. One of the future directions to reduce the dimension is to explore the man-made material or metamaterials [67].

Atakaramians et al. [68–70] and Ishikawa et al. [71] have shown the promising results with hollow-core and metamaterial cladding that such a material can guide the THz radiation and make the waveguide flexible, also the size reduces by 10 times to the wavelength.

The materials used for the fabrication of dielectric waveguides have the highest THz radiation absorption properties, as a result of which, the output wave will have a high loss when compared with the input wave. Apart from the transmission loss, dispersion will also be affected by the choice of waveguide material and its structure. From the following publications from Balakrishnan et al. [45], Fischer et al. [72], Jin et al. [73], and Cunningham et al. [74], it was remained that high-density polyethylene (HDPE) and polytetrafluoroethylene (best known as Teflon) materials absorb less THz radiation, i.e., low loss when compared with the polymethylmethacrylate and polycarbonate materials.

In the THz spectrum, cyclic olefin copolymer consumes the lowest material absorption loss among the available polymers and is also known as TOPAS and Zeonex. In case of THz bandgap waveguides, air is commonly used as a dielectric material with negligible absorption.

SOLID-CORE WAVEGUIDES/FIBERS

The solid-core waveguides are classified into three types: (1) microwires, (2) solid-core microstructure, and (3) single air hole discontinuity in the core.

MICROWIRE

Jamison et al. [75] have proposed the Sapphire fiber and Mendis and Grischkowsky et al. [76] have proposed the plastic ribbon waveguide and are the first two dielectric waveguides. The specialty of these materials is that they have a less absorption loss. This happens by the virtue of waveguide subwavelength dimension, where the transmitting mode is not firmly restricted to the waveguide material and enlarges to the air.

SOLID-CORE MICROSTRUCTURED WAVEGUIDE

The photonic bandgap effect is useful to achieve the low RI of photonic crystal fiber (PCF). The first experimental microstructured waveguides were demonstrated by Han et al. [77]. Within the 0.1–3 THz bandwidth, low loss and less dispersion were achieved with the HDPE tubes as a cladding and filament as a core, respectively. By decreasing the cladding material RI using innovative materials, Goto et al. [78] have proved that it is possible to reduce the absorption loss. Goto et al. [78] have experimentally shown this by replacing the PCF material with the Teflon in the THz regime.

WAVEGUIDES WITH A LOW-INDEX DISCONTINUITY IN THE CORE

The novel low-index discontinuity waveguides were proposed by Nagel et al. [79] to improve the electric field strength within the THz spectrum. This idea was borrowed from the works of Almeida et al. [80] optics field to THz field. The concept of electric field strength discontinuity at the boundary between two materials with no surface charge was explored to reduce the index of refraction.

POROUS-CORE WAVEGUIDES

The waveguiding mechanism of porous-core waveguides is also based on the principle of total interval reflection likewise in microstructured waveguides. Hassani et al. [81,82] have proposed a class of fiber-based porous-core waveguides to increase the actual material loss. Typical fiber-based porous-core examples with figures can be found at Ref. [83,84]. In these examples [83,84], most of the circular air holes were considered within the fiber, it leads to the reduction of THz loss and constrainment of THz radiation inside the air openings. PCF-based porous waveguides find numerous applications in biosensors due high birefringence due to asymmetrical discontinuity.

Most of the waveguides do not satisfy the required conditions for endoscopy applications, because of size and material loss. Miniaturization of waveguides both at the receiver and transmission modules with laser beam–guided endoscope systems are suitable other methods.

COMMERCIAL THZ SPECTROSCOPE SYSTEM

Many companies including Teraview, Picometric, and Zomega have produced the commercial THz spectroscopy systems for medical applications. These probes are based on the reflection imaging principle. One such a system is TPS Spectra 3000 from Teraview company.

Parrott et al. [85] have studied the effect of THz signal at five positions namely forehand, cheek, chin, forearm, and palm. From Fig. 12.4, it is evident that at first three positions the THz signal has shown similar response with a small variation in the initial peak signal followed by a large trough. But, in contrast, a more

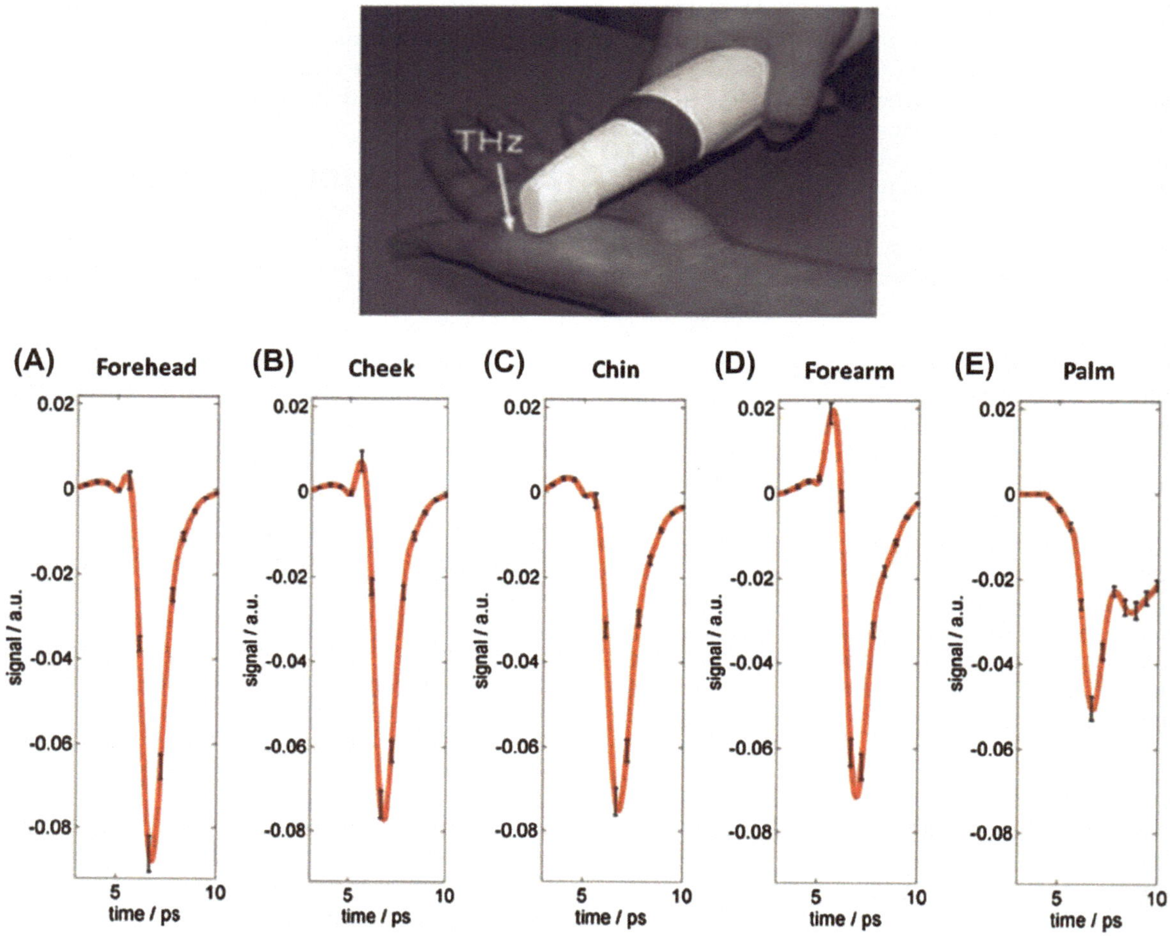

FIG. 12.4 Terahertz signal measured at **(A)** forehand, **(B)** cheek, **(C)** chin, **(D)** forearm, and **(E)** palm, respectively. (All images were reproduced with permission from E.P. Parrott, S.MY Sy, T. Blu, V.P. Wallace, E. Pickwell-MacPherson. Terahertz pulsed imaging in vivo: measurements and processing methods. Journal of Biomedical Optics 16(10) (2011) 106010.)

pronounced peak is observed in the THz signal for the dorsal forearm and palm.

HANDHELD THZ PROBE FOR INTRAOPERATIVE USE

Wallace et al. [86] have studied the breast tumor margins using the handheld THz imaging probe as an intraoperative tool. The system specifications are as follows: the bandwidth is between 0.1 and 2.0 THz and a scan length of 8 mm was achieved using a combination of silicon lens and Risley prims.

Ashworth et al. [87] have used a THz probe to study cancerous, adipose, and fibrous breast tissue types. The system shows a different response on fibrous and fat tissue. Thus, results demonstrated in this work prove the potential of THz imaging probe in identifying the various tissue types.

IN VIVO APPLICATIONS USING THZ ENDOSCOPE SYSTEM

The main requirement for the miniaturized THz endoscope probe is its size, the size should be less than 5 mm. Ji et al. [18] have demonstrated 26 mm long fiber ferrule miniaturized THz receiver and transceiver module. The schematic diagram of the THz endoscope with a miniaturized experimental setup was shown in Ref. [18] and the measured RI and power absorption of the mouth side wall, tongue, and water using the frequency-dependent magnitude and phase information of the measured THz pulses.

FUTURE DIRECTIONS

The above discussions clearly state that the handheld THz probes are highly promising for in vivo medical imaging of the malignant tissues from the benign tissues. The current THz market is now attractive and adequately flexible and it is possible to design and use it in the clinical environment. Already researchers around the world are working toward addressing the THz probe limitations, and we have seen few innovative solutions toward this direction in the form of new materials used for waveguides. These new waveguides not only reduce the physical size of the THz probe but also reduce the losses due to propagation by confining the wave within the cladding region.

Another major limitation of the THz probe is its small imaging region, by using which we can image only a small tissue volume. So as per the current clinical standards, it is expected to have high scan rate and could image the large tissue. One of the possible solutions could be the use of graphics processing unit–based solutions which will help us to do high rate volumetric imaging of the tissues.

One more major limitation is its shallow depth of imaging. Because of which tumors residing within the 1 mm depth cannot be imaged with high resolution. Therefore, one more possible future direction could be toward improving the penetration depth of THz imaging.

By using the computational techniques like deconvolution and noise reduction techniques, it is likely to enhance the signal to noise ratio of the current THz images. Also the errors in data registration should also be reduced. Once we get the clean data, it is also possible to machine learn all these features for automatic disease screening in the future and also the multimodal imaging with the same specimen is possible.

REFERENCES

[1] B.B. Hu, M.C. Nuss, Imaging with terahertz waves, Optics Letters 20 (16) (1995) 1716–1718.

[2] P.H. Siegel, Terahertz technology in biology and medicine, IEEE Transactions on Microwave Theory and Techniques 52 (10) (2004) 2438–2447.

[3] M. Walther, P. Plochocka, B. Fischer, H. Helm, P. Uhd Jepsen, Collective vibrational modes in biological molecules investigated by terahertz time-domain spectroscopy, Biopolymers: Original Research on Biomolecules 67 (4–5) (2002) 310–313.

[4] J.H. Son, Terahertz electromagnetic interactions with biological matter and their applications, Journal of Applied Physics 105 (10) (2009) 102033.

[5] E. Pickwell, V.P. Wallace, Biomedical applications of terahertz technology, Journal of Physics D: Applied Physics 39 (17) (2006) R301.

[6] P.U. Jepsen, D.G. Cooke, M. Koch, Terahertz spectroscopy and imagingemodern techniques and applications, Laser & Photonics Reviews 5 (1) (2011) 124–166.

[7] S.L. Dexheimer (Ed.), Terahertz Spectroscopy: Principles and Applications, CRC Press, 2007.

[8] D.F. Plusquellic, K. Siegrist, E.J. Heilweil, O. Esenturk, Applications of terahertz spectroscopy in biosystems, Chemical physics and physical chemistry 8 (17) (2007) 2412–2431.

[9] J.F. Federici, B. Schulkin, F. Huang, D. Gary, R. Barat, F. Oliveira, D. Zimdars, THz imaging and sensing for security applicationsdexplosives, weapons and drugs, Semiconductor Science and Technology 20 (7) (2005) S266.

[10] B. Ferguson, X.C. Zhang, Materials for terahertz science and technology, Nature Materials 1 (1) (2002) 26.

[11] D.L. Woolard, R. Brown, M. Pepper, M. Kemp, Terahertz frequency sensing and imaging: a time of reckoning future applications? Proceedings of the IEEE 93 (10) (2005) 1722–1743.

[12] T. Chen, S. Li, H. Sun, Metamaterials application in sensing, Sensors 12 (3) (2012) 2742–2765.

[13] H.T. Chugani, M.E. Phelps, J.C. Mazziotta, Positron emission tomography study of human brain functional development, Annals of Neurology 22 (4) (1987) 487–497.

[14] S. Ogawa, T.M. Lee, A.R. Kay, D.W. Tank, Brain magnetic resonance imaging with contrast dependent on blood oxygenation, Proceedings of the National Academy of Sciences 87 (24) (1990) 9868–9872.

[15] D.J. Brenner, E.J. Hall, Computed tomographydan increasing source of radiation exposure, New England Journal of Medicine 357 (22) (2007) 2277–2284.

[16] T.C. Kwee, H.M.Q. van Ufford, F.J. Beek, T. Takahara, C.S. Uiterwaal, M.B. Bierings, R.A. Nievelstein, Whole-body MRI, including diffusion-weighted imaging, for the initial staging of malignant lymphoma: comparison to computed tomography, Investigative Radiology 44 (10) (2009) 683–690.

[17] G. Antoch, A. Bockisch, Combined PET/MRI: a new dimension in whole-body oncology imaging? European Journal of Nuclear Medicine and Molecular Imaging 36 (1) (2009) 113–120.

[18] Y.B. Ji, E.S. Lee, S.H. Kim, J.H. Son, T.I. Jeon, A miniaturized fiber-coupled terahertz endoscope system, Optics Express 17 (19) (2009) 17082–17087.

[19] Y.B. Ji, S.H. Kim, K. Jeong, Y. Choi, J.H. Son, D.W. Park, S.K. Noh, T.I. Jeon, Y.M. Huh, S. Haam, S.K. Lee, Terahertz spectroscopic imaging and properties of gastrointestinal tract in a rat model, Biomedical Optics Express 5 (12) (2014) 4162–4170.

[20] P. Doradla, K. Alavi, C.S. Joseph, R.H. Giles, Detection of colon cancer by continuous-wave terahertz polarization imaging technique, Journal of Biomedical Optics 18 (9) (2013) 090504.

[21] S.J. Oh, J. Kang, I. Maeng, J.S. Suh, Y.M. Huh, S. Haam, J.H. Son, Nanoparticle-enabled terahertz imaging for cancer diagnosis, Optics Express 17 (5) (2009) 3469–3475.

[22] Y.C. Sim, J.Y. Park, K.M. Ahn, C. Park, J.H. Son, Terahertz imaging of excised oral cancer at frozen temperature, Biomedical Optics Express 4 (8) (2013) 1413–1421.
[23] A.J. Fitzgerald, V.P. Wallace, M. Jimenez-Linan, L. Bobrow, R.J. Pye, A.D. Purushotham, D.D. Arnone, Terahertz pulsed imaging of human breast tumors, Radiology 239 (2) (2006) 533–540.
[24] L.H. Eadie, C.B. Reid, A.J. Fitzgerald, V.P. Wallace, Optimizing multi-dimensional terahertz imaging analysis for colon cancer diagnosis, Expert Systems with Applications 40 (6) (2013) 2043–2050.
[25] H. Cheon, H.J. Yang, J.H. Son, Toward clinical cancer imaging using terahertz spectroscopy, IEEE Journal of Selected Topics in Quantum Electronics 23 (4) (2017) 1–9.
[26] T. Ito, Y. Matsuura, M. Miyagi, H. Minamide, H. Ito, Flexible terahertz fiber optics with low bend-induced losses, Journal of the Optical Society of America B 24 (5) (2007) 1230–1235.
[27] G. Gallot, S.P. Jamison, R.W. McGowan, D. Grischkowsky, Terahertz waveguides, Journal of the Optical Society of America B 17 (5) (2000) 851–863.
[28] R. Mendis, D. Grischkowsky, Undistorted guided-wave propagation of subpicosecond terahertz pulses, Optics Letters 26 (11) (2001a) 846–848.
[29] R.W. McGowan, G. Gallot, D. Grischkowsky, Propagation of ultrawideband short pulses of terahertz radiation through submillimeter-diameter circular waveguides, Optics Letters 24 (20) (1999) 1431–1433.
[30] R. Mendis, D. Grischkowsky, THz interconnectwith low-loss and low-group velocity dispersion, IEEE Microwave and Wireless Components Letters 11 (11) (2001b) 444–446.
[31] J. Werner, E. Kapon, A.C. Von Lehmen, R. Bhat, E. Colas, N.G. Stoffel, S.A. Schwarz, Reduced optical waveguide losses of a partially disordered GaAs/AlGaAs single quantum well laser structure for photonic integrated circuits, Applied Physics Letters 53 (18) (1988) 1693–1695.
[32] D.R. Grischkowsky, Optoelectronic characterization of transmission lines and waveguides by terahertz time domain spectroscopy, IEEE Journal of Selected Topics in Quantum Electronics 6 (6) (2000) 1122–1135.
[33] R. Mendis, D.M. Mittleman, Comparison of the lowest-order transverse-electric (TE 1) and transverse-magnetic (TEM) modes of the parallel-plate waveguide for terahertz pulse applications, Optics Express 17 (17) (2009a) 14839–14850.
[34] R. Mendis, D.M. Mittleman, An investigation of the lowest order transverse-electric (TE 1) mode of the parallel-plate waveguide for THz pulse propagation, Journal of the Optical Society of America B 26 (9) (2009b) A6–A13.
[35] T.I. Jeon, D. Grischkowsky, Direct optoelectronic generation and detection of sub-ps-electrical pulses on sub-mm coaxial transmission lines, Applied Physics Letters 85 (25) (2004) 6092–6094.
[36] T.I. Jeon, J. Zhang, D. Grischkowsky, THz Sommerfeld wave propagation on a single metal wire, Applied Physics Letters 86 (16) (2005) 161904.
[37] M. Wåchter, M. Nagel, H. Kurz, Frequency-dependent characterization of THz Sommerfeld wave propagation on single-wires, Optics Express 13 (26) (2005) 10815–10822.
[38] K. Wang, D.M. Mittleman, Metal wires for terahertz wave guiding, Nature 432 (7015) (2004) 376.
[39] A.L. Bingham, D.R. Grischkowsky, Terahertz 2-D photonic crystal waveguides, IEEE Microwave and Wireless Components Letters 18 (7) (2008) 428–430.
[40] T.I. Jeon, D. Grischkowsky, THz Zenneck surface wave (THz surface plasmon) propagation on a metal sheet, Applied Physics Letters 88 (6) (2006) 061113.
[41] M. Wächter, M. Nagel, H. Kurz, Metallic slit waveguide for dispersion-free low-loss terahertz signal transmission, Applied Physics Letters 90 (6) (2007) 061111.
[42] G. Goubau, Surface waves and their application to transmission lines, Journal of Applied Physics 21 (11) (1950) 1119–1128.
[43] H.A. Lorentz, A. Einstein, H. Minkowski, H. Weyl, A. Sommerfeld, The Principle of Relativity: A Collection of Original Memoirs on the Special and General Theory of Relativity, Courier Corporation, 1952.
[44] F.L. Wentworth, J.C. Wiltse, F. Sobel, Quasi-optical surface waveguide and other components for the 100-to 300-Gc region, IRE Transactions on Microwave Theory and Techniques 9 (6) (1961) 512–518.
[45] J. Balakrishnan, B.M. Fischer, D. Abbott, Sensing the hygroscopicity of polymer and copolymer materials using terahertz time-domain spectroscopy, Applied Optics 48 (12) (2009) 2262–2266.
[46] K. Nielsen, H.K. Rasmussen, P.U. Jepsen, O. Bang, Porous-core honeycomb bandgap THz fiber, Optics Letters 36 (5) (2011) 666–668.
[47] F. Benabid, P.J. Roberts, F. Couny, P.S. Light, Light and gas confinement in hollow-core photonic crystal fibre based photonic microcells, Journal of the European Optical Society-Rapid Publications 4 (2009).
[48] K.J. Rowland, Guiding Light in Low-Index Media via Multilayer Waveguides, 2010 (Doctoral dissertation).
[49] J.C. Knight, T.A. Birks, P.S.J. Russell, D.M. Atkin, All-silica single-mode optical fiber with photonic crystal cladding, Optics Letters 21 (19) (1996) 1547–1549.
[50] J.C. Knight, J. Broeng, T.A. Birks, P.S.J. Russell, Photonic band gap guidance in optical fibers, Science 282 (5393) (1998) 1476–1478.
[51] B. Temelkuran, S.D. Hart, G. Benoit, J.D. Joannopoulos, Y. Fink, Wavelength-scalable hollow optical fibres with large photonic bandgaps for CO_2 laser transmission, Nature 420 (6916) (2002) 650.
[52] T. Katagiri, Y. Matsuura, M. Miyagi, Photonic bandgap fiber with a silica core and multilayer dielectric cladding, Optics Letters 29 (6) (2004) 557–559.

[53] K.J. Rowland, S. Afshar, T.M. Monro, Bandgaps and anti resonances in integrated-ARROWs and Bragg fibers; a simple model, Optics Express 16 (22) (2008) 17935–17951.
[54] K.J. Rowland, S. Afshar, A. Stolyarov, Y. Fink, T.M. Monro, Bragg waveguides with low-index liquid cores, Optics Express 20 (1) (2012) 48–62.
[55] F. Couny, F. Benabid, P.S. Light, Large-pitch kagome structured hollow-core photonic crystal fiber, Optics Letters 31 (24) (2006) 3574–3576.
[56] A. Argyros, J. Pla, Hollow-core polymer fibres with a kagome lattice: potential for transmission in the infrared, Optics Express 15 (12) (2007) 7713–7719.
[57] F. Couny, P.J. Roberts, T.A. Birks, F. Benabid, Square lattice large-pitch hollow-core photonic crystal fiber, Optics Express 16 (25) (2008) 20626–20636.
[58] A. Argyros, S.G. Leon-Saval, J. Pla, A. Docherty, Antiresonant reflection and inhibited coupling in hollow-core square lattice optical fibres, Optics Express 16 (8) (2008) 5642–5648.
[59] T. Hidaka, H. Minamide, H. Ito, S.I. Maeta, T. Akiyama, Ferroelectric PVDF cladding terahertz waveguide, in: Optical Information, Data Processing and Storage, and Laser Communication Technologies, vol. 5135, International Society for Optics and Photonics, 2003, pp. 70–77.
[60] T. Hidaka, H. Minamide, H. Ito, J.I. Nishizawa, K. Tamura, S. Ichikawa, Ferroelectric PVDF cladding terahertz waveguide, Journal of Lightwave Technology 23 (8) (2005) 2469–2473.
[61] T. Hidaka, I. Morohashi, K. Komori, H. Nakagawa, H. Ito, THz wave hollow waveguide with ferroelectric PVDF polymer as the cladding material, in: Conference Digest. 2000 Conference on Lasers and Electro-Optics Europe (Cat. No. 00TH8505), IEEE, 2000, p. 1.
[62] Y.F. Geng, X.L. Tan, P. Wang, J.Q. Yao, Transmission loss and dispersion in plastic terahertz photonic band-gap fibers, Applied Physics B 91 (2) (2008) 333–336.
[63] P.J. Roberts, F. Couny, H. Sabert, B.J. Mangan, T.A. Birks, J.C. Knight, P.S.J. Russell, Loss in solid-core photonic crystal fibers due to interface roughness scattering, Optics Express 13 (20) (2005) 7779–7793.
[64] F. Couny, F. Benabid, P.J. Roberts, P.S. Light, M.G. Raymer, Generation and photonic guidance of multi-octave optical-frequency combs, Science 318 (5853) (2007) 1118–1121.
[65] L. Vincetti, Numerical analysis of plastic hollow core microstructured fiber for Terahertz applications, Optical Fiber Technology 15 (4) (2009) 398–401.
[66] Y.Y. Wang, N.V. Wheeler, F. Couny, P.J. Roberts, F. Benabid, Low loss broadband transmission in hypocycloid-core Kagome hollow-core photonic crystal fiber, Optics Letters 36 (5) (2011) 669–671.
[67] W. Withayachumnankul, D. Abbott, Metamaterials in the terahertz regime, IEEE Photonics Journal 1 (2) (2009) 99–118.
[68] S. Atakaramians, S. Afshar, T.M. Monro, D. Abbott, Terahertz dielectric waveguides, Advances in Optics and Photonics 5 (2) (2013a) 169–215.
[69] S. Atakaramians, A. Argyros, S.C. Fleming, B.T. Kuhlmey, Hollow-core waveguides with uniaxial metamaterial cladding: modal equations and guidance conditions, Journal of the Optical Society of America B 29 (9) (2012) 2462–2477.
[70] S. Atakaramians, A. Argyros, S.C. Fleming, B.T. Kuhlmey, Hollow-core uniaxial metamaterial clad fibers with dispersive metamaterials, Journal of the Optical Society of America B 30 (4) (2013b) 851–867.
[71] A. Ishikawa, S. Zhang, D.A. Genov, G. Bartal, X. Zhang, Deep subwavelength terahertz waveguides using gap magnetic plasmon, Physical Review Letters 102 (4) (2009) 043904.
[72] B.M. Fischer, M. Hoffmann, H.E.A. Helm, Broadband THz time-domain spectroscopy of biomolecules, Mathematics and Physics 246 (2005).
[73] Y.S. Jin, G.J. Kim, S.G. Jeon, Terahertz dielectric properties of polymers, Journal of the Korean Physical Society 49 (2) (2006) 513–517.
[74] P.D. Cunningham, N.N. Valdes, F.A. Vallejo, L.M. Hayden, B. Polishak, X.H. Zhou, R.J. Twieg, Broadband terahertz characterization of the refractive index and absorption of some important polymeric and organic electro optic materials, Journal of Applied Physics 109 (4) (2011) 043505.
[75] S.P. Jamison, R.W. McGowan, D. Grischkowsky, Single-mode waveguide propagation and reshaping of sub-ps terahertz pulses in sapphire fibers, Applied Physics Letters 76 (15) (2000) 1987–1989.
[76] R. Mendis, D. Grischkowsky, Plastic ribbon THz waveguides, Journal of Applied Physics 88 (7) (2000) 4449–4451.
[77] H. Han, H. Park, M. Cho, J. Kim, Terahertz pulse propagation in a plastic photonic crystal fiber, Applied Physics Letters 80 (2002) 2634–2636.
[78] M. Goto, A. Quema, H. Takahashi, S. Ono, N. Sarukura, Teflon photonic crystal fiber as terahertz waveguide, Japanese Journal of Applied Physics 43 (2B) (2004) L317.
[79] M. Nagel, A. Marchewka, H. Kurz, Low-index discontinuity terahertz waveguides, Optics Express 14 (21) (2006) 9944–9954.
[80] V.R. Almeida, Q. Xu, C.A. Barrios, M. Lipson, Guiding and confining light in void nanostructure, Optics Letters 29 (11) (2004) 1209–1211.
[81] A. Hassani, A. Dupuis, M. Skorobogatiy, Low loss porous terahertz fibers containing multiple subwavelength holes, Applied Physics Letters 92 (7) (2008a) 071101.
[82] A. Hassani, A. Dupuis, M. Skorobogatiy, Porous polymer fibers for low-loss Terahertz guiding, Optics Express 16 (9) (2008b) 6340–6351.
[83] A. Dupuis, J. Allard, D. Morris, K. Stoeffler, C. Dubois, M. Skorobogatiy, Fabrication and THz loss measurements

of porous subwavelength fibers using a directional coupler method, Optics Express 17 (2009) 8012–8028.

[84] A. Dupuis, A. Mazhorova, F. Desevedavy, M. Roze, M. Skorobogatiy, Spectral characterization of porous dielectric subwavelength THz fibers fabricated using a microstructured molding technique, Optics Express 18 (2010) 13813–13828.

[85] E.P. Parrott, S.M. Sy, T. Blu, V.P. Wallace, E. Pickwell-MacPherson, Terahertz pulsed imaging in vivo: measurements and processing methods, Journal of Biomedical Optics 16 (10) (2011) 106010.

[86] V.P. Wallace, A.J. Fitzgerald, B. Robertson, E. Pickwell, B. Cole, Development of a hand-held TPI system for medical applications, in: IEEE MTT-S International Microwave Symposium Digest, IEEE, 2005, p. 3.

[87] P.C. Ashworth, P. O'Kelly, A.D. Purushotham, S.E. Pinder, M. Kontos, M. Pepper, V.P. Wallace, An intra-operative THz probe for use during the surgical removal of breast tumors, in: 2008 33rd International Conference on Infrared, Millimeter and Terahertz Waves, IEEE, 2008, pp. 1–3.

CHAPTER 13

Prospects in Medical Applications of Terahertz Waves

AMIT BANERJEE, PHD • SAUMITRA VAJANDAR, PHD • TANMOY BASU, PHD

INTRODUCTION

The terahertz (THz) lies between 0.1 and 20 THz (10^{12} cycles per seconds) or from 3 to 0.02 mm wavelength range [1]. This frequency range is situated between infrared and microwave radiation in the electromagnetic spectrum and is largely untapped due to the lack of mature solid-state technologies (as well-established semiconductor technologies cannot be used to probe THz waves) for the generation, detection, and manipulation. Thus, this regime of frequency is commonly referred to as "THz technology gap" [2]. However, in recent years, a gamut of new studies opens new possibilities for materials characterization by THz. In fact, multitude of applications in semiconductor and superconductor characterization, tomographic imaging, genetic studies without labeling, biological cell imaging, and biosensing have revolutionized THz research.

Gebbie et al. first discovered the electrical discharge-pumped THz gas lasers in 1960 [3], which was followed by the development of optically pumped THz gas lasers [3]. In 1970s, development of magneto-optic-based and nonlinear optics-based THz sources took place [4,5]. Thereafter, attempts were made to develop new techniques for infrared spectroscopic measurements [6,7]. For next few decades, worldwide research efforts were made to overcome the technological challenges related to "terahertz gap" (e.g., generation and detection of THz radiation) [7]. One of the main goals of THz radiation-based technology is to develop an imaging method (like visible radiation) which started in 1960s. However, during this nascent stage, lack of suitable sources and compatible sensing mechanism were the main hindrances. However, very soon it gained the required momentum due to the advent of HCN laser-based THz generation at 1.12 THz [8]. In particular, during 1976s, Hartwick and his colleagues used far infrared gas lasers and Schottky diode harmonic mixer for imaging with THz which was further improvised by Cheo et al. to image air bubble defects in polymers [9,10]. After some intermediate efforts, picosecond optical pulse-based THz time-domain spectroscopy (THz-TDS) emerged by implementing nonlinear optical phenomena [11−13] and led to the pioneering work by Hu and Nuss of acquiring image using THz-TDS [14]. This has set the stage for further advancement of THz imaging and sensing. For instance, the possibility of THz-based tomography has been exploited by Mittleman et al. [15], later on, THz reflection imaging and synthetic aperture-based imaging have been demonstrated as well [16−18]. The comprehensive review of the evolution of THz sensing applications can be found in the review article by Siegel [19]. Around this time, chirped pulse beam was used by Sun et al. for THz measurements. They have shown that the spatiotemporal resolution of chirped pulse technique can be mathematically related to the square root of the product of unchirped probe pulse duration and chirped pulse duration [20]. The quest for an improved resolution has gotten a big boost after the implementation of near-field techniques [21−25]. Subsequently, continuous-wave (cw) THz radiation-based imaging got attention of the researchers which paved the way of THz quantum cascade lasers [26−31].

The THz imaging method has further been extended to quality control [32], detection of illegal drugs, etc. [33]. In 2008, single-pixel THz imaging was designed based on compressed sensing. This approach eliminates the need of raster scanning with the THz bean on the object [34]. Landy et al. presented the theory and experimental background of a polarization-insensitive metamaterial absorber imaging at THz frequencies [35]. In 2009, nanoparticle-enabled THz imaging was demonstrated by Oh et al. [36]. THz-TDS was used by Brun at al. for cancer diagnosis [37]. THz imaging, by self-mixing in quantum cascade laser with high sensitivity and faster response, was demonstrated by Dean

Terahertz Biomedical and Healthcare Technologies. https://doi.org/10.1016/B978-0-12-818556-8.00013-6

et al. [38] in 2011. Schuster et al. showed broadband THz imaging in a low cost silicon CMOS technology with high sensitivity [39]. In 2012, Busch et al. demonstrated optically controlled steering of THz beam by introducing optical grating structures [40]. In 2013, graphene modulator arrays were introduced for THz imaging which led to THz modulation with reflectance >50% with around 100% modulation depth [41]. This work has paved the way for developing low cost video rate THz imaging. Later, brain tissues were imaged using THz by Oh et al. showing its potential real-time brain tumors imaging [42]. Recently, Stantchev et al. has demonstrated noninvasive, subwavelength THz imaging of hidden features with single-pixel detectors [43]. Wade et al. performed real-time near-field THz imaging with atomic optical fluorescence with the potential of fast 2D image acquisition [44]. In 2018, subwavelength THz imaging by optical rectification has been shown by Sanjuan at al., where $\lambda/12$ resolution has been achieved [45]. A wide-ranging review on THz imaging can be found by Mittleman [46]. This year, Perraud et al. has proposed algorithm for 3D real-time THz imaging where the experimental reconstruction in 3D with a THz waves has been achieved by using a powerful source and a real-time THz camera [47]. In the following sections, we will confine the discussion within the usage of graphene and other 2D materials for THz applications.

TERAHERTZ IN BIOMEDICAL APPLICATIONS

In the past decade, there has been a strong need within biomedical fields to develop better, efficient, and nondestructive technologies for biomolecule sensitivities and medical imaging. The terahertz (THz $= 10^{12}$ Hz) frequency domain of the electromagnetic spectrum has gained a lot of research focus in this respect due to its unparalleled detection sensitivity and nondestructive nature leading to important developments in THz biomedical research (Fig. 13.1).

The THz region includes frequencies from 100 GHz to 10 THz on the electromagnetic spectrum. This region falls within a wavelength of 30–3000 μm or a wavenumber of 3.33–333 cm^{-1}. Applications of THz radiation include detection of various biomaterials such as nucleic acids, proteins, cells, and tissues.

Some of the properties that make THz ideal for biomedical research are listed below [49]:

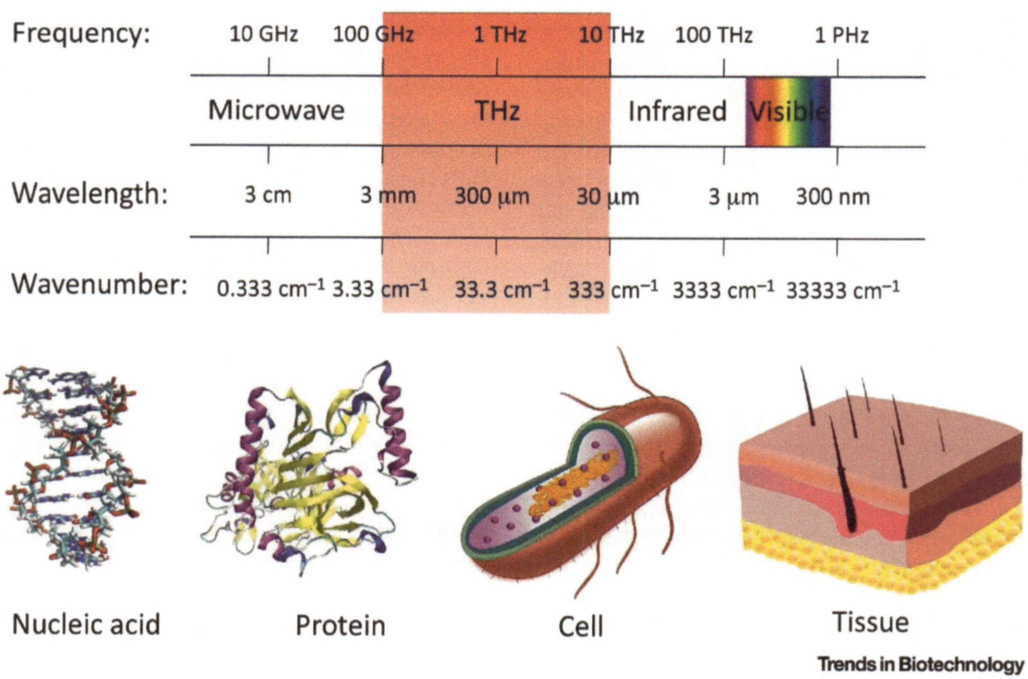

FIG. 13.1 The THz region includes frequencies from 100 GHz to 10 THz on the electromagnetic spectrum. This region falls within a wavelength of 30 μm – 3000 μm or a wavenumber of 3.33 cm^{-1} – 333 cm^{-1}. Applications of THz radiation include detection of various biomaterials such as nucleic acids, proteins, cells, and tissues. (Reproduced with permission from X. Yang, X. Zhao, K. Yang, Y. Liu, Y. Liu, W. Fu, Y. Luo, Biomedical applications of terahertz spectroscopy and imaging, Trends in Biotechnology 34 (2016) 810–824, Copyright 2016.)

- The vibrational, rotational, and translational motions (low-frequency motions) that occur in a molecule have energy levels matching that of a THz wave. This property gives a unique spectral THz signature to these molecular motions that can be used for biomolecule identification.
- THz radiation has a strong absorption coefficient in water. This makes it possible to use THz for precisely differentiating between normal and cancer tissues as these differ in their water content. Moreover, a bacteria's living condition can be determined using THz by monitoring their hydration levels.
- THz spectroscopy offers spatial resolutions on the order of several micrometers and time resolution on the order of subpicosecond to picosecond timescales. This enables detection of biomolecules with very high sensing capabilities.
- THz radiation consists of low energy waves of noninvasive and nonionizing nature. This makes it possible for in vivo medical imaging on a real-time scale. Furthermore, THz waves suffer negligible scattering losses in biological tissues due to their long wavelengths compared with infrared and visible light.

Technologies employing THz radiation are typically categorized into two kinds: THz spectroscopy and THz imaging. Here, we highlight few biomedical areas that use each of these two categories.

THz Spectroscopy for Biomedical Characterization

Since THz radiation excites the low-frequency molecular motions within a biomaterial, giving it a unique spectral fingerprint, using THz spectroscopy to recognize and characterize various biomolecules has gathered immense interest in the research community. Moreover, using the picosecond timescale frequencies of a THz wave, one can also use THz spectroscopy to detect the coupling between biomolecules and their hydration shells [50]. One important feature of THz spectroscopy is that it can measure not only the intensity of a spectral pulse but also the transient electric field associated with it. This implies that both the amplitude and phase of a pulse can be determined. Since these two parameters are directly associated with the absorption coefficient and the refractive index of a sample, the dielectric permittivity of the sample can be obtained. This is critical from the perspective of characterizing a biomaterial as it enables us to get a THz dielectric response of water, a major component of a biomaterial. Combining this with the high sensitivity that THz spectroscopy offers, this technique makes for an ideal tool for probing and characterizing various biomaterials. Listed below are two of the common examples of biomaterials that are the subject of THz spectroscopic investigations.

Tissues

THz spectroscopy, comprising of a broadband THz wave, has been used on freshly excised human tissue by Fitzgerald et al. [51]. They found that the refractive index and absorption coefficient were different for skin, adipose tissue, striated muscle, vein, and nerve. In another study on different human skin tissues, in vivo, Echchgadda et al. [52] showed a similar result. The absorption coefficients and refractive indices for the different skin tissues under their study varied significantly because of the disparate hydration levels associated with these tissues. THz radiation has been applied to differentiate between cancerous and normal tissues as well, as shown by Wahaia et al. [53] and Meng et al. [54], wherein they report that cancer tissues displayed a higher absorption coefficient and refractive index relative to normal tissues. On the other hand, results from the work of Ping et al. [55] on snap-frozen brain tissues they obtained from patients suffering from Alzheimer's disease revealed an opposite trend, the absorption coefficient was lower than that of a normal tissue. This implies that the THz signal is not only affected by a differing tissue water content but the tissue composition and structure also play a role in the final signal outcome. All these studies indicate a strong promise for THz spectroscopy to be used for early noninvasive diagnostic studies of tissues.

Proteins

Proteins routinely undergo extensive conformational changes as a prerequisite for functional activity, and tracing these changes is of paramount importance in understanding the biomolecular interactions associated with them. THz spectroscopy has been widely used as a tool of choice to study these protein conformational changes as they have a direct effect on the THz dielectric response of proteins [56]. For instance, Liu et al. have used THz spectroscopy to study the fibrillation of amyloid proteins and they found an increase in the absorption coefficient and refractive index spectra, associated with the corresponding change of alpha-helix to a beta-sheet [57]. This information is critically important in the clinical diagnosis of Alzheimer's disease. In another work, Mickan et al. have reported the use of THz time-domain spectroscopy to study bioaffinity sensing [58]. By measuring the transmission through a thin layer of biotin, they have observed binding of biotin to the sensor protein, avidin, with a sensitivity of 0.1 μg cm^{-2} of biotin. This outcome hints at a potential use of THz spectroscopy in cancer detection by identifying changes in the protein molecules, which are commonly used as markers for certain types of cancers.

THz Imaging for Biomedical Characterization

From a biomedical imaging standpoint, THz technology presents a distinct advantage. It enables concurrent collection of a spectrum and an image, thereby making it possible to extract intrinsic properties and morphological features of a biological system from the amplitude and phase information of a THz wave. While being noninvasive in nature, THz waves also have a penetration depth up to a few hundred microns making this technology superior to other imaging techniques such as X-rays, a potential radiation hazard, and MRI imaging, lacks depth information.

The primary mechanisms used in obtaining a THz biomedical image are changes in the structure and water content of a tissue. Structural changes such as mutation of biomolecules [59] in a tissue can result in contrast differences of an image, and nearly 50%–66% of this contrast change comes from the inner structural and compositional variations of a tissue [60]. Interstitial water content of a cancerous tissue differs significantly from that of a normal tissue due to abundant vascularity [61], and hence such tissues exhibit different THz absorption leading to differences in image contrast when compared with normal tissues. Here, we discuss few in vivo and ex vivo imaging applications of THz waves.

In vivo imaging

In vivo THz imaging has been used by Zaytsev et al. in a series of studies to detect skin melanoma, a type of cancer that is characterized by an abnormal mole (dysplastic nevus) [62–64]. They studied abnormal and normal skin samples from for patients using THz pulsed spectroscopy and observed distinct differences in the Cole-Cole diagrams between the two sets of samples. In their case, the differences between the abnormal and normal samples were more obvious from the real part of the dielectric permittivity than the imaginary part.

In a recent work performed on four subjects, the MacPherson group [65] have observed clear contrast in the refractive index of the scars and that of the skin surrounding these scars. They have also observed the healing process of a hypertrophic scar, post injury, over a span of 6 months. They have concluded that the refractive index contrast continues to show differences between the scarred and normal tissue, while the absorption coefficient contrast decreases with time. This work shows the potential of THz in vivo imaging in the noninvasive detection and observation of scarred tissues and their healing process, even when they are not easily visible to the naked eye.

Finally, THz imaging has been used toward the development of noninvasive in vivo glucose biosensors [66]. Attenuated total reflection (ATR) THz signals were reflected from the palms of six healthy subjects, and the results showed a dependency of blood glucose levels on the ATR amplitude.

Ex vivo imaging

Ex vivo THz imaging in biological samples holds equal significance to in vivo imaging as it constitutes a label-free method that complements pathological studies, which are used as a reference. Ex vivo THz imaging has been extensively used in the imaging of digestive systems [67–71], reproductive systems [72–75], respiratory system [37], and nervous system [42]. In early studies performed by Fitzgerald et al. on cancerous breast tissues [76], they have observed contrast between the diseased and healthy tissues using THz waves, the origin of which was affiliated to the differences in the water content and the cell densities between the tissues. In a more recent study, Bowman et al. [75] have imaged dehydrated breast cancer tissue samples that were formalin fixed, paraffin-embedded infiltrating ductal carcinoma. They observed a higher THz contrast from the cancerous cells as compared with the surrounding fatty and fibrous regions, which was attributed to a higher cell density in the diseased region of the tissue.

In the case of oral cancer, a form of cancer that can be easily overlooked in the early stages, it is critical to have a better method to obtain vital diagnostic information in the initial testing phase. THz imaging has shown potential in this regard as shown by Sim et al. [68,77] in their 2013 study. As part of their work, they obtained freshly excised oral cancer tissue samples and an oral malignant melanoma tissue, frozen at two temperatures: 20°C and −20°C, and imaged these using THz radiation. Their results showed a greater THz sensitivity at both temperatures and a bigger difference in the refractive index and absorption coefficient at −20°C between the diseased and healthy regions of the tissues. They concluded that the higher THz response was due to the removal of water from the tissues at the two temperatures.

TERAHERTZ NONINVASIVE MEDICAL SYSTEMS AND DEVICES

Recently, there have been several breakthroughs on high-power THz sources, highly sensitive detectors, and host of other devices for THz technologies for range of applications [78–81]. This part of the review deals with various type of THz instruments in spectroscopic, imaging systems for biological applications like in tissue detection or in biosecurity and also addresses strategies how to accelerate practical usage of THz in biosamples.

THz Spectroscopy

Instrument for THz detection, analysis, and imaging with the THz amplitude and phase information from the specimen is correlated with the optical parameters like refractive index and extinction coefficient [82]. Three main types of THz spectroscopic systems biological applications are described below.

Fourier transform spectroscopy

Substantial advancement on THz resonance spectroscopy was possible due to advent of new generation of THz sources and detectors. Recent THz Fourier transform spectroscopy can be useful for bacterial cell studies [81] with wide spectral coverage.

Photomixing spectrometer

A photomixing spectrometer system contains GaAs photoconductor laser-based THz generation (Fig. 13.2A) [83]. These spectrometers have resolution ~500 MHz which depends on the frequency step [84] and, however, has a long measurement time. This technique is highly accurate, simple, and commercially viable due [85].

THz time-domain spectroscopy

THz-TDS systems are designed with a femtosecond laser and has a spectral resolution ~50 GHz [1,12,86]. Schematic of a typical system is shown in Fig. 13.2B [1]. Here, THz electric field is obtained, with the amplitude and phase as time-resolved spectroscopic information avoiding common sources of noise.

THz Imaging Systems

Lately, there have been enormous developments in THz imaging systems considering various advantages mainly for use in medicine. Here, couple of standard THz imaging systems are introduced.

THz-pulsed imaging system

The THz pulsed imaging system (TPI) operates both mode (transmission and reflection, Fig. 13.3A) usually with a femtosecond pulse laser [88], along with lensing system to collect, collimated, focus THz and reflected and backscattered THz pulse from sample is collected by unbiased photoconductive antenna for the laser-gated THz detection and can provide three-dimensional information [88,89]. Though TPI system takes long time for scanning, it can provide time-domain THz waveforms including intensity and phase information giving detailed properties of the specimen [90].

Continuous-wave THz imaging system. The continuous-wave THz imaging system (CW THz) does imaging also in transmission and reflection mode. Fig. 13.3B shows CW THz reflection imaging system [91,92]. For CW system, only the intensity information is of importance, hence data processing is simple. Also it is possible to drive a whole CW system only by laser diodes, hence these can be compact and commercially viable.

Terahertz spectroscopy and imaging in tissue and cell detection

Medical investigation for early and accurate detection is critical in medical diagnosis and healthcare. However, he current cell detection techniques heavily rely on chemical or biological labeling technology (e.g., flow cytometry, fluorescence molecular tomography,

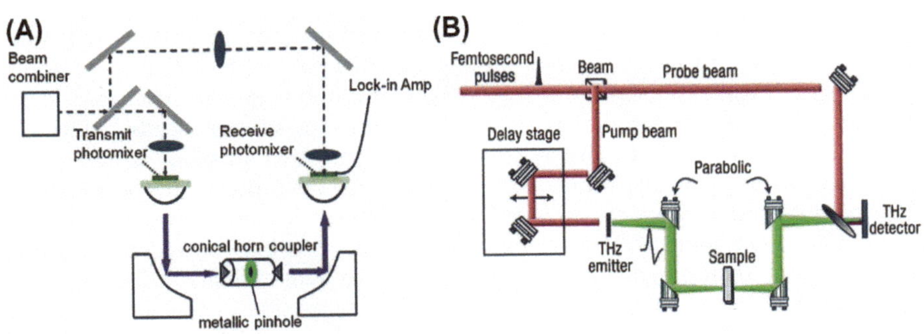

FIG. 13.2 The schematic of **(A)** photomixing spectrometer, with two photomixers (transmitter and receiver), and **(B)** a THz-TDS system. (Reproduced from L. Yu, L. Hao, T. Meiqiong, H. Jiaoqi, L. Wei, D. Jinying, C. Xueping, F. Weiling, Z. Yang, The medical application of terahertz technology in non-invasive detection of cells and tissues: opportunities and challenges, RSC Advances 9 (2019) 9354. https://doi.org/10.1039/C8RA10605C under creative commons attribution-noncommercial 3.0 unported licence.)

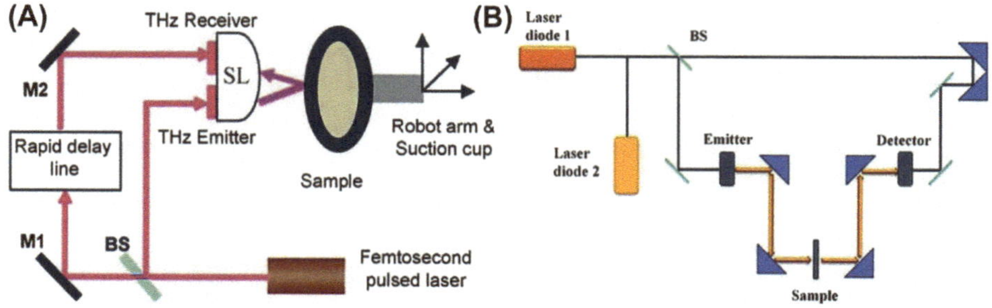

FIG. 13.3 Schematics of common THz imaging systems. **(A)** TPI reflection system. **(B)** The CW THz imaging system in transmission geometry. (Reproduced from L. Yu, L. Hao, T. Meiqiong, H. Jiaoqi, L. Wei, D. Jinying, C. Xueping, F. Weiling, Z. Yang, The medical application of terahertz technology in non-invasive detection of cells and tissues: opportunities and challenges, RSC Advances 9 (2019) 9354. https://doi.org/10.1039/C8RA10605C under creative commons attribution-noncommercial 3.0 unported licence.)

multiphoton microscopy), which may affect and interfere with live cells under study. Various label-free techniques also come with potential hazards and suffer poor sensitivity and detection speed. As discussed above, THz spectroscopy with various emerging highly sensitive and resolved spectroscopy systems can be developed for optical and label-free, reagent-free, noninvasive technique for identification of living cells and detection of any anomalies in their functionalities. THz spectroscopy is useful for detection and to differentiate a healthy from unhealthy (dehydrate, burned, pathological tissues) one. THz spectroscopy allows the study of time-resolved dynamics [26,93]. Table 13.1 gives the important features of THz spectroscopy for living cell detection.

It is important to note that large component tissue is water which has strong THz absorption [26], and various tissue preparation techniques are used to avoid the strong optical absorption of water (e.g., paraffin, frozen, formalin fixed tissues). However, they may have some reliability issues reported recently like cancer tissues embedded in paraffin displayed higher THz absorption than healthy tissues as shown in Fig. 13.4A [54]. Snap-frozen tissues are used to reduce the influence of water, but from various tissues' data from Alzheimer's patients it is observed to display less absorption than normal tissues [55]. As in biological tissues, strong optical absorption of water causes few millimeters' penetration; application of THz in vivo spectroscopy for biological tissues remains on the surface of the specimen. Interestingly, the strong water absorption is useful providing sensitive soft-tissue contrast. Different dielectric parameters, absorption coefficients, and refractive indexes are observed [52,63] among various skin tissues (Fig. 13.4B).

The study of THz spectroscopy and transmission imaging on dynamics of water, biomolecules, and tissues [94,95] is affected by the hydration level and morphology, hence both in vivo and in vitro reflection-based THz imaging systems are used (e.g., comparing water content, diagnose cancer, severity of burned tissues). THz imaging shows distinct features from healthy tissue to cancerous and diseased tissues with higher water content due to increased vascularity or edema. Simulation study reported InN-enhanced THz imaging for ultrasensitive skin cancer diagnosis which is based on water content variation [96]. It is possible to resolve the water contents in blood vessel and corneal tissue by THz imaging for in vivo long-term monitoring in blood and corneal tissue water content [97–99]. From higher THz reflection, gastric cancer tissues can be separated from normal mucosa correlating well with pathological images [100] (Fig. 13.5A). Also human hepatocellular carcinoma tissue imaging was possible with CW THz digital in-line holography systems in the absorption and phase-shift distributions (Fig. 13.5B) [101]. It was also reported that cross-polarized THz image of nonmelanoma skin cancer without Fresnel reflections from the glass–air interface shows tumor clearly [102].

THz in vivo imaging is still mainly applied to epidermal tissue due to low penetration depth; in addition, issues with water absorption need consideration in the THz spectrum for variable angle ellipsometry or polarized reflectometry [103,104]. However, in the future, integration of endoscopic system to THz imaging will be useful for clinical application [105,106] which is promising. However, there are still many issues with THz tissue detection mainly imperfect and nonstandardized sampling [94].

TABLE 13.1
Various Characteristics of THz Spectroscopy for Cell Detection.

Features	Explanation	Benefits	References
Low photon energy	THz radiation is insufficient to cause chemical damage to molecules, or knock particles out of atoms	Noninvasive method	C. Yu et al. Quantitative Imaging in Medicine and Surgery, 2012, 2, 33–45.
Sensitive to water molecules	Water molecules are significantly more absorptive than common macromolecules	Monitoring cellular activity and accessing the living state of cell according to different hydration	X. Yang et al. Journal of Biophotonics, 2016, 9, 1050–1058.
Precision of data analysis	Both amplitude and phase of the THz radiation can be obtained simultaneously	Precision analysis of spectral parameters	J.E. Haddad et al. Trends in Analytical Chemistry, 2013, 44, 98–105.
Spectral fingerprint	THz spectroscopies of different cells are unique and can be utilized as fingerprint	Distinguish different cells	C. Wang et al. Journal of Biophotonics, 2010, 3, 641–645.

Reproduced from L. Yu, L. Hao, T. Meiqiong, H. Jiaoqi, L. Wei, D. Jinying, C. Xueping, F. Weiling, Z. Yang, The medical application of terahertz technology in non-invasive detection of cells and tissues: opportunities and challenges, RSC Advances 9 (2019) 9354. https://doi.org/10.1039/C8RA10605C under creative commons attribution-noncommercial 3.0 unported licence.

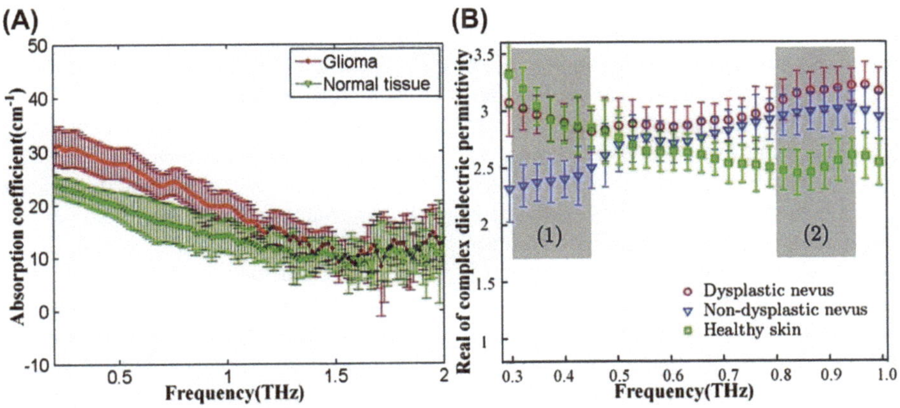

FIG. 13.4 THz absorption coefficients of tissues. **(A)** For glioma and normal tissue. **(B)** The real of the THz dielectric permittivity of dysplastic nevus, nondysplastic nevus, and healthy skin. (Reproduced from L. Yu, L. Hao, T. Meiqiong, H. Jiaoqi, L. Wei, D. Jinying, C. Xueping, F. Weiling, Z. Yang, The medical application of terahertz technology in non-invasive detection of cells and tissues: opportunities and challenges, RSC Advances 9 (2019) 9354. https://doi.org/10.1039/C8RA10605C under creative commons attribution-noncommercial 3.0 unported licence.)

On-Chip Integratable Terahertz Detectors

The advancement of the modern thermal radiation detectors combined with semiconductor device processing and materials science for on-chip integratable devices has created new opportunities in the electromagnetic frequency region ~1 THz for remote and nondestructive sensing and biomedical applications. THz waves are used for screening of tooth, skin cancer, tumors, analysis of DNA and gene, drug testing, environmental and homeland security, material defects, food diagnostics, investigating chemical compositions from planetary atmospheres, interstellar materials and mediums, among many other applications. Some interesting development was observed in recent time in high-power THz sources, uncooled detector, and real-time imaging and further improvisation on powerful and compact sources, detectors, with high-speed solid-state devices and may be flexible electronics is underway.

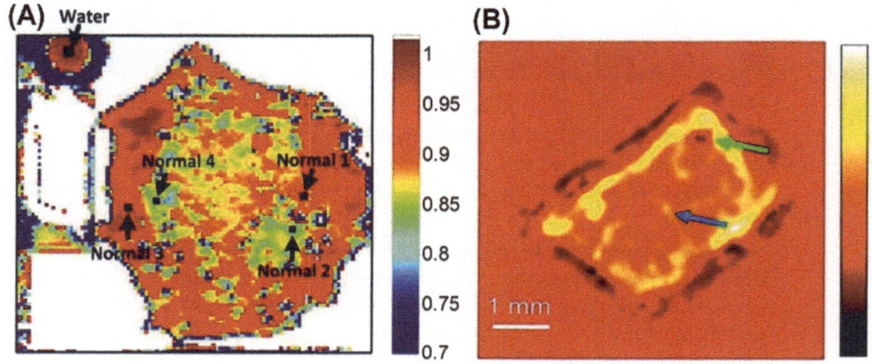

FIG. 13.5 Example of THz tissue imaging: **(A)** image from early gastric cancer tissue, **(B)** human hepatocellular carcinoma tissue from THz in-line hologram by phase-shift distribution reconstructing. (Reproduced from L. Yu, L. Hao, T. Meiqiong, H. Jiaoqi, L. Wei, D. Jinying, C. Xueping, F. Weiling, Z. Yang, The medical application of terahertz technology in non-invasive detection of cells and tissues: opportunities and challenges, RSC Advances 9 (2019) 9354. https://doi.org/10.1039/C8RA10605C under creative commons attribution-noncommercial 3.0 unported licence.)

Microbolometer is a THz detector which does not need cryogenic support; however, its room temperature detectivity is limited by thermal noise along with other performance limitations. With a large absorber for THz a structurally sustainable design is an antenna-coupled microbolometer; however, the thermistor and heater need to be independently optimized for higher sensitivity and a reasonable performance enhancement is expected for an optimum heater resistance. For microbolometer the key factors are responsivity and noise equivalent power (NEP) which are dependent on temperature coefficient of resistance (TCR) of the thermistor material. Hence, TCR of thermistor is the most important parameter in microbolometer design. Ti as a thermistor heater material has many advantages to fabricate uncooled antenna-coupled microbolometer at the 1-THz band with moderate to high responsivity [107−110]. A meander structure for integrated Ti heater thermistor yields higher responsivity than straight line thermistors [110]. Here, microbolometer design with meander shape Ti thermistor with increased effective length (hence higher electrical resistance resulting in enhanced responsivity) with narrow design width (DW = 0.1 μm or 0.2 μm) was found to have one-third of the TCR value of bulk Ti material [111] due to narrow-width effect. The microbolometers (Fig. 13.6) were fabricated with integrated heater/thermistor/half-wave dipole gold (Au) antenna with titanium (Ti) heater, SiO_2/SiN_x interlayer, and Ti thermistor on substrate (SiO_2/SiN_x). The microbolometer arrays are with meander-shaped Ti thermistor, with design width ~0.1 and 0.2 μm, with an integrated heater/thermistor/half-wave dipole antenna designed for 1 THz range. This design is based on our previous studies where process steps are discussed in details [109−113].

A comparative idea about these detectors with other related devices is given in Table 13.2. It is interesting to note that VO_x or VO_2 devices have far responsivity due to higher bulk TCR; however, they are not naturally abundant and are not compatible standard semiconductor manufacturing technologies. One study by Saxena et al. [115] has similar layout with short meander structure with design width ~ 2 μm with responsivity ~ 30 V/W. A few related studies on THz imaging and sensing can also be highlighted here for a comprehensive understanding of imaging using these devices [116−118]. However, these microbolometer devices in the study above stand out in terms of performance of the unit device and scope for further miniaturization and suited to state-of-the-art semiconductor fabrication technology as on-chip integrable detector arrays.

OUTLOOK

Although THz technology has undergone several impressive advancements over the past decade, there remains a gap between the technology and the ability to use it. Some of the challenges that need to be addressed are in the areas of THz sources, detectors, and manipulators. However, recent research has pointed toward 2DMs, with their unique properties, as a promising solution to bridge this gap [119,120].

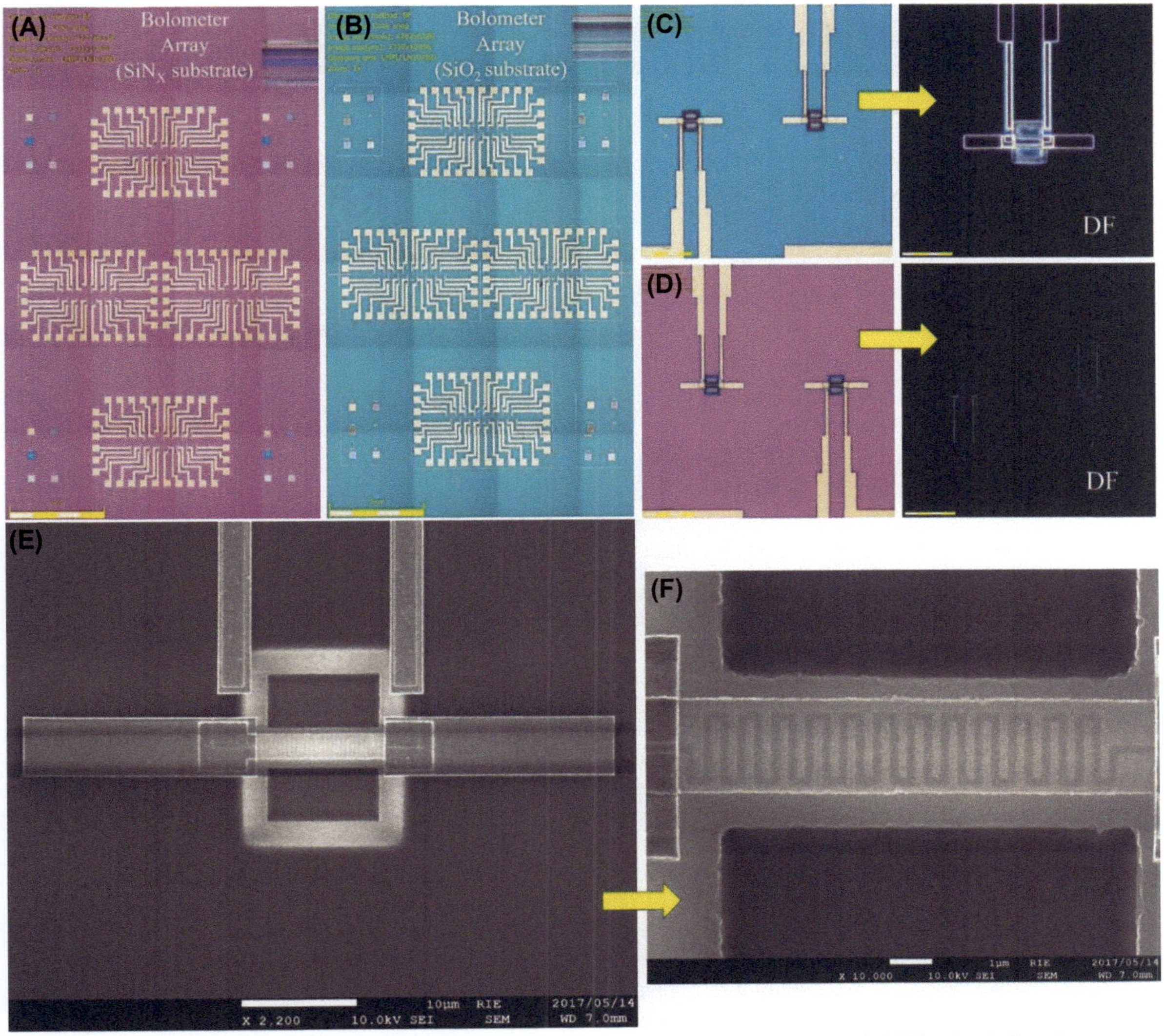

FIG. 13.6 (**A** and **B**) Optical microscope images of Ti-based uncooled antenna-coupled THz microbolometer arrays with design width of the thermistor ~ 0.1 and 0.2 μm on SiN_x and SiO_2 substrate. (**C** and **D**) Enlarged optical microscope images of a set of microbolometers with dark-field view. (**E** and **F**) FE-SEM enlarged view microbolometer device with heater and the meander–structured thermistor floating above the cavity. (Reproduced from A. Banerjee, H. Satoh, D. Elamaran, Y. Sharma, N. Hiromoto, H. Inokawa, Performance improvement of on-chip integrable terahertz microbolometer arrays using nanoscale meander titanium thermistor, Journal of Applied Physics 125 (2019) 214502.)

Of all the 2DMs, graphene has been the more explored option to fill the void [119,120]. Research outcomes by V. Ryzhii et al. [121,122] and F. Rana et al. [123] have shown that graphene plasmonic oscillators can be used as THz sources since graphene is known to possess intrinsic plasmons that can be manipulated [124]. Using an electron–hole plasma from an optically pumped graphene plasmonic oscillator, they were able to generate a 1 THz wave.

In another effort highlighting the applicability of 2DMs for THz applications, Zak et al. [125] have shown an enhanced THz detection response from graphene field effect transistors (GFET). Their THz detectors, fabricated from antenna-integrated GFETs using CVD-grown single-layer graphene on Si/SiO_2 substrates, were able to attain room temperature rectification of a THz signal and achieve an optical response of higher than 14 V/W with a minimum optical NEP of

TABLE 13.2
Comparative Performance of Devices.

S. No.	Detector Type	Responsivity (V/W)	NEP ($W/Hz^{1/2}$)	Detector Array Size	TCR Thermistor (%/K)
1	Absorber type VO_x	12.6k	…	32 × 32	−1.9
2	Absorber type polycrystal mixed thin VO_x film	9k	1.67×10^{-11}	…	−1.5
3	Absorber type thin VO_x film	5k	…	64 × 2	−0.02
4	Absorber type thin VO_2 film	17k	…	…	…
5	Absorber type Ti	1.6k	…	256 × 256	0.26
6	Half-wave antenna-coupled Ti	90	4.6×10^{-10}	…	0.03
7	Polycrystalline SiGe	975	…	…	…
8	Absorber type Ti	30 (meander DW = 2 μm)	…	16 × 16	0.27
9	Half-wave dipole antenna-coupled Ti	787 (meander DW = 0.1 μm)	1.85×10^{-10} (electrical)	Unit device	0.16

Reproduced from A. Banerjee, H. Satoh, D. Elamaran, Y. Sharma, N. Hiromoto, H. Inokawa, Performance improvement of on-chip integrable terahertz microbolometer arrays using nanoscale meander titanium thermistor, Journal of Applied Physics 125 (2019) 214502.

515 pW/Hz. Their basis for replacing the metal gate with graphene is because of the high carrier mobility in graphene leading to longer carrier scattering times.

On active manipulation of THz waves, there have been several approaches over the last decade to fabricate THz devices having reconfigurable optical and electrical components, with electrical manipulation being the most reliable option [126–130]. However, all of the electrically tunable THz devices have suffered from high insertion loss that defeats the very purpose of achieving reconfigurability. Graphene has shown a huge potential in this regard because of its unique ability to tune THz waves while adding negligible insertion loss [131,132]. It becomes an even more attractive option as an on-chip solution because of its structural integrity, easy availability, and low cost. Much work in this domain has been done by Sensale-Rodriguez et al. at the University of Notre Dame and their results on predicted and measured performances of graphene-based THz devices have been remarkable. For instance, in one of their works, they have achieved an enhancement in THz modulation depth of an AlGaAs/GaAs two-dimensional electron gas structure from less than 30% to more than 90% just by replacing the metal gate with a single layer of graphene [132]. They have further demonstrated that 100% THz transmission is possible from graphene-based THz devices if one were to use two sheets of graphene separated by an insulator.

Other than graphene, transition metal dichalcogenides (TMDs) have also been explored for novel THz devices, although not much work has been pursued in this regard. Of the few literature studies, Docherty et al. [133] have measured ultrafast carrier dynamics in monolayer and trilayer MoS_2 and WSe_2 using time-resolved photoluminescence and THz spectroscopy. Their results indicate that the response times for photoconductivity and photoluminescence is 350 fs for monolayer MoS_2 and 1 ps for trilayer MoS_2 and monolayer WSe_2. These are very promising results hinting at the potential of TMDs being applied in high-speed THz devices and thereby promoting the progress of 2DMs for THz applications.

With many ongoing research efforts in the 2DM and THz domain, we should expect to see more interesting and comprehensive outcomes in the very near future. Integration of 2DMs with existing THz technology has the potential to open a pathway into unique THz phenomena leading to novel THz devices having breakthrough performances than those of conventional devices. While this is true, there are still some hurdles that need to be overcome. Defects and contaminations that can creep in through 2DM growth or deposition need to be kept in check as they can cause sample degradation affecting device stability over time. Device cost is also a concern and a trade-off between THz performance and the related expenditure would need to be addressed too.

REFERENCES

[1] B. Ferguson, X.C. Zhang, Materials for terahertz science and technology, Nature Materials 1 (2002) 26–33, https://doi.org/10.1038/nmat708.

[2] C. Sirtori, Bridge for the terahertz gap, Nature 417 (2002) 132–133, https://doi.org/10.1038/417132b.

[3] D.M. Mittleman, Perspective: terahertz science and technology, Journal of Applied Physics 122 (2017), https://doi.org/10.1063/1.5007683.

[4] J. Button, D.R. Cohn, M. Von Ortenbert, B. Lax, Physical Review Letters 28 (1972) 1637–1639.

[5] K.H. Yang, P.L. Richards, Y.R. Shen, Generation of far-infrared radiation by picosecond light pulses in $LiNbO_3$, Applied Physics Letters 19 (1971) 320–323, https://doi.org/10.1063/1.1653935.

[6] K. Sakai, T. Fukui, Y. Tsunawaki, H. Yoshinaga, Metallic mesh bandpass filters and Fabry-Perot interferometer for the far infrared, Japanese Journal of Applied Physics 8 (1969) 1046.

[7] L. Genzel, K.-L. Barth, F. Keilmann, Precise determination of high metallic reflection in the far-infrared: the reflection-Fabry-Perot, International Journal of Infrared Millim Waves 11 (1990) 1133–1161.

[8] H.A. Gebbie, N.W.B. Stone, F.D. Findlay, A stimulated emission source at 0.34 millimeter wave-length, Nature 685 (169) (1964) 4933.

[9] T.S. Hartwick, D.T. Hodges, D.H. Barker, F.B. Foote, Far infrared imagery, Applied Optics 15 (1976) 1919–1922.

[10] P.K. Cheo, Far-infrared laser system for detection of defects in polyethylene-insulated power cables, Optics Letters 2 (1978) 78–80.

[11] A.P. DeFonzo, M. Jarwala, C. Lutz, Transient response of planar integrated optoelectronic antennas, Applied Physics Letters 1155 (1987) 1–4, https://doi.org/10.1063/1.97947.

[12] C. Fattinger, D. Grischkowsky, Point source terahertz optics, Applied Physics Letters 53 (1998) 1480–1482, https://doi.org/10.1063/1.99971.

[13] C. Fattinger, D. Grischkowsky, Terahertz beams, Applied Physics Letters 54 (1989) 490–492.

[14] B.B. Hu, M.C. Nuss, Imaging with terahertz waves, Optics Letters 20 (1995) 1716–1718.

[15] D.M. Mittleman, et al., T-ray tomography, Optics Letters. 22 (12) (1997) 904–906.

[16] K. McClatchey, M.T. Reiten, R.A. Cheville, Time resolved synthetic aperture terahertz impulse imaging, Applied Physics Letters 79 (2008) 4485–4487, https://doi.org/10.1063/1.1427745.

[17] T.D. Dorney, J.L. Johnson, J. Van Rudd, R.G. Baraniuk, W.W. Symes, D.M. Mittleman, Terahertz reflection imaging using Kirchhoff migration, Optics Letters 26 (2001) 1513–1515.

[18] J. Pearce, H. Choi, D.M. Mittleman, J. White, D. Zimdars, Terahertz wide aperture reflection tomography, Optics Letters 30 (2005) 1653–1655.

[19] P.H. Siegel, Terahertz technology, IEEE Transactions on Microwave Theory and Techniques 50 (2002) 910–928.

[20] F.G. Sun, Z. Jiang, X.-C. Zhang, Analysis of terahertz pulse measurement with a chirped probe beam, Applied Physics Letters 73 (1998) 2233–2235, https://doi.org/10.1063/1.121685.

[21] S. Hunsche, M. Koch, I. Brener, THz near-field imaging, Optics Communications (1998) 22–26.

[22] O. Mitrofanov, I. Brener, R. Harel, J.D. Wynn, L.N. Pfeiffer, K.W. West, J. Federici, Terahertz near-field microscopy based on a collection mode detector, Applied Physics Letters 77 (2000) 3496–3498, https://doi.org/10.1063/1.1328772.

[23] H. Chen, R. Kersting, G.C. Cho, Terahertz imaging with nanometer resolution, Applied Physics Letters 83 (2003) 3009–3011, https://doi.org/10.1063/1.1616668.

[24] U. Schade, K. Holldack, P. Kuske, G. Wustefeld, H.W. Hubers, THz near-field imaging employing synchrotron radiation, Applied Physics Letters 84 (2004) 1422–1424, https://doi.org/10.1063/1.1650034.

[25] K. Wang, D.M. Mittleman, N.C.J. Van Der Valk, P.C.M. Planken, Antenna effects in terahertz apertureless near-field optical microscopy, Applied Physics Letters 85 (2004) 2715–2717, https://doi.org/10.1063/1.1797554.

[26] K. Kawase, Y. Ogawa, Y. Watanabe, Non-destructive terahertz imaging of illicit drugs using spectral fingerprints, Optics Express 11 (2003) 2549–2554.

[27] J. Darmo, V. Tamosiunas, G. Fasching, J. Kröll, K. Unterrainer, M. Beck, M. Giovannini, J. Faist, C. Kremser, P. Debbage, Imaging with a Terahertz quantum cascade laser, Optics Express 12 (2004) 1879–1884.

[28] S.M. Kim, F. Hatami, J.S. Harris, A.W. Kurian, J. Ford, D. King, M. Giovannini, N. Hoyler, J. Faist, G. Harris, A.W. Kurian, J. Ford, D. King, G. Scalari, M. Giovannini, N. Hoyler, J. Faist, G. Harris, Biomedical terahertz imaging with a quantum cascade laser, Applied Physics Letters 88 (2008) 153903, https://doi.org/10.1063/1.2194229.

[29] A.W.M. Lee, Q. Qin, S. Kumar, B.S. Williams, Q. Hu, J.L. Reno, Real-time terahertz imaging over a standoff distance (>25 meters), Applied Physics Letters 89 (2008) 141125, https://doi.org/10.1063/1.2360210.

[30] A. Tredicucci, U. Pisa, E.H. Linfield, F. Rossi, Terahertz semiconductor-heterostructure laser, Nature 417 (2002) 156–159, https://doi.org/10.1038/417156a.

[31] K. Kawase, Y. Ogawa, H. Minamide, Terahertz parametric sources and imaging applications, Semiconductor Science and Technology 20 (2005) S258–S265, https://doi.org/10.1088/0268-1242/20/7/017.

[32] T. Yasui, T. Yasuda, K. Sawanaka, T. Araki, Terahertz paintmeter for noncontact monitoring of thickness and drying progress in paint film, Applied Optics 44 (2005) 6849–6856.

[33] M. Lu, J. Shen, N. Li, Y. Zhang, C. Zhang, L. Liang, X. Xu, Detection and identification of illicit drugs using terahertz imaging, Journal of Applied Physics 100 (2008) 103104, https://doi.org/10.1063/1.2388041.

[34] W.L. Chan, K. Charan, D. Takhar, K.F. Kelly, R.G. Baraniuk, M. Daniel, W.L. Chan, K. Charan,

D. Takhar, K.F. Kelly, R.G. Baraniuk, D.M. Mittleman, A single-pixel terahertz imaging system based on compressed sensing, Applied Physics Letters 93 (2008) 121105, https://doi.org/10.1063/1.2989126.
[35] N.I. Landy, C.M. Bingham, T. Tyler, N. Jokerst, D.R. Smith, W.J. Padilla, Physical Review 79 (2009) 125104, https://doi.org/10.1103/PhysRevB.79.125104.
[36] S.J. Oh, J. Kang, I. Maeng, J. Suh, Y. Huh, S. Haam, J. Son, Nanoparticle-enabled terahertz imaging for cancer diagnosis, Optics Express 17 (2009) 3469–3475.
[37] M.A. Brun, F. Formanek, A. Yasuda, M. Sekine, N. Ando, Y. Eishii, Terahertz imaging applied to cancer diagnosis, Physics in Medicine and Biology 55 (2010) 4615–4623, https://doi.org/10.1088/0031-9155/55/16/001.
[38] P. Dean, Y.L. Lim, A. Valavanis, R. Kliese, M. Nikoli, S.P. Khanna, M. Lachab, D. Indjin, Z. Ikoni, P. Harrison, A.D. Raki, E.H. Linfield, A.G. Davies, Terahertz imaging through self-mixing in a quantum cascade laser, Optics Letters 36 (2011) 2587–2589.
[39] F. Schuster, D. Coquillat, H. Videlier, M. Sakowicz, F. Teppe, L. Dussopt, B. Giffard, T. Skotnicki, W. Knap, Broadband terahertz imaging with highly sensitive silicon CMOS detectors, Optics Express 19 (2011) 7827–7832.
[40] S. Busch, B. Scherger, M. Scheller, M. Koch, Optically controlled terahertz beam steering and imaging, Optics Letters 37 (2012) 1391–1393.
[41] B. Sensale-rodriguez, S. Rafique, R. Yan, M. Zhu, D. Jena, L. Liu, H.G. Xing, Terahertz imaging employing graphene modulator arrays, Optics Express 21 (2013) 936–941.
[42] S.J. Oh, S. Kim, Y. Bin Ji, K. Jeong, Y. Park, J. Yang, D.W. Park, S.K. Noh, S. Kang, Y. Huh, J. Son, J. Suh, Study of freshly excised brain tissues using terahertz imaging, Biomedical Optics Express 5 (2014) 2837–2842, https://doi.org/10.1364/BOE.5.002837.
[43] R.I. Stantchev, B. Sun, S.M. Hornett, P.A. Hobson, G.M. Gibson, M.J. Padgett, E. Hendry, Noninvasive , near-field terahertz imaging of hidden objects using a single-pixel detector, Science Advances 2 (2016) e1600190.
[44] C.G. Wade, N. Šibalic, N.R. De Melo, J.M. Kondo, C.S. Adams, K.J. Weatherill, Real-time near-field terahertz imaging with atomic optical fluorescence, Nature Photonics 11 (2017) 40–44, https://doi.org/10.1038/nphoton.2016.214.
[45] F. Sanjuan, G. Gaborit, J. Coutaz, Sub-wavelength terahertz imaging through optical rectification, Scientific Reports 8 (2018) 13492, https://doi.org/10.1038/s41598-018-31970-w.
[46] D.M. Mittleman, Twenty years of terahertz imaging, Optics Express 26 (2018) 142–149.
[47] J.P. Erraud, J.G. Uillet, Shape-from-focus for real-time terahertz 3D imaging, Optics Letters 44 (2019) 483–486.
[48] X. Yang, X. Zhao, K. Yang, Y. Liu, Y. Liu, W. Fu, Y. Luo, Biomedical applications of terahertz spectroscopy and imaging, Trends in Biotechnology 34 (2016) 810–824.
[49] J. Qin, Y. Ying, L. Xie, The detection of agricultural products and food using terahertz spectroscopy: a review, Applied Spectroscopy Reviews 48 (2013) 439–457.
[50] B. Born, S.J. Kim, S. Ebbinghaus, M. Gruebele, M. Havenith, The terahertz dance of water with the proteins: the effect of protein flexibility on the dynamical hydration shell of ubiquitin, Faraday Discussions 141 (2009) 161–173.
[51] A.J. Fitzgerald, E. Berry, N.N. Zinovev, S. Homer-Vanniasinkam, R.E. Miles, J.M. Chamberlain, M.A. Smith, Catalogue of human tissue optical properties at terahertz frequencies, Journal of Biological Physics 29 (2003) 123–128.
[52] I. Echchgadda, J.A. Grundt, M. Tarango, B.L. Ibey, T.D. Tongue, M. Liang, H. Xin, G.J. Wilmink, Using a portable terahertz spectrometer to measure the optical properties of in vivo human skin, Journal of Biomedical Optics 18 (2013) 120503, https://doi.org/10.1117/1.JBO.18.12.120503.
[53] F. Wahaia, I. Kasalynas, D. Seliuta, G. Molis, A. Urbanowicz, C.D.C. Silva, F. Carneiro, G. Valusis, P.L. Granja, Study of paraffin-embedded colon cancer tissue using terahertz spectroscopy, Journal of Molecular Structure 1079 (2015) 448–453.
[54] K. Meng, T. Chen, T. Chen, L. Zhu, Q. Liu, Z. Li, F. Li, S.C. Zhong, Z.R. Li, H. Feng, J.H. Zhao, Terahertz pulsed spectroscopy of paraffin-embedded brain glioma, Journal of Biomedical Optics 19 (2014) 77001.
[55] G.M. Png, R. Flook, B.-H. Ng, D. Abbott, Terahertz spectroscopy of snap-frozen human brain tissue: an initial study, Electronics Letters 45 (2009) 343–345.
[56] L. Xie, Y. Yao, Y. Ying, The application of terahertz spectroscopy to protein detection: a review, Applied Sepctroscopy Reviews 49 (2014) 448–461.
[57] R. Liu, M. He, R. Su, Y. Yu, W. Qi, Z. He, Insulin amyloid fibrillation studied by terahertz spectroscopy and other biophysical methods, Biochemaical and Biophysical Research Communications 391 (2010) 862–867.
[58] S.P. Mickan, A. Menikh, H. Liu, C.A. Mannella, R. MacColl, D. Abbott, J. Munch, X.C. Zhang, Biology, Label-free bioaffinity detection using terahertz technology, Physics in Medicine and Biology 47 (2002) 3789.
[59] C.S. Joseph, A.N. Yaroslavsky, M. Al-Arashi, T.M. Goyette, J.C. Dickinson, A.J. Gatesman, B.W. Soper, C.M. Forgione, T.M. Horgan, E.J. Ehasz, Terahertz spectroscopy of intrinsic biomarkers for nonmelanoma skin cancer, in: Terahertz Technology Applied II, International Society for Optics and Photonics, 2009, p. 72150I.
[60] S. Sy, S. Huang, Y.-X.J. Wang, J. Yu, A.T. Ahuja, Y. Zhang, E. Pickwell-MacPherson, Biology, Terahertz spectroscopy of liver cirrhosis: investigating the origin of contrast, Physics in Medicine and Biology 55 (2010) 7587.
[61] H. Chen, T.-H. Chen, T.-F. Tseng, J.-T. Lu, C.-C. Kuo, S.-C. Fu, W.-J. Lee, Y.-F. Tsai, Y.-Y. Huang, E.Y. Chuang, High-sensitivity in vivo THz transmission imaging of

early human breast cancer in a subcutaneous xenograft mouse model, Optics Express 19 (2011) 21552–21562.
[62] K.I. Zaytsev, K.G. Kudrin, I.V. Reshetov, A.A. Gavdush, N.V. Chernomyrdin, V.E. Karasik, S.O. Yurchenko, In vivo spectroscopy of healthy skin and pathology in terahertz frequency range, Journal of Physics: Conference Series, IOP Publishing 584 (2015) 012023.
[63] K.I. Zaytsev, K.G. Kudrin, V.E. Karasik, I.V. Reshetov, S.O. Yurchenko, In vivo terahertz spectroscopy of pigmentary skin nevi: pilot study of non-invasive early diagnosis of dysplasia, Applied Physics Letters 106 (2015) 53702.
[64] K.I. Zaytsev, N.V. Chernomyrdin, K.G. Kudrin, A.A. Gavdush, P.A. Nosov, S.O. Yurchenko, I.V. Reshetov, In vivo terahertz pulsed spectroscopy of dysplastic and non-dysplastic skin nevi, Journal of Physics: Conference Series, IOP Publishing 735 (2016) 12076.
[65] S. Fan, B.S.Y. Ung, E.P.J. Parrott, V.P. Wallace, E. Pickwell-MacPherson, In vivo terahertz reflection imaging of human scars during and after the healing process, Journal of Biophotonics 10 (2017) 1143–1151.
[66] O. Cherkasova, M. Nazarov, A. Shkurinov, Noninvasive blood glucose monitoring in the terahertz frequency range, Optical and Quantum Electronics 48 (2016) 217.
[67] C.B. Reid, A. Fitzgerald, G. Reese, R. Goldin, P. Tekkis, P.S. O'Kelly, E. Pickwell-MacPherson, A.P. Gibson, V.P. Wallace, Terahertz pulsed imaging of freshly excised human colonic tissues, Physics in Medicine and Biology 56 (2011) 4333–4353, https://doi.org/10.1088/0031-9155/56/14/008.
[68] Y.C. Sim, J.Y. Park, K.-M. Ahn, C. Park, J.-H. Son, Terahertz imaging of excised oral cancer at frozen temperature, Biomedical Optics Express 4 (2013) 1413–1421, https://doi.org/10.1364/BOE.4.001413.
[69] H. Chen, S.H. Ma, X. Wu, W. Yang, T. Zhao, Diagnose Human Colonic Tissues by Terahertz Near-Field Imaging, SPIE, 2015, https://doi.org/10.1117/1.JBO.20.3.036017.
[70] P. Doradla, K. Alavi, C.S. Joseph, R.H. Giles, Detection of Colon Cancer by Continuous-Wave Terahertz Polarization Imaging Technique, SPIE, 2013, https://doi.org/10.1117/1.JBO.18.9.090504.
[71] F. Wahaia, I. Kasalynas, R. Venckevicius, D. Seliuta, G. Valusis, A. Urbanowicz, G. Molis, F. Carneiro, C.D. Carvalho Silva, P.L. Granja, Terahertz absorption and reflection imaging of carcinoma-affected colon tissues embedded in paraffin, Journal of Molecular Structure 1107 (2016) 214–219, https://doi.org/10.1016/j.molstruc.2015.11.048.
[72] B. St Peter, S. Yngvesson, P. Siqueira, P. Kelly, A. Khan, S. Glick, A. Karellas, Development and testing of a single frequency terahertz imaging system for breast cancer detection, IEEE Transactions of Terahertz Science and Technology 3 (2013) 374–386, https://doi.org/10.1109/TTHZ.2013.2241429.
[73] H. Chen, W.-J. Lee, H.-Y. Huang, C.-M. Chiu, Y.-F. Tsai, T.-F. Tseng, J.-T. Lu, W.-L. Lai, C.-K. Sun, Performance of THz fiber-scanning near-field microscopy to diagnose breast tumors, Optics Express 19 (2011) 19523–19531, https://doi.org/10.1364/OE.19.019523.
[74] E.-A. Jung, M.-H. Lim, K.-W. Moon, Y.-W. Do, S.-S. Lee, H.-W. Han, H.-J. Choi, K.-S. Cho, K.-R. Kim, Terahertz pulse imaging of micro-metastatic lymph nodes in early-stage cervical cancer patients, Journal of the Optical Society of Korea 15 (2011) 155–160. http://www.osapublishing.org/josk/abstract.cfm?URI&=josk-15-2-155.
[75] T.C. Bowman, M. El-Shenawee, L.K. Campbell, Terahertz imaging of excised breast tumor tissue on paraffin sections, IEEE Transactions on Antennas and Propagation 63 (2015) 2088–2097, https://doi.org/10.1109/TAP.2015.2406893.
[76] A.J. Fitzgerald, V.P. Wallace, M. Jimenez-Linan, L. Bobrow, R.J. Pye, A.D. Purushotham, D.D. Arnone, Terahertz pulsed imaging of human breast tumors, Radiology 239 (2006) 533–540, https://doi.org/10.1148/radiol.2392041315.
[77] Y.C. Sim, K. Ahn, J.Y. Park, C. Park, J. Son, Temperature-dependent terahertz imaging of excised oral malignant melanoma, IEEE Journal of Biomedical and Health Informatics 17 (2013) 779–784, https://doi.org/10.1109/JBHI.2013.2252357.
[78] D.H. Auston, M.C. Nuss, Electrooptical generation and detection of femtosecond electrical transients, IEEE Journal of Quantum Electronics 24 (1988) 184–197, https://doi.org/10.1109/3.114.
[79] I. Duling, D. Zimdars, Revealing hidden defects, Nature Photonics 3 (2009) 630–632, https://doi.org/10.1038/nphoton.2009.206.
[80] V. Petrov, J. Kokkoniemi, D. Moltchanov, J. Lehtomäki, Y. Koucheryavy, Enabling simultaneous cooling anddata transmission in the terahertz band for board-to-board communications, Physical Communication 22 (2017) 9–18, https://doi.org/10.1016/j.phycom.2016.11.002.
[81] T. Globus, A.M. Moyer, B. Gelmont, T. Khromova, M.I. Lvovska, I. Sizov, J. Ferrance, Highly resolved sub-terahertz vibrational spectroscopy of biological macromolecules and cells, IEEE Sensors Journal 13 (2013) 72–79, https://doi.org/10.1109/JSEN.2012.2224333.
[82] P. Sun, Y. Zou, Complex dielectric properties of anhydrous polycrystalline glucose in the terahertz region, Optical and Quantum Electronics 48 (2015) 27, https://doi.org/10.1007/s11082-015-0273-4.
[83] W. Zhang, E.R. Brown, M. Rahman, M.L. Norton, Observation of terahertz absorption signatures in microliter DNA solutions, Applied Physics Letters 102 (2013) 23701, https://doi.org/10.1063/1.4775696.
[84] W. Zhang, E.R. Brown, L. Viveros, K.P. Burris, C.N. Stewart Jr., Narrow terahertz attenuation signatures in *Bacillus thuringiensis*, Journal of Biophotonics 7 (2014) 818–824, https://doi.org/10.1002/jbio.201300042.
[85] S. Preu, G.H. Döhler, S. Malzer, L.J. Wang, A.C. Gossard, Tunable, continuous-wave Terahertz photomixer sources and applications, Journal of Applied Physics 109 (2011) 61301, https://doi.org/10.1063/1.3552291.
[86] A. Redo-Sanchez, N. Laman, B. Schulkin, T. Tongue, Review of terahertz technology readiness assessment and

applications, Journal of Infrared, Millimeter, and Terahertz Waves 34 (2013) 500–518, https://doi.org/10.1007/s10762-013-9998-y.

[87] L. Yu, L. Hao, T. Meiqiong, H. Jiaoqi, L. Wei, D. Jinying, C. Xueping, F. Weiling, Z. Yang, The medical application of terahertz technology in non-invasive detection of cells and tissues: opportunities and challenges, RSC Advances 9 (2019) 9354–9363, https://doi.org/10.1039/C8RA10605C.

[88] Y.-C. Shen, Terahertz pulsed spectroscopy and imaging for pharmaceutical applications: a review, International Journal of Pharmceutics 417 (2011) 48–60, https://doi.org/10.1016/j.ijpharm.2011.01.012.

[89] P.C. Ashworth, E. Pickwell-MacPherson, E. Provenzano, S.E. Pinder, A.D. Purushotham, M. Pepper, V.P. Wallace, Terahertz pulsed spectroscopy of freshly excised human breast cancer, Optics Express 17 (2009) 12444–12454, https://doi.org/10.1364/OE.17.012444.

[90] K. McClatchey, M.T. Reiten, R.A. Cheville, Time resolved synthetic aperture terahertz impulse imaging, Applied Physics Letters 79 (2001) 4485–4487, https://doi.org/10.1063/1.1427745.

[91] P. Doradla, K. Alavi, C.S. Joseph, R.H. Giles, Single-channel prototype terahertz endoscopic system, Journal of Biomedical Optics 19 (2014) 1–3, https://doi.org/10.1117/1.JBO.19.8.080501.

[92] C.S. Joseph, A.N. Yaroslavsky, V.A. Neel, T.M. Goyette, R.H. Giles, Continuous-wave terahertz reflection imaging of ex vivo nonmelanoma skin cancers, Proceedings of SPIE (2012), https://doi.org/10.1117/12.909135.

[93] D. Russo, G. Hura, T. Head-Gordon, Hydration dynamics near a model protein surface, Biophysical Journal 86 (2004) 1852–1862, https://doi.org/10.1016/S0006-3495(04)74252-6.

[94] G.M. Png, J.W. Choi, B.W.-H. Ng, S.P. Mickan, D. Abbott, X.-C. Zhang, The impact of hydration changes in fresh bio-tissue on THz spectroscopic measurements, Physics in Medicine and Biology 53 (2008) 3501–3517, https://doi.org/10.1088/0031-9155/53/13/007.

[95] Z.D. Taylor, R.S. Singh, D.B. Bennett, P. Tewari, C.P. Kealey, N. Bajwa, M.O. Culjat, A. Stojadinovic, H. Lee, J. Hubschman, E.R. Brown, W.S. Grundfest, THz medical imaging: in vivo hydration sensing, IEEE Transactions on Terahertz Science and Technology 1 (2011) 201–219, https://doi.org/10.1109/TTHZ.2011.2159551.

[96] M. Ney, I. Abdulhalim, Ultrahigh polarimetric image contrast enhancement for skin cancer diagnosis using InN plasmonic nanoparticles in the terahertz range, Journal of Biomedical Optics 20 (2015) 1–14, https://doi.org/10.1117/1.JBO.20.12.125007.

[97] T.-F. Tseng, S.-C. Yang, Y.-T. Shih, Y.-F. Tsai, T.-D. Wang, C.-K. Sun, Near-field sub-THz transmission-type image system for vessel imaging in-vivo, Optics Express 23 (2015) 25058–25071, https://doi.org/10.1364/OE.23.025058.

[98] Z.D. Taylor, J. Garritano, S. Sung, N. Bajwa, D.B. Bennett, B. Nowroozi, P. Tewari, J.W. Sayre, J. Hubschman, S.X. Deng, E.R. Brown, W.S. Grundfest, THz and mm-wave sensing of corneal tissue water content: in vivo sensing and imaging results, IEEE Transactions on Terahertz Science and Technology 5 (2015) 184–196, https://doi.org/10.1109/TTHZ.2015.2392628.

[99] D.B. Bennett, Z.D. Taylor, P. Tewari, R.S. Singh, M.O. Culjat, W.S. Grundfest, D.J. Sassoon, R.D. Johnson, J.-P. Hubschman, E. Brown, Terahertz sensing in corneal tissues, Journal of Biomedical Optics 16 (2011) 1–9, https://doi.org/10.1117/1.3575168.

[100] Y. Bin Ji, C.H. Park, H. Kim, S.-H. Kim, G.M. Lee, S.K. Noh, T.-I. Jeon, J.-H. Son, Y.-M. Huh, S. Haam, S.J. Oh, S.K. Lee, J.-S. Suh, Feasibility of terahertz reflectometry for discrimination of human early gastric cancers, Biomedical Optics Express 6 (2015) 1398–1406, https://doi.org/10.1364/BOE.6.001398.

[101] L. Rong, T. Latychevskaia, C. Chen, D. Wang, Z. Yu, X. Zhou, Z. Li, H. Huang, Y. Wang, Z. Zhou, Terahertz in-line digital holography of human hepatocellular carcinoma tissue, Scientific Reports 5 (2015) 8445, https://doi.org/10.1038/srep08445.

[102] C.S. Joseph, R. Patel, V.A. Neel, R.H. Giles, A.N. Yaroslavsky, Imaging of ex vivo nonmelanoma skin cancers in the optical and terahertz spectral regions optical and Terahertz skin cancers imaging, Journal of Biophotonics 7 (2014) 295–303, https://doi.org/10.1002/jbio.201200111.

[103] M. Ney, I. Abdulhalim, Does human skin truly behave as an array of helical antennae in the millimeter and terahertz wave ranges? Optics Letters 35 (2010) 3180–3182, https://doi.org/10.1364/OL.35.003180.

[104] M. Ney, I.A. II, Modeling of reflectometric and ellipsometric spectra from the skin in the terahertz and submillimeter waves region, Journal of Biomedical Optics 16 (2011) 1–16, https://doi.org/10.1117/1.3592779.

[105] P. Doradla, Book - Terahertz Endoscopic System for Cancer Detection, Lambert Publishing, Germany, 2015. https://www.morebooks.de/store/gb/book/terahertz-endoscopic-system-for-cancer-detection/isbn/978-3-659-68155-4.

[106] P. Doradla, C. Joseph, R.H. Giles, Terahertz endoscopic imaging for colorectal cancer detection: current status and future perspectives, World Journal of Gastrointestinal Endoscopy 9 (2017) 346–358, https://doi.org/10.4253/wjge.v9.i8.346.

[107] Y.L. Cheng, B.J. Wei, F.H. Shih, Y.L. Wang, Stability and reliability of Ti/TiN as a thin film resistor, ECS Journal of Solid State Science and Technology 2 (2013) Q12–Q15.

[108] A. Tanaka, S. Matsumoto, N. Tsukamoto, S. Itoh, K. Chiba, T. Endoh, A. Nakazato, K. Okuyama, Y. Kumazawa, M. Hijikawa, Infrared focal plane array incorporating silicon IC process compatible bolometer, IEEE Transactions on Electron Devices. 43 (1996) 1844–1850.

[109] A. Tiwari, H. Satoh, M. Aoki, M. Takeda, N. Hiromoto, H. Inokawa, Fabrication and analytical modeling of integrated heater and thermistor for antenna-coupled bolometers, Sensors and Actuators A Physical 222 (2015) 160–166.

[110] A. Tiwari, H. Satoh, M. Aoki, M. Takeda, N. Hiromoto, H. Inokawa, THz antenna-coupled microbolometer with 0.1-μm-wide titanium thermistor, International Journal of ChemTech Research 7 (2015) 1019–1026.

[111] A. Banerjee, H. Satoh, A. Tiwari, C. Apriono, E.T. Rahardjo, N. Hiromoto, H. Inokawa, Width dependence of platinum and titanium thermistor characteristics for application in room-temperature antenna-coupled terahertz microbolometer, Japanese Journal of Applied Physics 56 (2017) 04CC07.

[112] A. Banerjee, H. Satoh, D. Elamaran, Y. Sharma, N. Hiromoto, H. Inokawa, Optimization of narrow width effect on titanium thermistor in uncooled antenna-coupled terahertz microbolometer, Japanese Journal of Applied Physics 57 (2018) 04FC09.

[113] A. Banerjee, H. Satoh, Y. Sharma, N. Hiromoto, H. Inokawa, Characterization of platinum and titanium thermistors for terahertz antenna-coupled bolometer applications, Sensors and Actuators A Physical 273 (2018) 49–57.

[114] A. Banerjee, H. Satoh, D. Elamaran, Y. Sharma, N. Hiromoto, H. Inokawa, Performance improvement of on-chip integrable terahertz microbolometer arrays using nanoscale meander titanium thermistor, Journal of Applied Physics 125 (2019) 214502.

[115] R.S. Saxena, R.K. Bhan, P.S. Rana, A.K. Vishwakarma, A. Aggarwal, K. Khurana, S. Gupta, Study of performance degradation in titanium microbolometer IR detectors due to elevated heating, Infrared Physics & Technology 54 (2011) 343–352.

[116] N. Nemoto, N. Kanda, R. Imai, K. Konishi, M. Miyoshi, S. Kurashina, T. Sasaki, N. Oda, M. Kuwata-Gonokami, High-sensitivity and broadband, real-time terahertz camera incorporating a micro-bolometer array with resonant cavity structure, IEEE Transactions on Terahertz Science and Technology 6 (2015) 175–182.

[117] J. Oden, J. Meilhan, J. Lalanne-Dera, J.-F. Roux, F. Garet, J.-L. Coutaz, F. Simoens, Imaging of broadband terahertz beams using an array of antenna-coupled microbolometers operating at room temperature, Optics Express 21 (2013) 4817–4825.

[118] P. Hillger, J. Grzyb, R. Jain, U.R. Pfeiffer, Terahertz imaging and sensing applications with silicon-based technologies, IEEE Transactions on Terahertz Science and Technology 9 (2018) 1–19.

[119] M. Wang, E.H. Yang, THz applications of 2D materials: graphene and beyond, Nano-Structures and Nano-Objects 15 (2018) 107–113, https://doi.org/10.1016/j.nanoso.2017.08.011.

[120] J. Shi, Z. Li, D.K. Sang, Y. Xiang, J. Li, S. Zhang, H. Zhang, THz photonics in two dimensional materials and metamaterials: properties, devices and prospects, Journal of Materials Chemistry C. 6 (2018) 1291–1306, https://doi.org/10.1039/c7tc05460b.

[121] V. Ryzhii, M. Ryzhii, T. Otsuji, Negative dynamic conductivity of graphene with optical pumping, Journal of Applied Physics 101 (2007) 83114.

[122] V. Ryzhii, A. Satou, W. Knap, M.S. Shur, Plasma oscillations in high-electron-mobility transistors with recessed gate, Journal of Applied Physics 99 (2006) 084507.

[123] F. Rana, Graphene terahertz plasmon oscillators, IEEE Transactions on Nanotechnology 7 (2008) 91–99.

[124] A.N. Grigorenko, M. Polini, K.S. Novoselov, Graphene plasmonics, Nature Photonics 6 (2012) 749.

[125] A. Zak, M.A. Andersson, M. Bauer, J. Matukas, A. Lisauskas, H.G. Roskos, J. Stake, Antenna-integrated 0.6 THz FET direct detectors based on CVD graphene, Nano Letters 14 (2014) 5834–5838.

[126] C. Liu, J. Ye, Y. Zhang, Thermally tunable THz filter made of semiconductors, Optics Communications 283 (2010) 865–868.

[127] C.W. Berry, J. Moore, M. Jarrahi, Design of reconfigurable metallic slits for terahertz beam modulation, Optics Express 19 (2011) 1236–1245.

[128] D. Shrekenhamer, S. Rout, A.C. Strikwerda, C. Bingham, R.D. Averitt, S. Sonkusale, W. Padilla, High speed terahertz modulation from metamaterials with embedded high electron mobility transistors, Optics Express 19 (2011) 9968–9975.

[129] H.-T. Chen, J.F. O'hara, A.K. Azad, A.J. Taylor, R.D. Averitt, D.B. Shrekenhamer, W.J. Padilla, Experimental demonstration of frequency-agile terahertz metamaterials, Nature Photonics 2 (2008) 295–298.

[130] T. Kleine-Ostmann, M. Koch, P. Dawson, Modulation of THz radiation by semiconductor nanostructures, Microwave and Optical Technology Letters 35 (2002) 343–345.

[131] B. Sensale-Rodriguez, R. Yan, M.M. Kelly, T. Fang, K. Tahy, W.S. Hwang, D. Jena, L. Liu, H.G. Xing, Broadband graphene terahertz modulators enabled by intraband transitions, Nature Communications 3 (2012) 780.

[132] B. Sensale-Rodriguez, T. Fang, R. Yan, M.M. Kelly, D. Jena, L. Liu, H. Xing, Unique prospects for graphene-based terahertz modulators, Applied Physics Letters 99 (2011) 113104.

[133] C.J. Docherty, P. Parkinson, H.J. Joyce, M.-H. Chiu, C.-H. Chen, M.-Y. Lee, L.-J. Li, L.M. Herz, M.B. Johnston, Ultrafast transient terahertz conductivity of monolayer MoS_2 and WSe_2 grown by chemical vapor deposition, ACS Nano 8 (2014) 11147–11153.

Index

Note: Page numbers followed by "f" indicate figures and "t" indicate tables.

U

V

W

Z

Kolibri 360 GmbH
Ferdinand-Jühlke-Straße 7
99095 Erfurt, Deutschland
produktsicherheit@kolibri360.de